Midwives, Research
and Childbirth

VOLUME 2

Midwives, Research and Childbirth

VOLUME 2

Edited by

Sarah Robinson

*Senior Research Fellow, Nursing Research Unit
King's College, London University*

and

Ann M. Thomson

*Clinical Lecturer, Department of Nursing
University of Manchester
Midwife, St Mary's Hospital, Manchester*

CHAPMAN AND HALL

LONDON • NEW YORK • TOKYO • MELBOURNE • MADRAS

UK   Chapman and Hall, 2-6 Boundary Row, London SE1 8HN

USA   Chapman and Hall, 29 West 35th Street, New York NY 10001

JAPAN   Chapman and Hall Japan, Thomson Publishing Japan, Hirakawacho
              Nemoto Building, 7F, 1-7-11 Hirakawa-cho, Chiyoda-ku, Tokyo 102

AUSTRALIA   Chapman and Hall Australia, Thomas Nelson Australia, 480 La Trobe
              Street, PO Box 4725, Melbourne 3000

INDIA   Chapman and Hall India, R. Seshadri, 32 Second Main Road, CIT East,
              Madras 600 035

First edition 1991

© 1991 Sarah Robinson and Ann M. Thomson

Typeset in $9\frac{1}{2}$/11 Times Roman by
Leaper and Gard Ltd, Bristol
Printed in Great Britain by St Edmundsbury Press,
Bury St Edmunds, Suffolk

ISBN 0 412 31650 1

British Library Cataloguing in Publication Data

Midwives, research and childbirth.
Vol. 2
1. Women, Pregnancy & childbirth
I. Title   II. Thomson, Ann M., *1944-*
618.2
ISBN 0-412-31650-1

Library of Congress Cataloging-in-Publication Data
Available

Preface

This volume is the second in a series which brings together studies of particular relevance to the care provided by midwives for childbearing women and their families. The series is intended primarily for midwives but we hope that other health professionals involved in the provision of maternity care, as well as those who use the services, will also find the series interesting and useful.

In editing this series we have been fortunate in the encouragement and support received from colleagues, friends and family. In particular we should like to record our thanks to the editorial and production staff at Chapman and Hall in London, all the authors who have contributed to the series, our colleagues at the Nursing Research Unit of London University and the Department of Nursing at Manchester University, and Paul and Rachel Robinson. Special thanks are due to Keith Jacka for his statistical advice.

Sarah Robinson, *London*
Ann M. Thomson, *Manchester*
February 1990

Contributors

Rosamund Bryar   Senior Lecturer in Nursing, Teamcare Valleys, School of Nursing Studies, College of Medicine, Cardiff

Jean Davies   Community Midwife, Newcastle Health Authority

Frances Evans   Regional Adviser, Community Care, Northern Regional Health Authority

Caroline Flint   Independent Midwife and Consultant Midwife, London

Jo Garcia   Social Scientist, National Perinatal Epidemiology Unit, Oxford

Sally Garforth   Midwife, formerly Research Midwife, National Perinatal Epidemiology Unit, Oxford

Paul Lewis   Midwife Teacher, Queen Charlotte's Maternity Hospital, London

Margaret Logue   Midwifery Sister, Northwick Park Hospital, London

Tricia Murphy-Black   Research Fellow, Nursing Research Unit, University of Edinburgh

Sarah Robinson   Senior Research Fellow, Nursing Research Unit, King's College, University of London

Jennifer Sleep   Research Coordinator, Berkshire College of
                      Nursing and Midwifery

Ann M. Thomson   Clinical Lecturer, Department of Nursing,
                      University of Manchester and Midwife, St Mary's
                      Hospital, Manchester

CHAPTER ONE

Research and midwifery; moving into the 1990s

Sarah Robinson and Ann M. Thomson

RESEARCH AND PROFESSIONAL INDEPENDENCE

As stated in the introductory chapter to Volume 1, this series is based on the premise that midwives in Britain are qualified to provide care on their own responsibility throughout pregnancy, labour and the puerperium, to recognize those signs of abnormality that require referral to medical staff, and to provide advice, information and support from early pregnancy to the end of the postnatal period. This is the yardstick against which the acquisition and deployment of midwifery skills and knowledge must be judged. First, does the education of midwives equip them with the ability and confidence to practise with this range and degree of responsibility? And secondly, does the organization and management of maternity services in general and the midwifery services in particular enable them to do so once qualified?

The history of the midwifery profession in the last two decades has to some extent been dominated by concerns that its members have not been able to practise fully and effectively (Walker, 1976; Thomson, 1980; Cowell and Wainwright, 1981; Robinson, Golden and Bradley, 1983; Towler and Brammall, 1986; Robinson, 1989). Fragmentation of care, increasing involvement of medical staff in normal maternity care, short staffing and lack of control over education and management structures have all been identified as constraints that have contributed to loss of professional independence and to a decline in the quality of some aspects of care provided. However, the 1980s have also witnessed some progress on the part of midwives not only in regaining lost ground but also in developing and expanding their role to meet the varying needs of today's childbearing women.

A major component of this progress has been the recognition that if midwives are to be in a position to provide women with the best care possible then all aspects of midwifery – practice, education and management

– must have a knowledge-base grounded in research (Ball, 1983; Thomson, 1985; Houston and Weatherstone, 1986; Murphy-Black, 1987; Thomson, 1988). The efficacy of policies and practices must be evaluated; those long established as well as those introduced more recently. Interaction and communication between midwives and women in their care must be documented and assessed and there is a continuing need to monitor the extent to which midwives are able to exercise the level of responsibility and decision-making for which they are qualified. Systems of care based on midwives as the prime care-givers must be compared, in terms of perinatal outcome and women's satisfaction, with systems in which medical staff are the prime care-givers. Moreover innovative ways of deploying midwifery skills need to be implemented and evaluated. If midwives are to have a sound basis for competent and confident practice then attention must also be given to evaluating teaching methods and assessment strategies in classroom and clinical settings and the curriculum content of first-level and continuing education courses. If sufficient numbers of midwives are to be available to staff the service then opportunities for professional development must be monitored, career intentions and paths must be documented, deterrents to retention must be identified and methods for calculating work loads and staffing levels must be devised.

The recognition of this need for research has been translated into action and during the last decade the volume and range of studies undertaken has steadily increased. A recent review of the resulting body of literature (Murphy-Black, 1989) has shown that while the greater proportion of studies have focused on midwifery policies and practices and the way in which the delivery of midwifery care is organized, a growing number of researchers have concerned themselves with education, management, career development and inter-professional relationships.

Considerable diversity exists in the size and scope of these research projects, reflecting to some extent the varying circumstances under which they were undertaken. In educational settings these have included the following: projects undertaken by student midwives and by midwives on a variety of continuing education courses (e.g. diplomas, management courses); dissertations submitted in part fulfilment of undergraduate degrees; studies undertaken while in receipt of a Scottish Home and Health Department (SHHD) Nursing Research Training Fellowship; and research submitted for the postgraduate degrees of MPhil, MSc and PhD (some of which have been funded by SHHD or DHSS, (now the DOH)). Much research has been carried out by midwives in full-time practice, education or management posts: this includes working on a project by themselves and in their own time; working in collaboration with colleagues from other disciplines; holding an NHS research post; and participating in an innovative scheme and its evaluation. Other midwives have held posts as members of teams based in research units; these include the National Perinatal

Epidemiology Unit (NPEU) at Oxford and the Nursing Research Units of Edinburgh University and London University. Staff of the NPEU have worked with midwives on a number of studies and funding was made available by the DHSS in 1988 for a midwife to be appointed to a core post in the unit and to lead a programme of research.

Funding for research into midwifery has come from a variety of sources. Midwives have received awards through the Royal College of Midwives/ Maws Scholarship scheme and through Government Health Department fellowships. Charitable sources include the Iolanthe Trust, Birthright, the Wellington Foundation, the Wellcome Institute and the Wolfson Foundation. Funding has also been provided by a range of professional and statutory bodies; these include the National Boards for Nursing, Midwifery and Health Visiting, the Health Education Council, and District and Regional Health Authorities. The Government Health Departments have funded many projects including most of those based in the research units.

Running parallel with the steady accumulation of research findings the 1980s also witnessed a growing emphasis on developing appreciation and knowledge of research among the profession as a whole. Greater emphasis was placed on research in first level and continuing education courses, and an increasing number of conferences, study days and courses on research methods, and findings were made available. These developments have been facilitated by a steady increase in the range of publications (reports, books, journals, journal articles, conference proceedings, information services, and chapters in edited volumes from other disciplines). By the end of the 1980s considerable progress had been achieved towards the goal of midwifery becoming a research based profession.

THE AIMS OF THE *MIDWIVES, RESEARCH AND CHILDBIRTH* SERIES

In addition to the range of publications noted above we felt that there was also a need for studies to be brought together in a series of volumes concerned specifically with midwifery and so instituted the series of which this volume forms part. We have included some of the earliest studies undertaken as well as more recent work, so that in due course the series will constitute a reasonably comprehensive record of research in this area.

In the broadest sense our criteria for inclusion is research that is of particular relevance to the care provided by midwives. This includes studies concerned with clinical procedures, with the provision of advice, information and support, with responsibility for decision-making about the management of care, and with women's views and experiences of the care that they receive. However, midwives are only able to provide care to a high standard if they receive an education that equips them to do so, if career structures and conditions of service exist that encourage them to stay, and if the maternity service is organized in a way that facilitates the effective deployment of their unique combination of skills and knowledge. Consequently research on all these issues is included in this series of books. Having said this there is clearly an enormous volume of research that is not included but that is relevant to the care provided by midwives and of which midwives should be aware.

First, there is the body of research on clinical interventions in pregnancy and childbirth, recently the subject of an extensive review (Chalmers, Enkin and Keirse, 1989). Our first approach in deciding which studies to include from this field was to consider whether the aspect of care investigated could be regarded as coming within the sphere of obstetric practice and thus the study could be classified as obstetric research, or whether it came within the sphere of midwifery practice and the study could be classified as midwifery research. However, we concluded that this distinction is often not clear cut nor indeed particularly helpful or relevant at a time of increasing multidisciplinary collaboration. Our policy therefore has been to include studies on those aspects of care that midwives themselves have regarded as their sole or shared responsibility and have been sufficiently motivated to initiate research into their efficacy.

Turning to studies of women's views about childbirth and their experiences of the maternity services, these have long been the subject of study by social scientists. Although increasingly midwife researchers have explored these subjects often as part of a wider investigation we nonetheless felt that some of the social scientists' work was of considerable relevance to midwives as it documents experiences to which midwives can respond; these include communication during pregnancy, pain in labour, and conflicting advice during the postnatal period and so we have included some of these studies in the series (e.g. MacIntyre and Porter and McIntosh in Volume 1, this series; Niven in Volume 3). Our overall aim is to bring together as much research as possible relating to midwifery practice, education and management, but we are of course aware that others might well have used different criteria and included other studies.

Our policy is to give authors sufficient space to write at length not only about their findings but also about their choice of research strategy and instruments and the wider context in which their work is located. Therefore each volume contains only ten studies. In choosing which studies to include in each volume, our policy is for each to reflect not only the wide range of subjects that are relevant to midwifery but also the diversity of research methods that are appropriate for their study.

For two reasons we rejected an approach that brought together studies pertaining, for example, to antenatal care in one volume, labour in another, and education in a third. First, we believe that this approach is completely at odds philosophically with the holistic way in which midwifery should be developing and indeed is doing with developments such as 'team midwifery'.

This is not to deny that much research focuses on one specific issue, or that some midwives may wish to specialize in a particular area of practice, while others concentrate on education or management. Second, many studies do not fit neatly into one category or another; they encompass for example care in pregnancy, labour and the postnatal period or relate to experiences of education as well as to subsequent careers.

As in Volume 1 and re-stated at the beginning of this chapter we have worked on the premise that midwives are qualified to provide care for normal childbearing women. We have therefore presumed these women not to be sick and have not labelled them as 'patients'. We have followed the tradition that uses the term obstetrics as applied to care in childbirth provided by doctors, and midwifery as applied to care in childbirth provided by midwives. The term booking is a shorthand phrase used in mid-wifery and obstetrics and refers to the woman's first visit to the antenatal clinic to book (i.e. reserve) a bed. At the beginning of the 1980s it became practice within the midwifery profession to refer to 'midwifery education' and 'midwifery teacher' instead of 'midwifery training' and 'midwifery tutor'. In order to keep to the historical context we have used the terms training and tutors for events before the end of the 1970s, and education and teacher when referring to events from 1980 onwards.

Turning now to the research included in this volume, three kinds of studies relating to midwifery practice are represented; those that evaluate specific procedures, those that document the wider context of policy-making within which midwives practise, and those that focus on innovative schemes for the deployment of midwifery skills. Studies of the first kind, evaluation procedures, are represented by two chapters on perineal care. Jennifer Sleep (Chapter 8) describes a series of five randomized controlled trials which she and colleagues undertook to evaluate the following: liberal versus restricted use of episiotomy; different kinds of suture material used for perineal repair; varying bath additives; programmes of postnatal exercises; and electrical therapies for the relief of perineal trauma. Margaret Logue (Chapter 9) first discusses a study which examined the relationship between perineal muscle function one year after delivery and perineal management at delivery, and the value of postnatal exercise. She then describes attempts made in the light of the findings to reduce the episiotomy rate in the unit in which she works.

Much discussion in the profession in recent years has been concerned with constraints experienced by midwives as a consequence of increased medical involvement in policy-making and practice in maternity care (for example Towler and Brammall, 1986; Robinson, 1989). Jo Garcia and Sally Garforth (Chapter 2) report on the first major study to investigate the mechanisms of policy formulation and decision-making in maternity care, and to determine how much influence midwives have and indeed want in this process.

As noted at the outset of this introductory chapter, recent years have witnessed a resolve on the part of many midwives not only to restore but also develop and expand their role. This has been demonstrated in a number of innovative schemes, most of which are characterized by a commitment to provide women with individualized and continuous care by midwives. However, if such schemes are to be more widely adopted then midwives must also take up the challenge of evaluating their outcomes. Studies of four such schemes are included in this volume. Rosamund Bryar (Chapter 3) describes the process whereby a system of individualized care was introduced into a maternity unit and the evaluation that she undertook to assess the extent to which it had been achieved. The Know Your Midwife scheme based at St George's Hospital in London was one of the most imaginative and ambitious schemes of recent years to investigate the feasibility and benefits of midwife-based care, and in Chapter 4 Caroline Flint, the scheme's instigator, describes the philosophy behind the scheme, its implementation, and its evaluation by means of a randomized controlled trial. Concern for women deemed to be at high risk of perinatal mortality and morbidity was the driving force behind the scheme discussed in Chapter 5 by Jean Davies and Frances Evans. A team of community midwives provided enhanced support on a neighbourhood basis to childbearing women living in areas with a concentration of high risk factors and a social scientist evaluated the effectiveness of this intervention in terms of outcome, client satisfaction and relationships between hospital and community services. Re-establishment of midwives' clinics has been one of the most frequent developments in the move to deploy midwifery skills more effectively, and in Chapter 6 Ann Thomson describes her investigation into the extent to which this was achieved in one such clinic.

As discussed earlier, research into midwifery education has been much less in evidence than research into midwifery practice. Nonetheless the number of studies of both first-level and continuing education for midwives is now increasing and a body of findings is accumulating upon which the profession can draw. Two of the earliest pieces of research into midwifery education are included in this volume. Tricia Murphy-Black (Chapter 7) describes an evaluation of a post-basic course that aimed to encourage antenatal teachers to strive for greater interaction between themselves and the women attending their classes. Much of the existing work on course evaluation focused only on participants' assessment of the experience. However Murphy-Black also attempted the more difficult task of assessing the extent to which course attendance was associated with changes in subsequent teaching styles. The decision to extend the length of the midwifery education course from 12 to 18 months for the registered general nurse was taken in the hope that it would lead to an increase in the proportion of newly qualified midwives who felt confident to practise and indeed wished to do so. The extent to which these hoped-for outcomes were achieved was investigated by staff of the Nursing Research Unit, London

University, and in Chapter 11 Sarah Robinson discusses the findings of the study and some of their implications for present-day developments in midwifery education.

An issue that caused considerable controversy among midwives in the 1970s was whether men should be allowed to enter the profession. Men were in fact allowed to train from 1977 onwards and in 1987 Paul Lewis surveyed all those who were students at that time or had qualified. In Chapter 10 he describes the experiences of these men as midwifery students and as practitioners, focusing in particular on their acceptability to women and their partners, and their career patterns within the profession.

This volume, in association with the others, demonstrates the relevance to midwifery of descriptive and evaluative research; the former to obtain information on subjects on which little exists but much is needed, and the latter to assess the relative merits of alternative policies and practices. Descriptive research in this volume includes surveys and case studies. Evaluative research in this volume includes randomized controlled trials, comparative studies using matched group analysis, and action research. Both approaches have employed a diversity of research instruments.

Questionnaires, for example, have been used to obtain information from large and often widely dispersed groups; these include heads of midwifery service (Chapter 2), newly qualified midwives (Chapter 11), male midwives and staff of midwifery schools (Chapter 10), women allocated to different perineal care policies (Chapter 8) and women allocated to different styles of midwifery care (Chapters 4 and 5). Observation of interaction between givers and receivers of care formed part of three studies: in labour wards (Chapter 2), in antenatal clinics (Chapter 3) and in antenatal classes (Chapter 7). Several studies included interviews with midwives and with women about care given and received (Chapters 2,3 and 5). The studies in this volume also demonstrate the use in research of two kinds of documents: first, those designed for a particular project – midwives' assessment and care plans (Chapter 3) and midwives' assessments of trauma and healing (Chapter 8); the second type of documents studied were those designed for another purpose but whose analysis can provide information relevant to midwifery practice – policy documents (Chapter 2) and medical records (Chapters 4,5 and 6). Some authors employed just one method, such as a survey by questionnaire, but most adopted a multi-method approach to their investigation; for example interviewing and observing midwives and also analysing their care plans. All describe their choice of research strategy in some detail.

In looking to the future all the authors discuss the implications of their findings for midwifery practice, education and/or management. Directions for change as indicated by findings are outlined as well as identifying constraints that may militate against the implementation of such changes.

The authors also draw attention to the need for further research; either replication of their own study or investigation of certain issues in more depth. This volume, along with others in the series, demonstrates that a vigorous programme of research into many aspects of midwifery is being pursued.

CHALLENGES FOR THE 1990s

Much remains to be done however if achievements to date are to be con-solidated and expanded in the future: many areas of midwifery remain unresearched; the number of midwives with research skills and experience, although growing, is still relatively small; qualified staff need more oppor-tunities to develop an appreciation of the importance of research and an awareness of existing findings; information about completed projects needs to be more widely and effectively disseminated, and the profession needs to mount a concerted and co-ordinated programme of action to implement findings.

Midwives' views on how these diverse challenges might be faced have recently been brought together in two papers; the first representing views of selected midwives in Scotland and England, was prepared for a conference concerned with developing priorities for nursing and midwifery research (Murphy-Black, 1989); the second resulted from an analysis of views expressed by the 500 attenders at the 1988 Research and the Midwife Conferences (Robinson, Thomson and Tickner, 1989).

Both papers included participants' views on areas that they felt should be researched. Turning first to those related to practice, the topics specified most frequently included determining the place and type of care most beneficial for women who experience problems during pregnancy; ensuring that antenatal education is appropriately geared to women's needs, evalu-ating the effectiveness of different methods of pain relief in labour, strategies to encourage women to start and to continue breast feeding, prevention of incontinence after delivery and improving communication between midwives and women, particularly in relation to the latter's request for the kind of care which they desire. Midwifery education was regarded as con-siderably under-researched by comparison with midwifery practice. Educa-tion issues identified as requiring urgent investigation included different teaching methods and assessment strategies; development needs of midwife teachers; factors that facilitate or hinder continuing education; demand for direct entry courses; and the process of merging midwifery schools. Midwives themselves were the subject of many proposed areas of research. These included measures to calculate staffing levels, measures to audit standards of care, policies for recruitment and retention strategies including those to attract mature entrants, how best to divide responsibility for the various aspects of maternity care between the different professions involved, and how to organize midwifery care effectively in rural areas.

This study of proposals for research into midwifery practice, education and management does not indicate the order of priority in which the proposals were held by the respondents. Moreover it does not necessarily represent the views of the profession as a whole. Maybe the next step should be a 'Delphi' survey of midwifery research priorities of the kind that have been undertaken with regard to nursing research priorities (Lindeman, 1975; Bond and Bond, 1982; Goodman, 1986; Nursing Research Unit, Edinburgh, 1988). As well as identifying areas for research the midwives whose views were represented in these two papers also expressed views about the conduct of research in the future. Firstly, there is a need for larger collaborative studies to enhance validity and generalizability of findings. Secondly, researchers should replicate earlier work to determine whether findings can be corroborated. Thirdly, consideration should be given to how a programme of midwifery research might best be co-ordinated in the future. Clearly it is undesirable for this to be over-centralized and directed as motivation to undertake research often springs from an individual midwife's particular interests and concerns. On the other hand, lack of co-ordination may result in a less than effective use of resources. For example studies may be carried out on the same subject but in such a way that findings obtained are not comparable because the researchers were not in contact at the design stage of their studies. The answer probably lies somewhere in between. Maximum dissemination of information about research in progress will increase chances of collaborative and complementary efforts and similarly widespread availability of completed findings will indicate areas in which new or further research is required. The development of core programmes of research into specific aspects of midwifery based in particular teaching departments, in research units, and in midwifery units and schools should provide foci to which others interested in researching into the same area may be attached and obtain advice and support. This in turn will lead to a more co-ordinated approach. Such a development is to some extent already under way but could be greatly expanded.

The midwives who took apart in the study reported by Robinson, Thomson and Tickner (1989) were also asked for their views on how to increase a commitment to research in the profession and facilitate the would-be researcher, and improve dissemination and implementation of findings. Analysis of the numerous and diverse comments made demonstrated a cycle of needs and responsibilities in relation to research. In essence, when a profession is in the relatively early days of establishing the research component of its knowledge-base and developing the skills of its practitioners, it faces the problem of only a small minority of its members possessing the requisite skills, not only to undertake research but also to teach others about research methods. It is difficult, for example, for teachers to base teaching on research if they themselves have had little grounding in research methods and in evaluation of findings. Similarly if managers are to ensure that practice in their units is based on research, they too need knowledge of methods and of evaluation and for existing findings to be widely available. Those who wish to undertake research may be hampered by lack of adequate supervision, and may need help in preparing findings for publication. If the latter is not forthcoming then material is less likely to be available upon which practice and teaching can subsequently be based. Midwives can only discharge their responsibilities in relation to research if their own needs are met, in terms of information, education and/or funding. The many suggestions for action made by the participants are briefly summarized here. First in relation to responsibilities, second in relation to needs.

All midwives – in education and management as well as in practice – have five areas of responsibility: 1. A commitment to base their work on available research findings; 2. To develop skills in evaluating literature and marshalling arguments to defend a particular course of action; 3. Commitment to keep up-to-date with research literature; 4. To support and facilitate colleagues carrying out research; 5. To be receptive to identifying areas for research in their own area of work. Specific areas of responsibility were attributed to managers, teachers and midwife-researchers. Ensuring that practice is research based was seen as the responsibility of managers in the first instance. The respondents saw it as the managers' responsibility to motivate and stimulate staff to be interested in research, send them on research courses, and take a lead in setting up regular research discussion sessions in the workplace. Encouraging and supporting staff who want to carry out research was regarded as vital, so that initiative and enthusiasm is nurtured rather than stifled. Midwife teachers were seen to have a responsibility to base their teaching on research findings, and include sessions on research methods in their courses. An awareness of research and educational strategies and the need to base teaching on findings in this area were also emphasized.

Closer links between managers and teachers over what is taught and what is practised was identified as one way of ensuring maximum effectiveness of the research endeavour in a district. Students get a poor start in relation to research if teachers base teaching about practice on research findings, but managers adhere to practices that have been shown to be ineffective.

A number of responsibilities to be discharged by midwife researchers were identified. These included making their work widely known through publication and through public speaking at national and local levels. Requests were made for writing to be clear and jargon-free, although it was also recognized that midwives have a responsibility to learn research terminology in the same way that they have to learn the terminology of their practice. Once experience has been gained and subsequent projects undertaken, midwife researchers have a responsibility to supervise colleagues who are starting on their first project.

Participants also specified a number of organizations with responsibilities associated with midwifery research. These included funding research and, in the case of health authorities, funding course provision and attendance as well. It was suggested that midwives, as individuals and in groups, should approach a far wider range of charities and trusts for research funds than they have hitherto. Statutory bodies were deemed to have a responsibility to ensure that practice is research-based in units in which students are taught. All organizations that run courses, from basic education for the RM qualification to single study days, should ensure that the content is research based as far as is presently possible. Staff of research units and/or teaching departments in higher and further education were urged to devote time to supervising midwifery researchers and providing information on methods and relevant literature, and midwifery managers were urged to identify appropriate people in their district (or region) to whom they could send their staff for help in this respect.

A wide range of responsibilities have been identified for midwives as they go into the 1990s; some concerned specific groups, others related to the profession as a whole. In order to discharge these, however, midwives have many needs to be fulfilled, and this also was the subject of numerous and diverse comments. The subject that featured most frequently was the inclusion of an appreciation and understanding of research, at all levels of midwifery education. Much has already been achieved in this direction, although progress to date may well be uneven across the country. Comments made concerned both the structure and content of first-level and continuing education.

The respondents stated that much more emphasis on research is needed in first-level education. All practices taught should be based on research findings whenever possible; research modules should include teaching about research methods and critical evaluation of literature; students should have the opportunity to carry out small scale projects in order to give them 'hands on' experience of research. However there were those who did not agree with the latter. It was felt by some that staff and clients of local units could be inundated with requests to complete questionnaires or be interviewed for projects whose findings may be of doubtful validity and of little use to practitioners or consumers. In considering continuing education the respondents stated that the content of in-service courses should be research based whenever possible, and more courses, seminars and workshops should be provided on the appreciation and understanding of research. The structure of refresher courses should include the option of several individual research study days, and the content of all refresher courses should be research based. The content of midwifery diplomas and management courses should be research based and include more sessions on appreciating and understanding research.

If research increasingly becomes a core component of education at all

levels in midwifery, then the proportion of midwives who have a commitment to base practice on research and are able to critically evaluate the
literature will increase throughout the 1990s.

As well as increasing the research component of officially approved
courses, many midwives said that they would also like to see an increase in
the number and type of meetings at which they could get together to discuss
research. Their suggestions included a midwifery research society, with
meetings held at national and local level; more research conferences;
district-based research interest groups; meetings held in midwifery units at
which staff could discuss research relevant to their practice (the types of
meeting mentioned included quality circles and journal clubs).

The widespread availability of published material on research methods
and findings was identified by many of those who participated in the study
as an essential pre-requisite to base teaching and practice on research. A
number of suggestions were made to counteract what some saw as an
unsatisfactory situation at present. Those who undertook research were
exhorted to publish their findings as soon as possible in a range of journals,
that would reach all those to whom they were relevant, and this included
medical as well as midwifery staff.

It was recommended that as well as publishing in journals, midwife
researchers should send copies of their report (or at least a summary of its
main findings) to heads of midwifery services and to senior teachers so that
they would have material on hand on which to base practice and teaching.
Moreover, it was suggested that this material should be circulated to consultants and to family practitioner committees. Circulation of findings on
this scale to midwifery and medical staff would of course have considerable
financial implications, and some felt that reports should only be circulated
after submission to peer review. An alternative suggestion to increase the
dissemination of findings was for researchers to send their findings to
various centralized organizations that in turn could send out research
bulletins that summarized and commented on research findings. Researchers
were also exhorted to send reports on projects in progress and projects
completed to MIDIRS, the Midwives Information and Resource Service, as
they have an extensive nationwide membership, and to the Midwifery
Research Database (MIRIAD) currently being developed at the National
Perinatal Epidemiology Unit in Oxford.

Another group of comments related specifically to the needs of those
who wished to carry out research themselves. Obviously they require finance
and facilities for the project and the necessary time within which to carry it
out. They need access to literature and, particularly at the start of their
involvement in research, to people who can provide help in formulating and
designing the project and regular supervision during its progress. Help for
midwifery researchers in developing skills in writing and speaking about
their work was also mentioned as an important aid to the process of dis-

semination. Means whereby researchers can get together at national and at local level to discuss their common objectives and problems were mentioned as a pressing need, as were more advanced research courses for those who already had some experience.

Funding is of course central to the whole enterprise and was mentioned in relation to many of the needs already described: these included project costs, short-term replacement of staff undertaking research, sending staff on existing research courses, providing more in-service courses, making journals, conference reports, etc. available in all midwifery units and/or education departments. The latter was stressed as particularly important to aid dissemination; busy midwives need research information easily to hand if it is to be read, evaluated and considered for implementation. MIDIRS was specifically cited as making a major contribution in this respect.

A suggestion for facilitating and promoting the 'research mindedness' of midwifery units and schools was to appoint people for whom this would be a particular responsibility. It was argued that it was unrealistic to expect managers, teachers and staff who had had little or no training in research methods, to evaluate literature, to devise ways of implementing findings and/or base teaching on research. They could be helped in this respect by other midwives who did have the necessary expertise. Two kinds of posts were suggested, first that one (or more) of the managerial posts (or teaching posts if there is a midwifery school) should have a research component, and the appointee(s) would be responsible for bringing relevant research to the attention of colleagues; this would of course entail a concomitant reduction in the post holders' managerial or teaching responsibilities.

The other suggestion was for each unit to have a research midwife who would not only be responsible for encouraging 'research mindedness' among the staff and bringing research findings to their attention, but also carry out some research herself and guide others (students and staff who wished to do so). Midwives who have carried out research in their unit have helped to raise the level of research awareness among their colleagues, particularly when the latter are involved in data collection for the project. This awareness however may decrease again when the project is completed or the midwife leaves the unit. If there is a permanent research post in each unit and/or school of the kinds described then research is less likely to be seen as a rarefied activity carried out by a few, and instead a commitment to research and to keeping up-to-date will become part and parcel of every midwife's professional responsibilities. Posts such as these will require not only funding but also the existence of sufficient numbers of midwives with the research expertise to fill them. Such posts do exist in some districts but the creation of many more was identified as an essential development by many of the participants in this study.

As noted earlier various organizations were specified as having responsibilities in relation to midwifery research. If these are to be discharged then the organizations need resources and staff with relevant expertise. Thus government departments, companies, charities and health authorities require not only sufficient funding if they in turn are to finance research, but also personnel with appropriate expertise to assess research proposals and findings. Statutory and professional bodies also require expertise if they are to provide courses, information and support in relation to research. Staff of academic departments and research units require sufficient time to provide supervision. All these organizations need regular input from midwifery researchers in the form of proposals, findings and information about their needs.

In conclusion, the views about research into midwifery expressed by participants in these two studies (Murphy-Black, 1989; Robinson, Thomson and Tickner, 1989) and by the contributors to this volume indicate that there is much to be done at all levels, national, local and individual, if the momentum and progress of the 1980s is to be sustained and expanded in the 1990s.

REFERENCES

Ball, J.A. (1983) A midwifery practice research unit. *Midwives Chronicle and Nursing Notes*, **96**, 213.
Bond, S. and Bond, J. (1982) *Clinical nursing research priorities: a Delphi survey.* Health Care Research Unit report, University of Newcastle upon Tyne.
Chalmers, I., Enkin, M. and Keirse, M.J.N.C. (1989) *Effective care in pregnancy and childbirth.* Oxford University Press, Oxford.
Cowell, B. and Wainwright, D. (1981) *Behind the blue door: a history of the Royal College of Midwives 1881–1981.* Bailliere Tindall, London.
Goodman, C. (1986) *A Delphi survey of clinical nursing research within a Regional Health Authority.* Unpublished MSc dissertation, King's College, London University.
Houston, M. and Weatherstone, L. (1986) Creating change in midwifery: integrating theory and practice through practice-based research groups. *Midwifery*, **2**(2), 65–70.
Lindeman, C.A. (1975) A Delphi survey of priorities in clinical nursing research. *Nursing Research*, **24**, 434–41.
Murphy-Black, T. (1987) Developments in midwifery research. *Senior Nurse*, **6**(5), 7.
Murphy-Black, T. (1989) Research needs and priorities in midwifery. In *Proceedings of the Consensus Development Conference on Priorities for Nursing Research in Scotland.* (ed. Tierney, A.J.) Nursing Research Unit, University of Edinburgh, Edinburgh.
Nursing Research Unit, Edinburgh (1988) A Delphi survey of nursing research priorities. Report in *Unit's Biennial Report 1987–88.* Nursing Research Unit, University of Edinburgh.
Renfrew, M. (1989) Developing midwifery research: the role of the midwife researcher in the National Perinatal Epidemiology Unit. In *Research and the*

Midwife Conference Proceedings for 1988. (eds Robinson, S. and Thomson, A.M.) Department of Nursing, University of Manchester, Manchester.

Robinson, S. (1989) The role of the midwife: opportunities and constraints. In *Effective care in pregnancy and childbirth.* (eds Chalmers, I., Enkin, M. and Keirse, M.) Oxford University Press, Oxford.

Robinson, S., Golden, J. and Bradley, S. (1983) *A study of the role and responsibilities of the midwife.* NERU Report No.1, Nursing Research Unit, King's College, University of London, London.

Robinson, S., Thomson, A. and Tickner, V. (1989) Midwives' views on directions and developments in midwifery research. In *Research and the Midwife Conference Proceedings for 1988.* (eds Robinson, S, Thomson, A. and Tickner, V.) Department of Nursing, University of Manchester, Manchester.

Thomson, A.M. (1980) Planned or un-planned? Are midwives ready for the 1980s. *Midwives Chronicle and Nursing Notes,* 93(1106), 68–72.

Thomson, A.M. (1985) Research and midwifery (editorial) *Midwifery,* 1(2), 73.

Thomson, A.M. (1988) What is clinical significance? (editorial) *Midwifery,* 4(2) 47.

Towler, J. and Brammall, J. (1986) *Midwives in history and society.* Croom Helm, London.

Walker, J. (1976) Midwife or obstetric nurse? Some perceptions of midwives and obstetricians of the role of the midwife. *Journal of Advanced Nursing,* 1(2), 129–38.

CHAPTER TWO

Midwifery policies and policy-making

Jo Garcia and Sally Garforth

INTRODUCTION

Decisions about the ways that maternity care is organized and the details of midwifery policies and procedures at District and hospital level, have an important influence on the working conditions for midwives at all levels and on the sort of care that women receive. The decision, for example, to close an outlying general practitioner maternity unit affects the workload of midwives both in the community and in the central consultant unit. Similarly, a new labour ward protocol for the care of first-time mothers can change the ways that midwives work and the relations between midwives and medical staff. Both these decisions also affect the sort of care that women receive. What part do midwives play in making decisions of this kind? How do midwives work together and how do they relate to their medical colleagues? What are their views about the proper scope for policies and procedures in midwifery care? This chapter attempts to address these questions using data from a national study of policy and policy-making in midwifery.

With the exception of three important studies discussed below, very little research attention has been given to either the details of maternity policies or the mechanisms for policy-making.

The Chelsea College study of the Role and Responsibilities of the Midwife (Robinson, Golden and Bradley, 1983; Robinson, 1985; Robinson, 1989a,b), based on a national survey of the main professional groups in maternity care, has been an important influence on the work reported in this chapter. The Chelsea College study did not include a detailed examination of policies, but its findings on the balance of responsibility between midwives and doctors and on the levels of satisfaction expressed by midwives about aspects of their work, throw light on maternity policy-making.

Two other studies are also of particular value in understanding the way that maternity units work. The Cambridge-based Maternity Services Research Group explored the consequences of alternative medical staffing structures for midwives and doctors working in the labour ward (Green, Kitzinger and Coupland 1986; Volume 3 in this series, in preparation). They compared three hospitals which had a traditional three-tier medical staffing structure with three hospitals where there was no registrar grade – a two-tier structure. They observed care and interviewed staff and also asked some doctors to keep diaries about the pattern of their work. They concluded that midwives and doctors did relate differently in the two systems.

A Scottish study of the midwife's role (Askham and Barbour, 1987a,b) involved observation and interviews in a range of different maternity units and the community. This was followed by a questionnaire sample-survey of Scottish midwives in order to be able to generalize from the results of the in-depth studies. Their findings cover all aspects of maternity care and look at the ways that midwives work and at the division of responsibility between doctors and midwives. The authors explore the ways that midwives and doctors work together in practice and include evidence about midwives' views about their work.

The study reported here – The Policy and Practice in Midwifery Study – was set up to investigate various aspects of the work of midwives in England. In this chapter we concentrate on those aspects of the study that concern midwifery policy-making. Because midwives provide the majority of maternity care, we felt that the policies and procedures that they adopt and their relationships with other care givers were very important. The debate about the role of the midwife as team member or independent practitioner was one of the influences on the study. We were also interested in documenting routine aspects of maternity care, which have tended to be overlooked by researchers and which are usually the responsibility of the midwife. A third strand in the study was an interest in the relationship between the midwife and parents, and in the ways in which hospital policies can meet the varying needs of those who use the services.

In the next section we describe the origins of the study and the methods that we used. Then our findings are reported in two sections: the first deals with the making of midwifery policies at District level, with the role of the Director of Midwifery Services and with the part she plays in policy making; the second looks at midwifery policies within maternity units and discusses the attitudes of midwives towards policy, the division of responsibility between midwives and doctors and the links between policy and practice. These two sections giving details of our findings are followed by a comparison of our findings with those of the three studies mentioned above.

STUDY DESIGN AND METHODS

The Policy and Practice in Midwifery Study was a national study of midwifery policy and policy-making for normal labour and postnatal care. The initial idea for the study came from discussions between the National Perinatal Epidemiology Unit and the Royal College of Midwives. More detailed research proposals were then discussed with a very wide range of groups and individuals including other researchers in the midwifery area, midwives' professional bodies, the Department of Health, and advisors from other professional groups involved in the maternity services. These discussions covered both the contents of the study and also questions of access. Gaining permission to approach the potential respondents was quite complex, and that stage of the study took up a considerable amount of time.

The study was funded from the following sources: 1. The Department of Health funds the National Perinatal Epidemiology Unit and so provided both a salary for the first author and also the accommodation; 2. Birthright, the charity attached to the Royal College of Obstetricians and Gynaecologists, provided the main project funds; 3. The Iolanthe Trust, at the Royal College of Midwives, enabled the research midwife (SG) to carry out extra work on the findings about breastfeeding.

The study was made up of two parts – a national survey involving the Directors of Midwifery Services in all the English Health Districts and an in-depth study of a small sample of Health Districts using interviews and observation of care. A fuller description of the aims and methods is given elsewhere (Garcia, Garforth and Ayers, 1987) but the aspects of the study that are most relevant to this chapter will be outlined here.

The national survey was carried out in 1984 following a pilot study in one Region. Directors of Midwifery Services (DMSs) in the English Health Districts were sent a set of questionnaires. The set included a questionnaire about organization of midwifery services in that Health District, and individual questionnaires about midwifery policies in each NHS consultant and general practitioner maternity unit in the District. We asked the DMSs to arrange for the maternity unit questionnaires to be filled in by whichever senior midwife they thought most appropriate. The response rate was 93%, representing 180 out of 193 Health Districts, and covering 220 consultant units and 175 general practitioner units. The general practitioner units included those that comprised units or wards situated within a consultant obstetric unit and those that were sited separately from a consultant obstetric unit; they are referred to as integral and isolated general practitioner units respectively.

The in-depth study was carried out in the first half of 1985 and involved eight Health Districts from among those that had taken part in the national survey, selected in order to provide a range of work circumstances and approaches to policy. Its aim was to complement the survey data and to find out more about the links between policies and practice. In each of the eight Districts, individual interviews were carried out with the DMS and with her senior midwife colleagues. Thirty such interviews took place, and covered the respondent's role in policy-making, as well as her views about policies in midwifery. In addition, policy and procedure documents were collected. Finally, labour ward care was observed in the nine consultant maternity units in the eight study Districts.

Two aspects of care were observed: admission in labour, and routine care immediately after a normal delivery. This observation involved a three-way look at each event. During an admission, for example, the researcher recorded what she saw and heard on a semi-structured observation form. After the admission a short interview was carried out with the midwife responsible for the care and, on the next day, with the woman whose care had been observed. In this way it was possible to take into account the perceptions of three individuals about what had taken place. Although these short interviews were mainly concerned with the events that had been observed, midwives were also asked some general questions about their views on policies in their unit. In total, 80 labour ward midwives were interviewed in the nine maternity units.

The two researchers spent two weeks in four Districts each. We visited each District together on one occasion to arrange the details of the fieldwork and to inform staff about the project, but then we worked separately. We were made very welcome by the staff in all the Districts, although it was sometimes necessary to dispel initial doubts about our purpose. Midwives at all levels gave us a great deal of their time and were very hospitable to us. The time we spent in each place was extremely useful, but also frustrating, because we realized how long we would need to stay to obtain a proper understanding of what was happening.

The observation of care was rewarding, and has produced useful findings (Garforth and Garcia 1987, 1989a; Garcia and Garforth, 1989). It was also very taxing, both methodologically and personally. Our aim, as far as possible, was to avoid doing anything which would affect what was happening. We had to decide how much we could participate in conversations, how to respond to requests for information from parents and how to be helpful and sociable without getting too involved. For the research midwife it was probably more difficult because the staff knew that she was a midwife and so expected her to have views about the care being provided. It is inevitable that our presence in the labour ward had some effect on the care that we were there to observe – some midwives told us that this was so. On balance, though, midwives tended to get used to us quite quickly and we felt that we were usually able to get a good idea of what normal care involved.

This chapter is based on the findings from the various elements of the study, used in the following ways. Policies at District level are considered first, drawing on data from two sources:

1. The questionnaire about District-wide maternity services completed by the Directors of Midwifery in the national survey;
2. The interviews with senior midwives carried out in the eight Health Districts in the in-depth study.

Policies at hospital level are then considered, drawing on data from:
1. The questionnaires about consultant and general practitioner maternity units in the national survey;
2. Observation of care and interviews with labour ward midwives in the eight Districts in the in-depth study;
3. Interviews with senior midwives in the in-depth study;
4. Policy documents collected in both stages of the study.

POLICIES AT DISTRICT LEVEL AND THE ROLE OF THE DIRECTOR OF MIDWIFERY SERVICES

In a District in which the Director of Midwifery is responsible for midwives in the community as well as in hospital, she has a unique responsibility for the provision of maternity care to all the women in a particular geographic area. No other professional has quite this wide a concern. In practice, the findings from this study show that not all Districts have a midwife with overall responsibility for hospital and community services, and decision making about maternity care varies considerably between Districts. At present many Districts are making crucial decisions about the way that maternity care is to be provided – for example, whether to close general practitioner maternity units, or to adjust hospital postnatal length of stay. These decisions have consequences for those who use the services and for the midwives providing care, and so it is important to find out more about the part that midwives play in decision-making.

In the questionnaire about policies at district level in the national survey, DMSs were asked for information about their own job and about their involvement in policy-making in the District. Table 2.1 gives some details about the respondents.

Table 2.1 Characteristics of respondents in 180 Health Districts

	No.	%
Responsible for all midwifery services in the District	151	84
A supervisor of midwives	169	94
In Director of Services post	156	87

In the majority of Districts a midwife held a Director's post and was responsible for all midwifery services. The exceptions form a rather mixed group. In a few Districts our respondent indicated that she was not a practising midwife and usually held a Director of Nursing Services (DNS) (Community) post. Other respondents were heads of midwifery, but held less senior positions. In some cases our respondent managed most of the midwives in the District with a few falling under a DNS (Community) or another manager in a remote hospital.

We also asked which additional specialties were managed by our respondents. A minority, 26%, managed midwifery only. A further 54% were also in charge of nursing in the related specialties of neonatal paediatrics, family planning and gynaecology. The remaining 19% were responsible for other services including paediatrics, community nursing and health visiting, as well as some less obvious ones like ophthalmology and geriatrics. Just over half our respondents had been in post for less than four years.

In the in-depth study, Directors of Midwifery were asked about the advantages and disadvantages of working 'on the management side of midwifery'. Several mentioned the satisfaction of having overall responsibility for an aspect of care. For example, one said:

I enjoy the overall picture. I was quite naive until I started.

and another said:

It's lovely to make your own policy and put it into action.

One liked the fact that midwifery was about positive health rather than illness. Two mentioned their interest in advising the midwives for whom they were responsible. Problems of the job were quite varied. Pressure of time and the need to compete for resources were both mentioned, as was the lack of everyday contact with those using the services.

In the in-depth study we also asked about the division of responsibility between the senior midwives. In three of the eight Districts there were midwives in Assistant DMS posts between those at Nursing Officer grade and the DMSs in the management structure. In one such District the DMS was responsible for overall management while the two consultant maternity units in the District were each run by Assistant Directors of Midwifery. The remaining five Districts had Nursing Officers who were responsible to the DMS and took charge of specific aspects of care. Of these, one rather small District had a DMS who acted as 'matron' of the free-standing small consultant maternity unit and was assisted by one Nursing Officer. The division of roles seemed to be less formalized here than in some of the larger Districts.

In the national survey, respondents were asked about their membership of committees in which maternity service policies are made. Sixty-six percent (119/180) attended meetings of the Division of Obstetrics and Gynaecology and 35% (63/180), the Division of Paediatrics. In the interviews with the eight Directors of Midwifery in the in-depth study, it was found that all six who attended meetings of the Division of Obstetrics and Gynaecology felt that they played an active part in the meetings, in some cases initiating meetings when there was something important to discuss and putting items on the agenda.

We asked about Maternity Services Liaison Committees (MSLCs) and found that almost all Districts had either set one up or planned to do so. Only 12 Districts (of the 180) had no MSLC or plans for one at the time of the study. We assumed that our respondents would be members of the MSLC if it existed, but in a few cases another midwife attended. Information about the composition and role of the MSLCs obtained in this study are given in another paper (Garcia, 1987). In theory, these committees should provide a very influential forum for decision-making about district level maternity care policies. Their brief, as specified in the first report of the Maternity Services Advisory Committee, includes:

> the agreement of generally applicable procedures and the monitoring of the effectiveness of these procedures as they apply to individual women.
>
> (Maternity Services Advisory Committee, 1982, para 1.13)

In practice, their role may be restricted by many factors. They may meet very infrequently and may limit the topics which they address. Other groups – formal or informal – may predate the formation of the MSLC and may have more power. Any proper assessment of their roles in different Districts would have required a separate research project. Even for those Districts in which the in-depth study took place, we only have material from our interviews with senior midwives to help us to place the MSLC in the context of local maternity decision-making.

In the eight Districts studied in depth, seven respondents were members of their MSLC and gave us some idea of the issues discussed and their own reactions to the way that the Committees were working. Several were evidently quite dissatisfied with their Committees but were reluctant to say too much because, as one said:

> ... it's a question of individuals really.

Another said:

> I'm trying hard not to be too negative ... It is slow and hard going.

Two respondents were pleased with the way their MSLCs were working, though one of these felt that the good progress was largely due to her efforts in preparing material for discussion. A third reported considerable tension between disciplines but called the Committee 'lively and vocal'. MSLCs certainly varied a great deal in what they saw as their task. Some seemed to run out of steam once they had discussed the Maternity Services Advisory Committee recommendations, while others took on a wide range of policy issues.

The national survey also asked respondents to list any local policy-making groups or committees of which they were members. This was obviously quite a difficult question to answer, probably because some Districts work in a much more formal way than others. Twenty-seven percent (48/180) of respondents recorded no relevant groups or committees other than the MSLC or Division of Obstetrics. The remainder mentioned attending one or more of a very wide range of bodies in which general or specific aspects of maternity care were discussed, and policies made. Thirty-seven percent (66/180) attended regular meetings with their midwife colleagues in the hospital or District; 33% (60/180) went to interdisciplinary meetings (of various degrees of formality) to consider general maternity care policies; 21% (38/180) recorded attendance at Unit Management Team meetings; and 19% (35/180) mentioned regular interdisciplinary meetings about specific aspects of care – usually the organization of general practitioner maternity care.

One respondent with a fairly typical pattern attended a monthly meeting of senior midwives; a weekly Unit Management Team (consisting of herself, a consultant, a general practitioner, an administrator and an accountant) and a quarterly meeting of obstetric, paediatric and midwifery staff. In addition, one of her senior midwives attended a quarterly meeting with general practitioners to discuss the general practitioner maternity unit.

Unfortunately, our knowledge of the involvement of senior midwives in policy-making groups and committees tells us very little about their real influence on decisions about the provision of services. As will be clear from the next section, there is wide variation in the way that hospital maternity policies are made, and in the power of the different professions in this respect. The present study has only given a very limited idea of the ways that maternity policies are made at District level. Research into the workings of the Maternity Services Liaison Committees, which have now been set up in nearly all Health Districts, would be a good way to start on the process of untangling the threads of influence and decision-making. Another approach would be to investigate the process whereby major decisions have been reached; the closure of outlying maternity units would be one example. Both these research ideas would be quite time-consuming to put into practice and would involve a considerable amount of interviewing and observation, but they would provide useful and interesting data.

POLICIES AT HOSPITAL LEVEL

Two interconnected themes recur throughout this section of the chapter. The first concerns the varying approaches to policy within midwifery, including the style of midwifery policy and procedure documents and the ways that they are seen and used by midwives; the second is the division of responsibility between midwives and doctors for care of women experiencing normal pregnancy and childbirth in both the details of policies, and in the ways that policies are made and implemented.

The first sub-section discusses the style of midwifery policy documents and the aspects of care that they cover. We then consider the key issue of who makes policy for care in normal labour. This leads on to two subsections; the first is a brief examination of the division of responsibility between midwives and doctors and the second is about midwives' varying attitudes towards policy and policy-making. The section concludes with an examination of the ways in which policies are translated into practice.

The scope and style of policies in midwifery

How would a newly appointed midwife encounter midwifery policies? Here is a typical example from information that we gained in the course of the in-depth study. The policy folder is kept at the desk in the labour ward and contains some very diverse material. There are standing orders for drugs for various consultants, a copy of the District policy on sick pay, detailed guidance on the care of mothers with rare medical or obstetric conditions, a list of local GPs, together with their preferences for being informed if a woman in their care arrives in labour; amongst these there are copies of recent and not so recent policy documents intended to guide midwives caring for women at admission and during labour and delivery.

In a minority of consultant units the pattern would be different because some obstetricians have adopted a new approach that involves the production of a unified labour ward policy book which covers both obstetric care and care which has traditionally been the concern of the midwife. This has the advantage of minimizing the extent to which different obstetricians have different policies for the women in their care, but may also place severe constraints on the midwife's scope for independent judgement. Although in this latter type of unit, obstetricians have a major influence on policies for care in normal labour, it should not be assumed that midwives have had no impact; nor should the former type of policy be seen as the product of purely midwifery decisions.

Why are policies needed for care in normal labour? Midwives are educated to provide this care and are governed by their own professional standards. Moreover, as Chalmers, Enkin and Keirse (1989) have recently demonstrated many of these policies are of unproven efficacy. Midwives' own views about this vary considerably and the justifications given for having more or less detailed policy documents include the presence of students and questions of safety and consistency (see midwives' attitudes towards policies, p. 32). An important influence that extends the scope of policy is the trend towards active management of labour since this requires predetermined responses to particular patterns of progress in labour.

The present study gave some indication of the scope of policy by asking questions in the national survey about the extent to which aspects of care were covered by policies at all, and then seeking details of the policy if one existed. We give here a few examples to illustrate the wide variations that we found. In the findings that follow the base numbers differ slightly because respondents were not always able to provide the information requested.

Policies concerning two routine admission procedures were studied: shaving and bowel preparation. Evidence from research does not support the routine use of either procedure (Garforth and Garcia, 1989a) and so the policies were of particular interest. In relation to shaving, we found that 42% (92/220) of consultant units had a policy of no shave, and 37% (82/220) a policy of a partial shave. In one in ten units (22/220) the policy was to leave the decision to the individual woman or midwife, in 6% (12/220) the policy of a particular consultant determined whether or not a woman had a shave, and one unit had a policy of a complete shave.

Findings on bowel preparation showed that 16% (36/220) of units had a policy of routine bowel preparation with either an enema or suppositories and 16% (36/220) had a policy of no bowel preparation. In 14% (31/220), the policy was to leave the decision to the midwife or the woman, and in 3% (7/220) policies varied between consultant obstetricians. In the largest percentage of units (48%, 106/220) the policy specified indications for bowel preparation – usually no bowel action in the last 24 hours or a 'loaded rectum' on examination. Similar policies were reported from the general practitioner units. Further findings from this study, on both shaving and bowel preparation, can be found in Garforth and Garcia (1987).

Policies concerning care in the first and second stages of labour were also investigated (for further details see Garcia, Garfoth and Ayers (1987) and Garcia and Garforth (1989)). We asked if there was a unit policy that specified when to rupture the membranes in normal labour. Thirty-eight percent (83/220) of consultant units had such a policy as did 13% (22/175) of general practitioner units. Similarly, 70% (154/219) of consultant units and 35% (62/175) of general practitioner units had a policy that specified how often vaginal examinations should be performed in labour. The 154 consultant units with a policy in this respect were almost equally divided into those that had a fixed time schedule (79/154), and those that had a flexible schedule (75/154). Of the former, 77% (61/79) had a policy that specified that vaginal examinations should be performed every four hours, 5% (4/79) specified three-hourly, 8% (6/79) every two hours, and in 10% (8/79) the schedule varied according to certain criteria (e.g. when epidural analgesia was in use).

Turning to another aspect of following the progress of labour, we investigated policies on the use of electronic fetal monitoring. The largest group of consultant units (49%, 107/218) adopted a selective policy, monitoring the heart rate of fetuses considered to be at risk in some way. In 20% (44/218) of the units the policy was to monitor all fetuses throughout labour, in 8% (18/218) the policy specified a period of electronic monitoring for all, and consultants varied in their policies in a further 11% (24/218) of units. There was a policy that specified the maximum length of second stage that should elapse before action was taken in just over half (119/220) the consultant units, compared to just under half (80/171) of the general practitioner units. Of those consultant units that specified a second stage time limit, around two-thirds gave a limit of one hour for primiparae and half an hour for multiparae.

Respondents in consultant units were also asked whether the circumstances in which an episiotomy should be performed were set out in a unit policy. Twenty-six percent (56/218) of consultant units and 15% (27/175) of general practitioner units had such a policy, though some of these specified circumstances which would not be included in our category of normal labour such as preterm delivery or hypertension. Respondents who said that there was no policy on episiotomy often added that this was a matter for the midwife's judgement. For example:

midwife judges need at delivery according to circumstances

and

midwives use their own professional judgement

In summary, this aspect of the study demonstrates that policies concerning care in labour can vary considerably from one unit to another, so that a midwife taking up a job in a different unit might find herself working with some policies that were diametrically opposed to those that she had been familiar with. In some units midwives also have to work in the context of a lack of agreement between consultants about some aspects of policy. In many of the examples discussed, general practitioner units were less likely to have a policy than were consultant units. On pp. 41–43, we discuss some of the reasons why policies do not always translate directly into practice.

Without looking at the contents of policies we can also identify fairly distinct styles of midwifery policy document; at one end of the spectrum is a reliance on detailed guidance for the midwife with little scope for judgement or decision-making, at the other is an approach that should allow the midwife to use her understanding of the basic principles and her own judgement in deciding what is best for the woman in her care. In many cases these two styles co-exist within the policies of one unit, perhaps because the more detailed policies were aimed at students or less experienced midwives, or because the work of reviewing and updating policy documents is very time-consuming so that old and new policies may both be found in the files.

An example of the traditional type of document is headed 'Normal Delivery' and begins with a list of the standard equipment in the delivery pack. The procedure is then described in detail, action by action, with some of the midwife's hand movements specified precisely. For example:

> The posterior shoulder and back are supported by one hand and the baby's body is brought up over the mother's abdomen.

The document also contains implicit references to policy as well as the details of procedure. For example:

> The patient is assisted into a dorsal position (for delivery).

and:

> ... as the anterior shoulder appears, the attendant gives IM syntometrine. . . .

From another unit comes a document entitled 'Normal delivery procedure for midwives' that has some features in common with the first but which allows more scope for choice. For example, it allows a choice of dorsal or left lateral for the woman's delivery position and offers two alternative hand positions for the midwife at delivery. However, these are described in detail. Under 'episiotomy' the document offers only a guide to the correct local analgesic and assumes that the midwife decides on the need for episiotomy:

> If an episiotomy is indicated the perineum should be infiltrated with. . . .

A rather different style of document, from another unit, concerns baby feeding and is headed 'Guidance Document'. It sets out the unit's approach to baby feeding in fairly general terms though it also includes some specific items of policy. The first item is:

> Breastfeeding should be encouraged by every sensible means. . . .

Suggestions for the promotion of breast feeding follow and include concern for the woman's comfort and privacy. Among these suggestions is the specific instruction to staff to avoid the use of formula feeds for breast-fed babies.

Maternity units have adopted various approaches in an attempt to meet the needs of students as well as staff. One unit has parallel documents for qualified staff and students for the same aspects of care. In the document for student midwives on labour care, the details of the observations to be carried out in labour are listed. The same document for qualified midwives merely states that 'regular observations are carried out'. In another hospital, policy documents for teaching purposes are made up of two columns, one of which specifies, in some detail, the action required while the other column gives reasons alongside the actions.

In practice, the style of midwifery policy documents may be more important because of what it says about attitudes within the unit towards responsibility and flexibility in midwifery care, than by the direct influence of documents on midwives' behaviour. As will be clear from the sections that follow, the documents themselves may be consulted relatively rarely, and midwives certainly do not always follow all procedures and policies to the letter. The process of producing and updating policies can itself be of importance as the following section shows.

Who makes policies for the care of 'normal' women?

Although the issue of who makes policy is a central one for the study we are reporting, the extent to which we have been able to provide clear answers is limited. In one unit the midwives may be completely free to make their own policies, but only over a narrow range of issues; the overall agenda may be set by the obstetric and paediatric staff. In another, all aspects of care may be governed by a joint labour ward policy document that was the result of an initiative by the obstetric staff but which was then worked out in detail in a collaboration between midwives and doctors. Even during the in-depth field work it was only possible to get a very limited idea of the politics behind the policy documents.

We asked several questions about policy documents in the national survey which give an indication of the process of producing policy. We asked respondents about the form in which policies and procedures were available to staff, and whether separate compilations of documents existed for midwives and doctors. We had information about this from three-quarters (164/220) of consultant units. Of these 30% (49/164) had policy documents only for midwives, 22% (36/164) had separate compilations for midwives and doctors and the largest group, 35% (57/164), had some form of joint policy folder or procedure book. Only a minority of these latter units actually had a single, jointly produced, labour ward policy and procedure book aimed at all staff. The rest probably had a single folder containing some midwifery policies, some medical policies and standing orders and some joint documents. There was also a final 'other' category represented by 22 units (13%) who were either in the process of deciding on policies, or who fell between the clear categories.

We asked who updated policies and procedures and found that of the 210 units where this information was available, just over half (107) said that this was done jointly by midwives and doctors. In the majority of these units, midwives devised policies and then had them approved by consultants, a few having joint committees and one or two indicating that doctors took the lead in developing policies. Of the remaining 103 units, all but 11 reported that midwives decided policies, either formally, as a midwifery procedure committee, or in some other way. Of the 11 units left, two stated that policies were made by the Maternity Services Liaison Committee, six said that procedures were made by midwives and policies were made jointly by midwives and doctors, and three gave other answers. Altogether, in 27% (56/210) of the consultant units in which this information was available, the existence of a midwifery procedure committee was mentioned.

The interviews with senior midwives that we carried out in the in-depth study in eight Districts also provide insights into the process of policy-making. In two of the eight Districts there had been consultation between midwives and doctors resulting in joint labour ward guidelines for normal care (in one case for first time mothers only). Midwives in these two places felt that their input into policy-making was significant, and that there were aspects of care in which doctors were not interested, and where midwives made the policies. In a third District the role of the consultant obstetricians was greater and this was the only one of the eight in which doctors appeared to be taking the lead in determining the policies for routine labour ward care. The obstetricians here seemed to work together closely and were, for example, far more interested in this research project than the doctors that we met in the other in-depth study Districts. A senior midwife in this District said:

> ... on delivery suite the working group of three consultants and two midwives are at present reviewing all policies. On the postnatal ward, policies ... are being updated ... by a Nursing Officer and sister. The consultants on the whole are not so bothered about postnatal care so we just ask them to verify them.

In the other five Districts, policies were basically initiated by midwives and then usually sent to consultant obstetricians and paediatricians for comment, or for information. Doctors did not have their own agreed policies and procedures and this sometimes caused problems for midwives. One senior midwife said:

> We've asked them to put down guidelines – even for locum doctors. Recently we had a meeting between the senior consultant, an administrator and myself, to put it very firmly that locums should be given some guidelines.

Another respondent put it rather less politely when asked about policy documents for medical staff:

> They haven't got any documents at all. I don't think it would occur to them. Their powers of communication are small.

In these five Districts the role of the Director of Midwifery in initiating changes in policies and procedures varied considerably. In some cases, midwifery procedure committees had been set up to evaluate and update existing policies and to propose new ones. In one such District the DMS was fairly new in her post and intended to oversee the updating of all midwifery procedures. She set up a committee with representation from different clinical areas and grades of staff and their proposals came to her. When she was asked what part she played in determining midwifery procedure she replied:

> It is overall control. If there's something in it I don't like, it is changed.
> I can say it's all very democratic but that's true if I'm in agreement.

In another District in which the DMS felt that she kept policy-making under her control, the pattern was different. Suggestions for policy came from the midwives with specialist clinical responsibility. She looked at them from the point of view of litigation and conformity with any District guidelines and then authorized them. Some DMSs were less concerned with the details of policy and procedure. One saw her role as facilitating the introduction of policies that had been developed by her staff, for example by obtaining the authorization of District level committees. The part played by midwifery tutors also varied considerably. In one District they took the lead in initiating changes in policy while in others they had little or no involvement.

In general, the different senior midwives interviewed in a particular District in the in-depth study tended to agree with each other in their account of how policies were made and by whom. Sometimes, however, the DMS said that she played the key role, while one of her senior staff saw herself as the person initiating policy. For example the DMS in one District said:

> I play a large part – my other managers might say too big! I actually issue policies – they go out from this office under my name.

One of her nursing officers said:

> Well, I do (prepare and update policies), for the consultant floor in conjunction with my senior staff.

And added:

> I am the correlator and facilitator. I get the information and shape it.

What these findings and those from the national survey tell us is that in most consultant maternity units, midwives take the lead in determining policies for the care of women who experience a normal pregnancy and labour but they do this within very varying constraints. In some places consultants do not confer together and may each issue their own standing orders for drugs and sometimes set out specific policies for the care of 'their' women. They may also wish to approve any midwifery policies and procedures that are developed. In other places consultants may reach agreement on policies that may impinge to a greater or lesser extent on the scope for midwives to set their own policies and guidelines. In only a few units had a comprehensive labour ward protocol for care in normal labour been developed.

The boundaries of midwifery responsibility

Some of the questions asked in the national survey dealt with the roles of midwives and doctors in making decisions about care. This is a topic that overlaps with the question of who makes policies for care, since the involvement of doctors in producing detailed procedures for care in normal labour tends, in practice, to lead to more direct involvement by doctors in care – giving and decision-making, even where there are no problems. In the tables that follow, figures are given separately for consultant units, integrated general practitioner units and isolated general practitioner units; all differences mentioned in the text are significant at the 0.01 level or higher, using the chi-square test. The findings from two questions about admission in labour are given in Table 2.2

These figures show that it was the policy in only a small minority of consultant units that a doctor had to see all women at admission. On the other hand midwives could rarely take the initiative in sending a woman home if she turned out not to be in labour. In general practitioner units doctors were rarely involved in admission in a routine way, and were less likely than their consultant unit colleagues to take the decision to send a woman home if she was judged not to be in labour. In two of the units in the in-depth study, women with ruptured membranes at admission had to have a vaginal examination performed by a doctor, but we did not ask specifically about this in the survey, so we cannot say how common a policy it was.

We asked whether units had a policy that a doctor should see each woman in labour at regular intervals. The findings are shown in Table 2.3.

In 20% of consultant units the policy was that all women should be seen by a doctor at regular intervals during labour. Such a policy was rare in general practitioner units. Quite a few respondents who answered 'no' to this question, mentioned that doctors did in fact visit the labour ward regularly. In at least one consultant unit the respondent added that a doctor had to be called to carry out every third vaginal examination in labour, though, again, we did not ask specifically about the existence of policies of this sort.

We also asked questions in the national survey about the roles of midwives and doctors in postnatal care and the findings are shown in Tables 2.4 and 2.5. In general the policy differences between different types of unit are not very great for this aspect of care. Routine examination of the baby

Table 2.2 Roles of midwife and doctor at admission in labour

Are women examined routinely by a doctor on admission?	*Consultant units*		*Integral GP units*		*Isolated GP units*	
	No.	*%*	*No.*	*%*	*No.*	*%*
No	67	31	62	89	88	89
Yes, all women	13	6	0	0	3	3
Yes, some women	134	61	6	8	8	8
Other	5	2	2	3	0	0
Total	219	100	70	100	99	100
Who can send a woman home if she has been admitted with intact membranes and judged not to be in labour?						
Midwife	19	9	11	16	13	13
Doctor	164	75	40	57	49	50
Midwife or doctor	14	6	4	6	13	13
Other	22	10	15	21	24	24
Total	219	100	70	100	99	100

Source: Compiled by the authors.

by a doctor was less common in general practitioner units, and midwives working there were somewhat more likely to make the decision on discharge of both mother and baby, than were midwives in consultants units. Women in isolated general practitioner units were more likely to be visited every day by a doctor than those in integral general practitioner units.

Midwives' attitudes towards policies

The study provided information on various aspects of midwives' attitudes towards policies, and these are described in this section. We consider first the views stated by the DMSs (who filled in the questionnaires in the

Table 2.3 Roles of midwife and doctor in normal labour

Is it unit policy that each woman in labour must be seen by a doctor at regular intervals?	*Consultant units*		*Integral GP units*		*Isolated GP units*	
	No.	*%*	*No.*	*%*	*No.*	*%*
No	168	76	65	93	85	87
Yes, all women	43	20	2	3	3	3
Yes, some women	4	2	0	0	0	0
Other	5	2	3	4	10	10
Total	220	100	70	100	98	100

Source: Compiled by the authors.

Table 2.4 Roles of midwife and doctor in postnatal care of women

How often are normal women examined by a doctor?	*Consultant units*		*Integral GP units*		*Isolated GP units*	
	No.	*%*	*No.*	*%*	*No.*	*%*
Not unless referred by a midwife	38	17	15	21	16	16
Routinely once or twice	136	62	51	73	59	60
Daily	43	20	1	1	16	16
Other	3	1	3	4	8	8
Total	220	100	70	100	99	100
Is the decision on fitness for discharge always made by a doctor?						
No	25	11	16	23	30	30
Yes	168	77	49	70	61	62
Other	27	12	5	7	8	8
Total	220	100	70	100	99	100

Source: Compiled by the authors.

Table 2.5 Roles of midwife and doctor in postnatal care of babies

Apart from an initial examination, how often are babies examined by a doctor?	Consultant units		Integral GP units		Isolated GP units	
	No.	%	No.	%	No.	%
Not unless referred by a midwife	63	29	36	51	51	52
Routinely once or twice	151	68	32	46	43	43
Daily	4	2	0	0	1	1
Other	2	1	2	3	4	4
Total	220	100	70	100	99	100
Is the decision on fitness for discharge always made by a doctor?						
No	22	10	15	22	27	27
Yes	182	83	51	74	64	65
Other	16	7	3	4	8	8
Total	220	100	69	100	99	100

Source: Compiled by the authors.

national survey) on the proper scope for policy and procedure documents, and the implications for the role of the midwife. The interviews with senior midwives in the in-depth study then provide some comments about the style of policies and procedures. Finally, the short interviews with midwives in the labour wards asked whether policies were restrictive and whether midwives would like to change any of them.

Views on the desirability of policies. Respondents in the national survey were asked to comment on one of the recommendations of the Maternity Services Advisory Committee's report on intrapartum care:

> To ensure a consistent standard of care and avoid any confusion over practice, each unit should have written operational policies which have been developed with all disciplines and which all staff understand.
> (Maternity Services Advisory Committee, 1984)

Altogether, 139 respondents (77%) made some comment on this quotation. Of these, 43% (60/139), made comments that were favourable to the recommendation. They referred to the benefits that such agreed policies would bring to midwives, for example, in defining their role more clearly, and to women by reducing conflicting advice and generally improving the quality of care. Here are two such positive comments:

I see policies and procedures as very important for the protection of midwife and patient.

It is to the midwife's advantage to have a clearly defined operational policy. It must be seen as an opportunity to establish her role.

Several respondents said that one advantage of the process of drawing up such policies would be that doctors would learn more about the midwife's role. Quite a few who were generally positive added qualifying comments which, for example, mentioned the need for midwives to be fully involved in the process of drawing up such agreed policies or emphasized the advantages of a flexible approach.

Ten percent of those who replied to this question (14/139) were against the idea set out in the Maternity Services Advisory Committee recommendation. They felt that such policies would be inflexible and would limit the scope for a midwife to exercise her judgement. Comments from two such respondents included:

My main concern is the erosion of midwives' skills in caring for normal births and the introduction of written policies will speed this up.

Operational policies could mean less flexibility if applied too rigidly.

And a third felt that there was a danger that during the process of drawing up policies, doctors would impose their views on midwives.

A further 21% of respondents (29/139) made comments about the recommendation, but did not come down as either for or against it. The views most often expressed emphasized the need for flexibility in any policies that were drawn up and stressed the need to safeguard the midwife's role. Finally just over a quarter (26%, 36/139) made comments that did not apply directly to the recommendation, but referred rather to their local situation. For example, some indicated that the development of agreed policies was already taking place in their District, or that there were local difficulties in achieving agreement about such a project.

The questionnaire for each consultant maternity unit in the national survey contained a section concerning policy-making in that unit. At the end of that part of the questionnaire, there was a request for comments about the purpose of the policy documents and the philosophy behind them. This information was provided in 164 units out of the 220 (75%). The most common justification for having written policy documents was that they were useful for students and new staff. This was mentioned by 35 (21%) of those who answered this question. Others said that they were useful to provide consistency, to protect against allegations of mismanagement and to make care safer.

Another group of comments, from 33 (20%) of the 164 responses, emphasized that policy and procedure documents should be guidelines only, to allow flexibility and to protect the midwife's role. For example:

> I have tended to get away from rigid 'thou shalt' procedures and provided guidelines to good working practice. I feel that midwives must think for themselves and not always work by rote.

and from another reply:

> Care must be taken in compiling these documents so that flexibility to meet individual patient's needs is possible.

There was a range of other comments, some dealing with particular difficulties encountered in specific maternity units. For example:

> All policies are affected by the clinical freedom of five consultant obstetricians.

and

> Polices are useful to avoid mistakes in a unit with many staff changes.

A few responses dealt with the disadvantages of having a large number of policy documents. This is one such comment:

> We do not have many written policy documents but we do have policies which we follow. I sometimes feel that written pieces of paper are ignored, especially if they appear in profusion, and I worry in case people cease to use their brains and rely on a piece of paper.

Overall, the senior midwives who filled in the consultant unit questionnaires in the national survey were torn between a desire to set up a safe and well-regulated environment in which students could see good, consistent practice, and their concern that the role of the midwife – as someone who assesses and responds to each situation individually – should be safeguarded. Some quotations indicate the range of opinions:

> I think the Midwives' Code of Practice is quite adequate as a policy document and along with the Midwives' Rules and agreed specific nursing guidelines which relate to the mother and her baby, I doubt if there could be any confusion about the standards of care, particularly

if the supervisor of midwives is doing her job and midwives are exercising their skills.

I think that good (i.e. up to date and agreed) policies leave the midwife clear as to her role and responsibilities as an individual and as a team member, and leave her mind free to concentrate on the woman's needs.

Originally I felt policies restricted individual practice, but I am becoming increasingly aware that policies protect staff rather than restricting them. Midwives have traditionally worked within the code of practice, but this does not give enough guidance in specific areas.

Views on the flexibility and detail of policies. Senior midwives interviewed in the in-depth part of the study were asked if they were happy with the style of their policies and procedures from the point of view of flexibility and detail. Quite a few respondents had taken on the task of revising the policies and this usually involved a move away from very detailed procedures. In some cases procedures were retained for students. Respondents sometimes felt that progress was not fast enough. In one District there was an interesting conflict between the needs of students and the trend towards more flexible policies. The DMS said:

I would prefer broader outlines to allow midwives some freedom. Conflicts always arise between the teaching and the service sides ... the school always wants more detail for the student.

And in her interview the senior tutor in the District said:

I would like some detail to be added. A student needs to know how to put her hands on and where, and when.

A senior midwife in another District also identified this conflict:

There are people who want every 'i' dotted and every 't' crossed. It does not allow for the individual mother or midwife or situation. To be honest I think we have too much detail – a blanket policy because we try to comply with the education department.

In a District in which the policies were being revised to make them more flexible, all the senior midwives interviewed were very positive about the process, though their perspectives differed. The DMS who had initiated the process of revision emphasized that progress had to be gradual.

I would much rather stage it [process of revision].... people have got to appreciate them which is why they have got to be staged gradually.

The senior tutor said the policies and procedures:

> ... form a good basis of guidance and are easily interpreted by new staff. We've got to finish updating them.... I think you can only take it slowly. No point in imposing things without discussion.

Two of the three nursing officers interviewed also said that policies would be good once the changes had been made, and the third said:

> ... as a newcomer I'm very impressed.... Patients really have the service they want.

Views on working within policies. Another perspective on midwives' attitudes to policies and procedures is provided by the interviews with labour ward midwives that we carried out following observation of care in the in-depth study. We asked the midwife about the care that we had just seen, about some specific policies and also about her views on working within that unit's framework of policies and procedures.

Midwives were asked 'Do you find the policies here useful as guidance or do you feel that they restrict your freedom to decide what's best for your patient?' Seventy midwives were asked this question and their replies are summarized in Table 2.6. Therefore, a majority of the labour ward midwives that we interviewed thought that policies were not restrictive. Their comments included:

> I'm quite happy with them. We've got a bit of our own leeway. We can use our own initiative.

> No, the policies are good. We are allowed to discuss things. [DMS] is very good and willing to make changes.

> I am happy to be protected by policies.

> Policies are useful. Protocol – we don't have to stick rigidly to it if patient requests. Need policies with students and medical students.

And here are some of the things said by those who found policies restrictive:

> Yes they do sometimes restrict. That's mainly to do with medical decisions. Midwifery – they are fairly flexible.

> Restrictive ... every third vaginal examination by doctor – housemen are less experienced. It's frustrating.

> The protocol restricts. It has been modified by midwives now and we have to prove it works.

Table 2.6 Midwives' views on policies

Midwives' views	No.	%
Useful	41	59
Restrictive	10	14
Mixed	17	24
Other answer	2	3
Total	70	100

Source: Compiled by the authors.

Some gave mixed replies:

> I think you've got to have a framework of policies initially. As a new midwife you just can't go doing your own thing entirely, it wouldn't be safe. But I do feel we are a bit restricted here. We have a very rigid consultant. We did once get a birthing chair but he saw it and said get rid of it. I've never seen it since.

> A bit of both. When the doctors did the protocol it was a bit rigid – new one is much better – we were consulted. So much change in the last 12 months. I often have to consult a procedure sheet.

> In general they are good ... they are broad. I don't like the business of routine monitoring, but that's not from the midwifery side, that's from the doctors.

Although the number of midwives interviewed in each hospital was quite small there are a few comparisons that can be made between places. The most negative comments usually came from the places in which doctors had had an important role in drawing up policies for care in normal labour. For example, in one hospital (already referred to) there was a policy that a doctor should carry out every third vaginal examination in labour, and midwives were unhappy about this.

In another large teaching hospital the midwives' replies were particularly interesting. Doctors had initiated the development of a protocol for some aspects of care in normal labour and midwives had felt that it was restrictive. They were now involved in negotiating a new, and more flexible protocol. These midwives' comments are fuller than those from many other places and though they contain many negative or mixed remarks the atmosphere is one of optimism and interest rather than resignation.

The only place in which all the midwives had positive things to say about the policies was one in which new policies were being developed at the instigation of the senior midwives, involving very thorough consultation with midwives at different levels. In answer to a later question, one midwife here implied that the pace of change was a little too fast for her.

As a contrast to these two hospitals in which morale was high and there was considerable interest in the policies, we can look at another District in which the midwifery policies were generally 'old fashioned', for example in the admission routines. Midwives there were asked a slightly different question in the interview – Have you any comments about working within hospital policies? The majority of midwives (5/9) replied that they were happy with the policies. One said:

> It is easy for me because I haven't worked anywhere else.

Two gave mixed replies, but two were very negative in their answers. One said:

> I find it hard working here. I am used to doing things very differently.

In answer to a later question she spelled out the aspects of care that upset her, and that were, in fact, unusual in terms of the national picture. The other was obviously unhappy:

> I hate working in a hospital like this but you have to work where your husband's job is, don't you.

In general, the atmosphere here was not one of participation in decision-making about policies and most midwives accepted the situation rather than actively supporting the style of care being provided.

Views on whether midwives wanted changes in policies. In the interviews with labour ward midwives in the in-depth study we also asked for more information about the aspects of policies and procedures that were of concern to midwives. Forty-six midwives were asked if there were any particular policies they would change if they could; their views were fairly evenly divided: 20 said 'yes' and 26 said 'no'. Some of those who did not have any changes to suggest took a positive view of existing policies. For example:

> We are lucky that our policies are worked out by us.

For other respondents the question was not one that they had thought about:

> I haven't thought about it really.

> Hard to think ... we have eased up a lot.

> Can't think of anything at the moment.

Those who wanted changes sometimes felt strongly and had obviously been thinking and talking about what they wanted:

> I don't like everyone on a monitor. I would like to see mums more mobile. I would like an early labour room with easy chairs. Doctors here have to do every third VE which I think is crazy. If we can't do a simple VE as midwives what on earth can we do?

> I don't agree with a full shave. I'm used to doing just the tiniest little perineal shave. When I question it they just say 'This is an obstetric unit with consultant care so we must prepare everyone for section.'

> Only thing is about rupturing the membranes – I think it is a shame to rupture them too early.

Others had to make more effort to come up with policies that needed changing:

> (pause) ... I don't think ... we wear masks for suturing and I don't think it makes any difference with infection.

> I don't know, I'd have to think ... Some things about equipment, maybe.

Policies in practice

In some of the other reports of findings from the Policy and Practice in Midwifery Study we have looked in some detail at the ways that policies relate to practice, and have tried to take into account the views of women about their care. Papers on admission to the labour ward (Garforth and Garcia, 1987), on breastfeeding (Garforth and Garcia, 1989b) and on the contact between the new baby and parents (Garcia and Garforth, 1989) show, for example, that policies do not always translate directly into practice and that senior midwives are not always aware of the details of practice in their labour wards. An understanding of some of the constraints under which midwives operate can help to explain the gaps between what is intended and what actually happens. For example, giving a woman help with the first breastfeed may be difficult to achieve in a relaxed way because of the many other tasks that the labour ward midwife has to undertake following delivery and the pressure to make the room available.

One of the obstacles to putting policy into practice is the extent to which midwives are informed about policies and policy changes. In the in-depth study we asked the labour ward midwives that we interviewed how they were informed about hospital policy. Some commented on the occasionally haphazard nature of the process:

> ... you find out the policy, probably by chance. Find it on a desk

saying 'Read, sign and return'. But you might be ill or on days off or just not see it. Most of it is by word of mouth.

Memos and bits and pieces. It's a bit hit and miss. Labour ward manual is out of date.

A lot of people don't look at the book.

... you are not always told, especially about minor changes.

Pick it up as you go along.

Some hospitals seemed better than others in this regard, judging by the midwives' comments.

In the interviews we also asked midwives for the details of some policies in their labour ward. For example, we asked whether a doctor had to see each woman admitted in normal labour and whether a midwife could send a woman home if she was not in labour and all was well. There was generally good agreement in the answers given to these questions by the different midwives within each unit. Only two midwives (in different hospitals) out of a total of 46, said that in their labour ward a doctor should see all women at admission. Quite a few, however, mentioned circumstances in which a doctor would be called at admission. In answer to the other question, six midwives out of a total of 33 said that a midwife could send a woman home if she turned out not to be in labour. Three of them came from one hospital in which that was the policy. The other three were probably mistaken. One further midwife thought that she was able to send a woman to the antenatal ward on her own authority but her colleagues disagreed.

Another aspect of policy on which agreement was less good, concerned bowel preparation on admission in labour. Midwives' replies are difficult to categorize because many of them described their practice rather than any agreed policy. In some hospitals, interpretations varied considerably between midwives. For example these four replies are from one hospital:

Optional.

You don't usually ask them – ask questions and if you think they need one you suggest it.

If she wants or if she hasn't had bowels open or if you examine her and her rectum is loaded – but it's really her request.

Not so very routine because we've got some radical midwives. I do explain to parents and they are happy to have one.

In another hospital with a policy of no routine bowel preparation there was much more agreement between midwives. Most replies indicated that an enema was not routine but would be given if the mother asked for it or might be advised by the midwife if the woman seemed very constipated. In units in which it was the routine, some midwives were unhappy with the policy and others were ardent supporters. For example one said:

> I believe in enemas. I prefer these water enemas to the disposables – much more effective.

A more subtle approach was expressed by someone from a hospital in which the policy had changed:

> Once it was for everyone, but now if the patient doesn't want it you don't give it. Sometimes with gentle persuasion you can get her to have an enema.... You can explain if she has a loaded rectum it may hold up her baby.

In their responses to some of the open questions in the national survey, many of the senior midwives mentioned the need for flexibility in policies, so that women's needs could be met. It may be that flexible policies are of greatest benefit when both midwives and parents are already well informed. A flexible policy on bowel preparation can allow midwives to recommend what they 'know' to be best for the mother, as some of the comments above make clear. This makes it all the more important for policy changes and the reasons for them to be fully discussed. One DMS said:

> I think that our feeding policy is quietly being abused at night by auxiliaries who think they know better.

COMPARISONS WITH OTHER STUDIES OF MIDWIFERY CARE

In this section a brief comparison of our findings is made with those of the three studies of midwifery care mentioned in the Introduction. This comparison can only be rather general because the studies had different objectives and did not use methods that would allow the findings to be directly comparable.

The findings from the Chelsea College study (Robinson, Golden and Bradley, 1983; Robinson, 1989a,b) about the extent to which care in normal labour is governed by policies, are broadly similar to our findings. In both studies, for example, the timing of vaginal examinations was more likely to be specified in a unit policy than was the timing of the decision to rupture the membranes in labour. In each study, few units had policies that specified when to perform an episiotomy in normal labour. The detailed figures vary but the questions were not asked in exactly the same ways in the two studies. In each study, unit policies were more likely in consultant, than in general practitioner maternity units.

Tables 2.2 and 2.3 show the answers to questions in the Policy and Practice in Midwifery Study about the role of doctors in care in normal labour. In 20% of consultant units, for example, the policy was that all women in labour should be seen by a doctor at regular intervals. The Chelsea College study also explored this subject in some detail. In a general question about labour ward care, midwives who currently or had recently worked in a labour ward were asked about the degree of responsibility taken by midwives for care in normal labour in the place in which they worked. Over 80% of respondents indicated that it was the midwife who took primary responsibility and that women in normal labour were not examined by a doctor unless requested to do so by the midwife. Ten percent of respondents said that all women were seen by a doctor at admission but then cared for by the midwife if all was normal. Only 4% indicated that in the unit in which they worked, a doctor saw all women regularly throughout labour and made decisions about their management. These respondents were more likely to work in consultant maternity units in teaching hospitals.

When the same question was put by the Chelsea College team to their sample of hospital medical staff in obstetrics, a very different picture emerged with less than half the medical respondents stating that the midwife had primary responsibility for care in normal labour and 22% stating that the doctor was responsible for decision making throughout labour. This difference in the perceptions of medical and midwifery staff also appears in the replies to their questions about responsibility for specific decisions on aspects of labour care. No comparable data exist from our study, which collected information from midwives only. The mismatch between the views of midwives and doctors found in the Chelsea College study should make us interpret the replies to some of our questions with some caution. Policies are sometimes vague and may be open to different interpretation by different staff. They do not always give a clear idea of what happens in practice.

The Chelsea College study also addressed the role of the doctor in the postnatal care of woman and baby and found that midwives working in consultant units in teaching hospitals were most likely, and those working in separate GP units least likely, to say that women were examined daily by a doctor in the postnatal period. Those working in separate GP units were most likely to say that babies were not examined by a doctor unless referred by a midwife. In our study we also found variation in these aspects of care (Tables 2.4, 2.5 pp. 33 and 34) with the routine role of the doctor being somewhat reduced in GP units when compared to consultant units. We did not, however, find a difference between integral and isolated GP units of the kind reported by Robinson and her colleagues.

The Scottish researchers on the midwife's role (Askham and Barbour, 1987a,b) showed that in some of the consultant units that they studied there were policies which led to a great deal of involvement of doctors in every labour; for example policies that specified that the first and each subsequent third vaginal examination should be carried out by a doctor. Routine involvement of a doctor in normal labour care, in consultant units, was more common than in Robinson's English and Welsh data. The Scottish researchers found that the midwives that they interviewed generally accepted the existing division of responsibility and were not especially keen to take on new areas of work like perineal suturing, though training programmes for this were in progress at the time of the study.

In the Cambridge study of different forms of medical staffing in obstetrics (Green, Kitzinger and Coupland, 1986, in preparation in Volume 3 of this series) the authors looked at the role of midwives in the labour ward and at their relationships with the different grades of medical staff. They found that in hospitals without a registrar grade, midwives were likely to carry out more tasks that are seen as an extension of their normal role, for example, suturing the perineum and setting up intravenous infusions. Midwives were also more likely to phone consultants in the two-tier setting; in the three-tier hospitals this was done by registrars. Midwives in the two-tier hospitals were also found to be more involved in some aspects of decision making about care. The researchers looked in some detail at the ways that midwives and doctors saw the boundaries of their respective roles. 'Normal' labour is certainly not a self-evident concept, and can refer either to what is common or usual, or some idea of natural progress in labour. Many interventions are part of a midwife's usual care and so the debate about extending the midwife's role to include, for example, the setting up of intravenous lines is not really about a radical departure from the essence of midwifery. Midwives in the Cambridge Group's study tended to use the idea of normality to defend the sort of practice that they wanted, but shifted the boundaries when they felt that a particular task should – for various reasons – fall within their remit.

Questions to midwives in the Chelsea College study also sought opinions about the extent to which midwives should be taking on new areas of practice. The range of opinion was quite wide, though, for example, a majority wanted midwives to be able to suture the perineum and set up intravenous infusions. The concept of normal labour was again raised by some respondents as a reason for limiting the tasks performed by midwives.

A common thread in these three studies, and in ours, is the wide variation both in midwives' actual level of responsibility for the provision of care in normal labour, and in their attitudes to the division of responsibility. Whether these factors contribute to midwives' career patterns or to the loss or retention of midwives is an important subject for further research.

CONCLUSION

Taken as a whole the findings of the Policy and Practice in Midwifery Study provide a picture of the very varied work circumstances of English midwives. Senior midwives, for example, are involved to very varying degrees in the processes of policy making in their District or maternity unit. Policies that affect the day-to-day work of midwives vary in several dimensions. They may consist of detailed instructions or broad guidelines; they may be rigid or flexible; they may assume that the midwife is the main decision-maker when all is normal or, alternatively, involve the doctor in regular checks on the progress of labour and the puerperium. Because of this there is no single answer to the question of whether policies are a good thing – for midwives, parents or other care givers. What may be very important, however, is the active involvement of midwives in the process of policy making and in the debates about the proper scope for policies in maternity care.

The study has suggested areas in which further research would be useful. There is certainly scope for more studies which look in detail at the ways that policies work out in practice. In some cases, research studies merge into audit, when, for example, the local care given to breastfeeding mothers is assessed (Renfrew, 1988). In other such studies the main focus is a research one, but the information collected may well be of value to managers (Henderson, 1984; 1985). As has already been mentioned, there is also a need for more work that explores the details of maternity policy-making. We hope that one result of our own and other research in this field will be a growing interest among midwives in the whole subject of their role and their influence on the ways that maternity services are provided.

For us, the most encouraging approach to policy in midwifery that we came across in some of the places that we visited and that appears in some of the national questionnaire replies, is an active involvement of midwives of all grades in the process of shaping policies and procedures for their work. If midwives are to safeguard their pre-eminent role in the care of the woman in normal labour they need confidence and a sound basis for the approaches that they take.

ACKNOWLEDGEMENTS

We would like to thank the mothers and midwives – too numerous to mention by name – who helped us by giving up their time to fill in our questionnaires or take part in our interviews. We are also grateful to all those who helped with the design and completion of the project, including our colleagues at the National Perinatal Epidemiology Unit, especially Sarah Ayers, and to the editors of this volume. Financial support for this project came from Birthright, from the Iolanthe Trust and from the Department of Health, which funds the National Perinatal Epidemiology Unit.

REFERENCES

Askham J. and Barbour R. (1987a) *The role and responsibilities of the midwife in Scotland.* The final report of a research project. Scottish Home and Health Department, Edinburgh.

Askham J., and Barbour R. (1987b) The role and responsibilities of the midwife in Scotland. *Health Bulletin.* **45**(3), 153–59.

Chalmers I, Enkin M. and Keirse M. (1989) (eds) *Effective care in pregnancy and childbirth.* Oxford University Press, Oxford.

Garcia, J. (1987) The role and structure of the Maternity Services Liaison Committee. *Health Trends,* **19**, 17–19.

Garcia J. and Garforth S. (1989) Parents and newborn in the labour ward. In Garcia, J., Kilpatrick, R. and Richards, M. (eds) *The Politics of Maternity Care,* Oxford University Press, Oxford.

Garcia, J. Garforth, S. and Ayers S. (1987) The Policy and Practice in Midwifery Study: Introduction and methods. *Midwifery,* **3**(1), 2–9.

Garcia J. and Garforth S. (1989) Labour and delivery routines in English consultant maternity units. *Midwifery,* **5**(4), 155–162.

Garforth, S. and Garcia, J. (1987). Admitting – a weakness or a strength? Routine admission of a woman in labour. *Midwifery,* **3**(2), 10–24.

Garforth, S. and Garcia J. (1989a) Hospital admission practices, in Chalmers I, Enkin M, Keirse M. (eds) *Effective care in pregnancy and childbirth,* Oxford University Press, Oxford.

Garforth, S. and Garcia J. (1989b) Breastfeeding policies in practice – No wonder they get confused. *Midwifery.* **5**(2), 75–83.

Green, J., Kitzinger, J. and Coupland, V. (1986) *The division of labour: Implications of medical staffing structure for doctors and midwives on the labour ward,* Child care and Development Group, University of Cambridge.

Green, J., Kitzinger, J. and Coupland, V. (in preparation) Midwives' responsibilities, medical staffing structures and women's choice in childbirth. In Robinson, S. and Thomson, A.M. (eds) *Midwives, Research and Childbirth, Vol 3,* Chapman and Hall, London.

Henderson, C. (1984) *Some facets of social interaction surrounding the midwife's decision to rupture the membranes,* MA Dissertation, University of Warwick.

Henderson, C. (1985) Influences and interactions surrounding the midwives' decision to rupture the membranes. In Robinson, S. and Thomson, A. (eds) *Research and the Midwife Conference Proceedings for 1984,* Nursing Research Unit, King's College, London.

Maternity Services Advisory Committee (1982) *Maternity Care in Action, Part 1: Antenatal Care.* HMSO, London.

Maternity Services Advisory Committee (1984) *Maternity Care in Action, Part II, Care during childbirth,* HMSO, London.

Renfrew, M.J. (1988) *Infant feeding survey,* Oxford District Health Authority, Submitted to Director of Midwifery Services.

Robinson, S., Golden, J., and Bradley, S. (1983) *A study of the role and responsibilities of the midwife,* Nursing Education Research Unit, Report No. 1, Chelsea College, University of London, London.

Robinson, S. (1985) Midwives, obstetricians and general practitioners: The need for role clarification. *Midwifery,* **1**(2) 102–13.

Robinson, S. (1989a) Caring for childbearing women: the interrelationship between midwifery and medical responsibilities. In Robinson, S. and Thomson, A. (eds) *Midwives Research and Childbirth, Vol 1,* Chapman and Hall, London.

Robinson, S. (1989b) The role of the midwife: opportunities and constraints. In Chalmers, I, Enkin, M. and Keirse, M. (eds) *Effective Care in Pregnancy and Childbirth,* Oxford University Press, Oxford.

CHAPTER THREE

Research and individualized care in midwifery

Rosamund Bryar

INTRODUCTION

The purpose of this chapter is to describe the experience as well as the processes of a research project that aimed to evaluate the extent to which individualized care had been introduced within a British maternity unit. It was initiated by senior midwives within this unit in collaboration with members of staff from a University Department of Nursing. A number of issues, of concern to midwives, provided the impetus for the project. These included consumer dissatisfaction with maternity services, effective use of midwives' skills and the need to identify appropriate staffing levels in maternity units.

During the 1970s there was increasing evidence of consumer dissatisfaction with maternity services. Dissatisfaction related to lack of individuality and continuity of care, and lack of responsibility felt by women for their own care (Garcia, 1982). Pregnancy and childbirth may be times of physical danger for the woman and her baby, but are also times of psychological and social growth and role change (Comaroff, 1977). Demands for changes in services to meet more adequately these psychological, as well as physical needs, come from consumers and professionals (Chard and Richards, 1977; Newton *et al.*, 1979; Kitzinger, 1983).

By 1979, 98.5% of women were delivered in hospital. The institutionalization of care of childbearing women has resulted in fragmented care (Cowell and Wainwright, 1981; Robinson, Golden and Bradley, 1983) and this in turn has contributed to consumer dissatisfaction and to dissatisfaction amongst midwives. The latter have expressed concern about loss of their expertise and exercise of decision-making (see for example Towler, 1982; Robinson, Golden and Bradley, 1983; Roch, 1983), and, as Thomson (1980) stated:

... we [midwives] have become assembly-line workers with each midwife doing a little bit to each woman who passes by.

The midwifery managers in the research hospital were keen to encourage the involvement of midwives in evaluating the quality of care that they provide and the procedures that they employ, as advocated by Chalmers (1978). The identification of appropriate staffing levels to provide a high standard of care also formed part of the background to this project. Earlier research had indicated a shortage of midwives in post nationally (Robinson, 1980) and the need for methods to determine appropriate staffing levels had been stressed (Moores, 1980).

During this period the nursing process with various forms of patient allocation was being developed within nursing (Kratz, 1979). The nursing process has been defined as:

... the problem-solving approach applied to nursing
(Ashworth, 1980, p. 26).

Or, more fully:

... A term applied to a system of characteristic nursing interventions in the health of families, individuals and/or communities. In detail, it involves the use of scientific methods for identifying the health needs of the patient/client/family or community and for using these to select those which can most effectively be met with nursing care; it also includes planning to meet these needs, provide the care and evaluate the results. The nurse, in collaboration with other members of the health care team and the individual or groups being served, defines objectives, sets priorities, identifies care to be given and mobilizes resources. She then provides the nursing services, either directly or indirectly. Subsequently, she evaluates the outcomes. The information feedback from the evaluation of outcomes should initiate desirable changes in subsequent interventions in similar nursing care situations. In this way, the nursing becomes a dynamic process lending itself to adaptation and improvement
(World Health Organisation, 1977, pp. 1–2).

Amongst the reasons for the development of the nursing process were the need to provide more individualized and continuous care and to define the role of the nurse (de la Cuesta, 1979). These issues were similar to the concerns of senior midwives in the study district and it was therefore decided that a project should be undertaken in which the effects of the nursing process and 'patient' allocation could be assessed. The author of this chapter was appointed as the research assistant to the project.

THE INTRODUCTION AND ASSESSMENT OF
INDIVIDUALIZED CARE IN MIDWIFERY

As shown in Figure 3.1, a project to introduce individualized care into the midwifery service took place over a three-year period and an assessment of the progress of this innovation was undertaken concurrently. This section describes both the methods employed to introduce changes and the design of the associated research.

Introducing individualized care

In the autumn of 1979 a project was initiated with the following broad aims:

1. To develop and implement midwifery care plans;
2. To improve communication with women, their families and the primary health care team.

Changes were gradually introduced within parts of the hospital and associated community midwifery service. The main method of introducing change was via an educational programme aimed primarily at midwifery staff.* A Midwifery Assessment and Care Plan was developed and brought into the care of all women attending the hospital with various types of midwife–woman allocation. The various aspects of the project were as follows:

1. In-service education was provided for midwifery staff, students and new staff who joined the hospital and involved discussion of the nursing process, midwifery care, methods of allocation, etc;
2. Development of documentation. Small groups of sisters and staff midwives developed initial midwifery assessment formats and care plan formats;
3. Pilot studies were undertaken of the various forms of allocation and documentation in the antenatal clinic, in the antenatal, labour and postnatal wards and in the community (Adams *et al.*, 1981);
4. Midwifery process meetings were held monthly for all midwifery staff and social workers. Attendance at these meetings was voluntary and aimed to provide staff with a place to discuss problems and issues relating to the changes being introduced;
5. A Midwifery Process Co-ordinating Group was set up during the second year of the project to monitor the changes being introduced.

---

*Midwifery staff was the term used within this study to describe collectively the team of midwifery and nursing staff, including midwives, student midwives, registered and enrolled nurses, nursery nurses, nursing auxiliaries, obstetric nurses and student nursery nurses.

Figure 3.1 Progress of the project to introduce and assess the introduction of individualized care with the methods of data collection used.

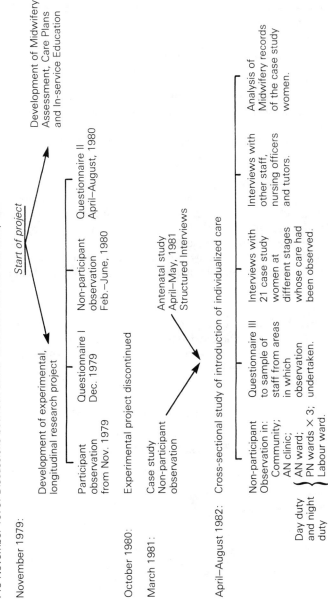

Time:
Pre-November 1979: Discussions between senior midwives and the university team

November 1979:

Start of project

Development of experimental, longitudinal research project

Development of Midwifery Assessment, Care Plans and In-service Education

Participant observation from Nov. 1979

Questionnaire I Dec. 1979

Non-participant observation Feb.–June, 1980

Questionnaire II April–August, 1980

October 1980: Experimental project discontinued

March 1981: Case study Non-participant observation

Antenatal study April–May, 1981 Structured Interviews

April–August 1982: Cross-sectional study of introduction of individualized care

Non-participant Observation in: Community; AN clinic; AN ward; PN wards × 3; Labour ward.

Day duty and night duty

Questionnaire III to sample of staff from areas in which observation undertaken.

Interviews with 21 case study women at different stages whose care had been observed.

Interviews with other staff, nursing officers and tutors.

Analysis of Midwifery records of the case study women.

October 1982: Report to hospital

Source: Bryar (1985)

This group consisted of the nursing officers and senior midwifery managers, the co-ordinating tutor and the research midwife.

6. Information to other staff was provided informally by the midwifery staff, the co-ordinating tutor and research midwife. One formal session was held with medical staff at which the project was described. Social workers attended the regular midwifery process meetings.

7. A Midwifery Assessment was designed, following the pilot studies, that commenced when the childbearing woman first made contact with hospital or community midwifery antenatal care and continued until discharge by the community midwives postnatally. In October 1980, this assessment was brought into the care of all women under the care of the hospital.

8. A care plan format was also brought into use at this time. Over the next two years the care plan format was changed, several times, by groups of staff.

9. Nursing Process Co-ordinators' Group. This was a group of staff from different districts, all of whom were involved in trying to introduce the nursing process. They met regularly to exchange ideas and information about their progress, and to provide each other with support. Some staff from the study district attended meetings of this group as well as outside study days. These meetings provided information about changes in other places and invaluable support for those involved in change during the project.

Following the pilot studies, 'patient' allocation was extended to the care of all women attending the antenatal clinic and was introduced in several wards in the hospital. The community midwives had reorganized their work to enable pairs of midwives to work together to provide continuity of care. Changes and new ideas were introduced in each area at different rates as staff in each area worked through the introduction of change. Further details can be found in Bryar and Strong (1983) and Bryar (1985).

The research project

The aim of the research project was to monitor the effect of the changes on:

1. Midwifery practice;
2. Women's perceptions of care.

Methven (1981) has discussed the need to evaluate existing patterns of care prior to the introduction of change. To enable such an evaluation to take place, the longitudinal study was designed as an experiment. The process and outcomes of care to two groups of women were to be contrasted. One group would receive care provided by a task-orientated system and the experimental group was to receive care by midwives using the nursing process and midwife allocation.

Three factors, however, prevented this project from being undertaken. Observation showed that it would have been extremely difficult to have separated out the care of the experimental and control groups of women. The project failed to secure funding and the university team withdrew. The third factor that militated against the experimental design was the rate of change within the research hospital. As part of the in-service education programme on the nursing process, a study day was held within three days of the start of the project, for all sisters and nursing officers at the hospital and in the community midwifery service. The project, the nursing process and various forms of allocation were discussed on this day. This illustrates the difficulty of conducting experiments in social settings, but also illustrates the pressure for change exerted by clinicians who, in anticipation of an improvement in a service, may be impatient of the rather long time scale of research (Schatzman and Strauss, 1973, p. 11).

During 1980–81, various research methods were tested and a cross-sectional study design was developed with the following aims:

1. To assess the extent to which a systematic approach to midwifery care, i.e. the nursing process approach with patient allocation, had been introduced into care provided by midwifery staff at the research hospital.
2. To examine the views of midwives, other staff and clients about this approach.

Specific questions that were considered during data collection and analysis were:

1. What was the knowledge of, the attitudes towards, and use of the nursing process and client allocation by midwifery staff?
2. What was the knowledge of and attitudes towards the nursing process and client allocation of other staff?
3. To what extent was care individualized to meet the needs of the individual woman/family?
4. To what extent did the woman and her family participate in her own care?

The purpose of the cross-sectional study was to provide a description at one point in time of the effects of change on midwifery practice. The work of several writers on the process of change, and particularly on change within organizations, was drawn upon in considering an appropriate framework for the research questions; this work is discussed prior to a description of methods of data collection employed in the study.

CHANGE AND THE ORGANIZATION OF THE SERVICE

Change and the nursing process

In a description of the dissemination of the nursing process in Britain, de la Cuesta (1979) argues that the nursing process was presented as a means of making good nursing more systematic rather than as a fundamental change in nursing. The development of the nursing process as an educational framework and method of providing more individualized care has been described by Ashworth (1982a) and Hayward (1986). Evidence of marked change in nursing practice through use of the nursing process is still rare (de la Cuesta, 1979; Hayward, 1986). While the speed of dissemination of the nursing process ideal is remarkable, the evidence of its effects appear less obvious (Dickinson, 1982). de la Cuesta (1979) suggests that lack of evidence of fundamental change may be due to the method by which the process was introduced in Britain; this focused on the need for change in the nurse–patient relationship rather than the need to make fundamental organizational changes:

> Thus, it seems that so far the Process is not of much use to the nurse practitioner. It does not represent a change in hospital organisation (the major source of the nurse's problems at work), but it operates entirely on the nurse/patient relationship.
>
> (de la Cuesta, 1979, p.77).

At whatever level, introduction of the nursing process is an attempt to make changes. Change has been classified by Marris (1974) as comprising three types: sudden and unexpected, revolutionary, or planned. Introduction of the nursing process usually falls into the third category, namely planned change, a process described by Hegyvary (1982) as follows:

> It starts with the first presentation of an idea to a group, and, if successful, it ends when the new idea is integrated into the culture of the group.
>
> (Hegyvary, 1982, p.12).

Three strategies for achieving change have been described (Chin and Benne, 1976; Hayward, 1986). The empirical-rational approach suggests that if people are presented with information they will change their behaviour if the new behaviour is seen as beneficial. The normative-re-educative approach considers that, although the presentation of information is important, people will not make changes unless their attitudes and values are altered. The third approach, power-coercive, depends on the exercise of power on those with less power to force them to change. It may be anticipated that the process of change in organizations will take a considerable time as it is dependent upon the reactions of individuals.

Marris (1974) also suggests that change may be understood as a type of bereavement and describes it in terms of the balance between continuity, growth and loss in relation to past experiences involved in the change. The first type of change is substitutional and does not disrupt the meaning of life. The second type represents growth but the changes can still be incorporated within the current meanings of life. The third type of change is potentially destructive, entailing loss and discontinuity. Different individuals will react to change in different ways but any change may be disruptive:

> Change threatens to invalidate this experience, robbing them of the skills they have learned and confusing their purposes, upsetting the subtle rationalisations and compensations by which they reconciled the different aspects of their situation.
>
> (Marris, 1974, p. 157).

The person who has been bereaved needs time to work through his feelings about the loss and Marris (1974) argues that those involved in change have a similar process to work through. Unless this process occurs the change may simply be ignored or integrated into current work routines with little or no noticeable effects:

> Most of these people have little part in the decisions which determine the policy of the organisation; but collectively they have great power to subvert, constrain or ignore changes they do not accept, because, after all, they do the work. If innovation is imposed on them, without the chance to assimilate into their experience, to argue it out, adapt it to their own interpretation of their working lives, they will do their best to fend it off. The changes may be tamed into conformity with familiar routines, or segregated as an extraneous adjunct of the organisation.
>
> (Marris, 1974, p.157).

It therefore appears that the individual's reaction to change, in this case the nursing process, is important but the context within which change occurs is also influential.

A model to illuminate change in organizations

Various models have been developed to describe the processes and actions of organizations and bureaucracies. The ideal type of formal organization described by Weber is characterized by hierarchical authority, division of labour, systematic rules and impersonality (Weber, 1957; Goss, 1963). Such organizations are described as having organizational goals and are structured in a way that these may be achieved.

Systems theory describes the processes of such organizations by relating their activities to the activities of biological systems (Silverman, 1972). Raw materials are taken-in by the organization which acts upon these materials to produce an output, the end product. Systems theory pays little attention to the purposes of individuals within organizations who, according to the bureaucratic model, are expected to have adopted the role of their hierarchical position.

Alternative models have been developed to take into account the purposes of individuals within organizations and are termed professional organizational models (Davies and Francis, 1976). Freidson, (1970), for example, describes organizations as consisting of professional groups that interrelate in terms of dominance and domination. In health care organizations, the dominant role of the medical profession has consequences for the work of members of other occupational groups and hospital organization has been described as an arena of negotiation between members of different professions for power and positions (Strauss *et al.*, 1964).

As Davies (1979) has argued, many of these models isolate the organization from the wider society rather than taking into account the interrelationships between an organization and the wider context within which it exists.

An alternative framework for the analysis of organizations that does take into account the purposes of individuals within the organization and the inter-relationship of the organization with the wider society has been provided by Silverman (1972). This action approach to organizations rests on the view that society and thus organizations are socially constructed and dependent on the meanings attached to them by members of society or the organization (Berger and Luckman, 1985). Silverman argues that the bureaucratic model, systems approach, and the professional organization models are unsatisfactory. Bureaucratic and systems-models emphasize the formal structure and role positions of members while ignoring their individual values. The professional organization models exaggerate the extent to which individuals seek to achieve their own ends and extend their own power while ignoring the existence of shared values (Silverman, 1972). Silverman describes a framework (Figure 3.2) for organizational analysis that consists of four inter-related elements: the changing stock of knowledge outside the organization, the organizational role system, the individual's attachments and definitions of the situation based on her wider experiences and experiences within the organization, and the actions of the individual that are a consequence of the other elements.

This approach emphasizes the importance of the organizational role system that has developed over time and the expectations that individuals will have about the behaviour of particular role occupants. Emphasis is also given to the changing body of knowledge within society and the effect that this will have both on individuals within the organization and those coming into contact with the organization. Both the internal relations of the organization and its relations with the wider society are considered.

Figure 3.2 Action analysis of organizations (from Silverman, 1972, p. 151).

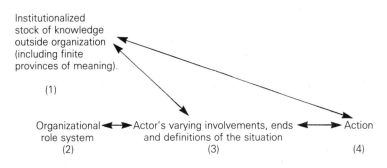

THE ACTION ANALYSIS FRAMEWORK AND MIDWIFERY

The study described here considered the introduction of change within one occupational group, the midwifery staff, within an organization. Silverman's framework for the action analysis of organizations was found useful in describing the process and effects of change, namely the introduction of individualized care, on the action – the care of the childbearing woman – and this is shown in Figure 3.3.

Aspects of each of these four elements that may affect the introduction of individualized care are considered in this section.

Figure 3.3 Inter-relationships of the four elements of the action framework in the context of introducing the nursing process into care of childbearing women.

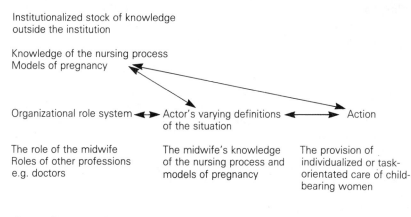

Source: Bryar (1985)

Knowledge in the wider society

Literature relating to two areas of knowledge was considered: models of pregnancy current in society, and the development of, and attitudes towards, the nursing process. Two contrasting models of pregnancy and childbirth are in evidence: the obstetric model and the model of pregnancy as a normal life event. The medical/obstetric model of pregnancy defines pregnancy as a potentially pathological condition requiring medical intervention, with emphasis on physical care rather than care of the whole person (see for example Chalmers, Oakley and MacFarlane, 1980; Weitz and Sullivan, 1985). The alternative model views pregnancy as a natural process and a period of growth:

> ... pregnancy and childbirth are 'natural' processes; as such, they are best managed by the woman herself, with assistance from, rather than control by, professional agents.

> (Comaroff, 1977, p. 115).

The model of pregnancy prevalent within an organization, or held by an individual midwife, it is suggested, will have consequences for the type of care provided by a midwife.

As discussed above, the nursing process had been developed to a great extent in nursing but to a much lesser extent in midwifery (Bryar, 1985). As Webb (1981) has demonstrated, the use of the nursing process approach requires fundamental changes in the sharing of knowledge and power within health care organizations. If the nurse, or midwife, is to undertake total patient care rather than task-orientated care, she needs the knowledge and skills to provide such care. If women are to be involved in care planning they have to be made fully aware of their choices. Both the childbearing woman and midwife using a nursing process approach need to be given responsibility. Such fundamental changes, advocated in the wider body of knowledge (nursing process literature), could have dramatic effects on the action of the organization – i.e. care of the childbearing woman.

Organizational role system

Systems of management vary considerably: Burns and Stalker (1961), for example, identify two contrasting styles – the mechanistic and the organic. The first is appropriate when the task is predictable and follows a routine: tasks are separated, relationships are vertical and responsibility rests at the top of the hierarchy. An organic system is appropriate when the nature of the task is unpredictable and changing: tasks are interrelated, communication is horizontal and the boundaries of jobs are continually re-negotiated (Burns and Stalker, 1961, p. 5). Considering these management systems in relation to nursing, Pembrey (1980) has described the work of the ward sister as being unpredictable but taking place within a mechanistic system with hierarchical relationships between professional groups and within nursing.

It has been suggested by Grant (1979) and Metcalf (1982) that the view taken of patient care requires an appropriate management system. If the care of the childbearing woman is considered to consist of meeting needs that are standard throughout the population, then a mechanistic system of management in which midwifery staff carry out particular tasks according to their competence may be appropriate. If, however, the care of the childbearing woman is viewed on an individual basis, with each woman having different and changing needs, then an organic system in which a particular midwife has in-depth knowledge of the woman, and skills to meet her needs, may be more appropriate.

Actors' definitions of the situation

It is suggested that psychological and sociological factors contribute to the individual's perception of herself and her behaviour, in this case the giving of midwifery care. Jourard (1971) and Menzies (1981) have described how nurses protect themselves from the different types of anxiety engendered by involvement with patients. They also describe the development of defence mechanisms, illustrated in the 'bedside manner' used by nurses to protect themselves from involvement with the patients. Such a defence system has been described for midwifery by Odent (1984):

> Then there are others, (staff) possibly more of them, who unconsciously protect themselves from over-involvement and will offer more impersonal, technical, brisk, mechanical and ultimately 'inhuman' care. They are a bad model for the mother to emulate. The behaviour of some professional staff who have grown too accustomed to the newborn can only be compared with the conscientious but loveless maternal rearing ...
>
> (Odent, 1984, p. 90).

The expectations that others within the organization have of the behaviour of people holding particular positions will also influence the individual. For example, Duff and Hollingshead (1971) found that the work of nurses was limited by the expectation held by doctors, that nurses would follow their orders and provide for the daily requirements of patients. Their work was also limited by patients' expectations that nurses were only able to make limited decisions. Arms (1981, p. 323) has illustrated the effect that the expectations of others can have on the actions of nurse-midwives.

> Despite the personal beliefs and intentions of residents and midwives alike, both are caught in a system that moves women through birth too quickly to permit closeness with any patient.

If nurse-midwives are ever to function as true midwives, they must be free from pressure to rush and alter the natural process. The average hospital is not conducive to normal birth experiences, even with the finest nurse-midwives and the finest intentions.

Other factors that contribute to the actor's definition of the situation in the present context are the model of pregnancy held by the individual and knowledge of the nursing process as discussed above.

Action. In the model developed by Silverman (1972) the interaction of the three elements contributes to the action, i.e. care of the childbearing woman; this may be task-orientated or individualized.

METHODS OF DATA COLLECTION AND ANALYSIS

As shown in Figure 3.1, a range of methods of data collection were used during this study and included participant and non-participant observation, questionnaires, interviews and examination of documents. Figure 3.4 shows the methods used in the cross-sectional study to obtain information on each of the four elements of the action framework that was used for design of this part of the project. (The findings from the literature review have been discussed in the preceding section.)

Figure 3.4 Methods of data collection used in the cross-sectional study.

Institutionalized stock of knowledge

Examination of the literature

Organizational role system	Actor's varying definitions of the situation	Action
Non-participant observation	Non-participant observation	Non-participant observation
Questionnaire III	Questionnaire III	Questionnaire III
Interviews with other staff	Interviews with other staff	Interviews with other staff
Interviews with Nursing Officers	Interviews with Nursing Officers	Interviews with Nursing Officers
	Record analysis	Record analysis

Source: Bryar (1985)

Midwifery is a complex practice, taking place within a complex organization, and the view was taken that no single method could adequately provide information on the process of introducing change to the way in which care is delivered. A combination of methods was therefore used. This strategy, advocated by Denzin (1970), is known as between method triangulation, and as well as providing a more complete picture of a complex situation, has the advantage of avoiding reliance upon a single method.

The rationale for this strategy is that the flaws of one method are often the strengths of another, and by combining methods, observers can achieve the best of each, while overcoming their unique deficiencies.

(Denzin, 1970, p. 308).

This multiple method approach to studying the process of introducing change has been advocated in relation to the nursing process (see for example, Hayward, 1986).

The initial research proposal and subsequent proposal were approved by the ethical committee of the study hospital. Access was granted to all areas of the hospital. Access to individual wards, general practitioners' surgeries and women's homes was obtained by discussion with the individuals concerned. Verbal consent to data collection was obtained from individual staff and from women seen in the hospital or community. No-one refused to consent, although some staff expressed their concern about data collection at particular times.

The methods were developed during the three years of the project. Each method was pilot-tested prior to the cross-sectional study as well as earlier in the course of the project's history. Throughout the period of data collection and analysis, the researcher received valuable support from the previously mentioned nursing process co-ordinators' group and also from a group of nurse researchers.

Participant observation

Data were collected by participant observation in the early part of the project. Participant observation has been defined as the collection of '... required data while taking part in the activity being studied.' (Abdellah and Levine, 1979, p. 701). Data were collected in notebooks in the presence of those being observed and written up in diary form the same or the following day.

My participant role during the study was as the research midwife helping to introduce staff to the use of the nursing process and individualized care, and undertaking research. The four key aspects of the oberver's role that were present in this study have been described by Schatzman and Strauss (1973) as follows:

the researcher is substantially an outsider to the organisation or setting
s/he studies; relationships between the researcher and host are entirely
voluntary; the identity of the researcher and the broad aims of the
study are known to the host, and the main interests of the researcher
are scientific: the purpose is to describe and analyse the activities of the
hosts

(p. ix).

The two main problems experienced with participant observation were
objectivity and isolation. Recording of information is inevitably selective and
interpretation is the interpretation of one researcher (Dingwall, 1976). To
increase objectivity, observations of similar events were compared and
individuals often provided me with their interpretation of events. The
observer is in a unique position within an organization, as Lofland (1971)
describes:

He is close enough to be one of them, but he can't. His job is to write
about their life, not live it. He cannot completely give himself over to
participation, because he has to be considering and remembering all
that occurs in order to record it. And what is most important, the
participants to whom he is close know all these things about him.
There is, then, a subtle separation between the observer and the
members that can be painful and poignant: 'You are here and you
know, but yet you are not really one of us'.

(Lofland, 1971, p. 97).

Data collected during participant observation were analysed as described
below and used to describe the introduction of change.

Non-participant observation

During the cross-sectional study the observer role was adopted exclusively
and I withdrew from any involvement with use of the nursing process and
methods of allocation. The main aim of this observation was to obtain
information about the use of the nursing process and methods of allocation
in relation to midwifery care. Non-participant observation was carried out
for periods ranging from three nights to 10 days in the community, antenatal
clinic, antenatal ward, three postnatal wards and the labour ward.
Midwifery staff including sisters, staff midwives, state enrolled nurses,
student midwives, obstetric students, nursery nurses and auxiliaries were
accompanied in their work during a period of duty. Information was
collected in relation to midwifery care, including the timing of events,
participants involved, activities and conversations. The information was
recorded by means of notes made at the time, which were then written out
fully on the same or the following day.

These records of my observations were examined and analytic notes made on the topics that they covered, (see Lofland, 1971 for a discussion of this process). Following the observation period, the notes were re-examined in relation to a set of pre-determined topics about aspects of the nursing process identified from the literature. During the course of analysis other topics emerged from the data, for example, the effects of hospital policies on use of the nursing process and I reorganized my original notes under the new topic headings. These data were then considered in relation to the data that had been collected using other methods.

Questionnaires

Following observation in each area, all midwifery staff (apart from auxilliary nurses) were asked to complete a questionnaire that contained a mixture of closed and open-ended questions. The purpose of the questionnaire was to collect information about their understanding of the nursing process and forms of allocation, and to obtain their views on the effects of these changes in practice.

The response rate to the questionnaire (which was distributed to 143 midwifery staff and nursing officers) was only 30%. Three main reasons are thought to be responsible for this low response rate. The questionnaire took over one and a half hours to complete and staff were not given time on duty to undertake this task. Some people found difficulty in putting thoughts into words and of understanding terms in the questionnaire, and this may indicate insufficient piloting of the instrument. Many staff felt that they had given their views on the nursing process during the period of observation and could see no point in repeating those comments in written form. It is probable that interviews with staff would have elicited more information than the questionnaire.

The completed questionnaires were analysed manually. Comments made in response to open-ended questions were subject to content analysis and this identified the main themes contained in the answers.

Interviews

Semi-structured interviews were held with a sample of women, other staff and nursing officers. In the semi-structured or focused interview:

> ... the interviewer works with a fixed list of questions or problems to be covered but alters that list and rephrases questions for each respondent. This is a strategy which has the benefits of eliciting common information grounded in the perspective of those observed.
>
> (Denzin, 1970, p. 172).

Interviews were held with a sample of 21 women (the case study women) who were at different stages of pregnancy, or who had delivered, and whose care had been observed. A sample of fifteen other staff was also interviewed; they included physiotherapists, social workers, doctors and ward clerks. Both samples were ones of convenience i.e. a sample consisting of subjects selected because they happened to be present in the study site at the time of sampling (Abdellah and Levine, 1979, p. 333). Interviews were also held with all the nursing officers and midwifery tutors at the hospital (a total of ten).

The aims of interviews with the case study women were to discover the following: to what extent the women had experienced continuity of care; what problems/needs (if any) had been experienced during the childbearing process and whether these needs had been recognized by the midwifery staff, and what help, if any, had been provided by the midwifery staff in relation to these needs. Interviews with other staff sought to discover their previous knowledge of the nursing process and forms of client allocation, their knowledge of, and views of, the use of these approaches in the study hospital and to what extent they used the nursing process documentation. Similarly, interviews held with nursing officers and tutors explored their views on the use of the nursing process and forms of client allocation. Notes were made during the interviews and these were written up immediately afterwards. A summary was made of responses to the main question areas, and these were then categorized according to themes emerging from the study and found in the literature.

Document analysis

New documentation in the form of a Midwifery Assessment and Care Plan was developed during the study period. Information relating to midwifery care from the time the woman 'booked' to the time of her discharge from the hospital (or community midwifery service – if she lived in the area served by the hospital) was recorded on this documentation. Care during labour was not recorded on this documentation. Content analysis of the midwifery records of the 21 case study women was now undertaken; a process described by Holsti (1968) as:

> ... any technique for making inferences by systematically and objectively identifying specified characteristics of messages.

Various researchers have developed methods to analyse nursing records and nursing process records (Hunt, 1979; Ashworth, 1982b; O'Neill, 1984). However, none of these was directly translatable to the analysis of midwifery records, and so a new content analysis schedule had to be developed. The purpose of the content analysis was to identify the following: the extent to which problems/needs were identified on the Midwifery Assessment and Care Plans; the number and content of problems/needs; the number and content of aims; the number and content of plan statements; the number and content of implementation (action) statements; the number and content of continuing assessment statements and their relation to problem statements, and the number and content of evaluation statements.

The documents were only analysed by myself; the validity of the categories and the allocation of data to them was thus dependent on the interpretation of one researcher. Content analysis was extremely time-consuming; this was due to the amount of documentation involved in covering the 21 pregnancies and the different methods by which different staff had completed the records.

Summary

The use of multiple methods of data collection provided information on the introduction of individualized care, from different perspectives. A vast amount of data were collected and it was only through the generosity of a bursary that time was made available for analysis. Given the constraints of time and manpower, a study using fewer methods might have been more appropriate. However, it is argued that any assessment of the nursing process must include observation of practice, information on the knowledge and attitudes of staff and those being cared for, as well as information from records. The attitudes of other staff and the context into which the nursing process is being introduced also need to be considered. Concentration on one aspect of the change to individualized care, for example record-keeping, may produce a distorted picture.

SELECTED FINDINGS

Findings relating to one aspect of the nursing process – care planning – are presented in this section. They illustrate the contribution that different methods of data collection can make to an understanding of a complex activity. Participant observation data from the beginning of the study showed that midwifery staff had little knowledge of the nursing process. Information from questionnaires showed that by the time of the cross-sectional study they had acquired considerable theoretical knowledge. Descriptions of the nursing process included the need to identify and plan for individual needs of women and to assess, plan, implement and evaluate in a systematic manner. The descriptions also showed that the majority viewed the nursing process as an activity to be carried out by midwifery staff rather than a collaborative process between staff, women and their families:

to enable the nursing staff to plan their care of the patients ... a way for mothers and babies to be worked on together ... establishing the needs of the patient.

When the documentation was examined by the researcher it was found that problems were identified by use of the Midwifery Assessment. However, of the 142 problems identified on the 21 Midwifery Assessments by the research midwife, only 27% were also recorded on the Care Plans allowing for care planning etc. to meet these problems. However, 230 problems were recorded on the Care Plans, although the majority had not been noted on the Midwifery Assessment. The majority of these (86%) were actual as opposed to possible problems. Eighty four percent referred to physical problems and 16% to emotional, educational and family problems, for example, 'cracked nipple' and 'looks tired, says she hasn't time for anything'.

In relation to care planning, it was found that only 58 aims were recorded that may have contributed to the problems of evaluation, as it was found that only 3% of statements on the Care Plans related to evaluation.

During the period of non-participant observation, use of the Care Plans was observed. In the antenatal clinic the plans were rarely referred to while care was being implemented. Problems and plans were usually recorded after all the women had been seen, making the recollection of problems difficult. In practice many more problems/needs were identified and care initiated to meet these problems than were recorded on the Care Plans. In the majority of cases these problems related to midwifery aspects of care, for example, providing information about different types of pain relief in labour.

Comments on the questionnaire indicated that staff considered that care was usually planned but that care was planned by other means than use of the Care Plans. This was borne out by observation. Verbal care-planning took place at ward reports and during the giving of care. Plans were recorded in the personal note books of midwifery staff, Treatment Books and on various ward lists. The almost universal use of supplementary personal notes suggests that in practice the Care Plans may be inadequate as a source for up-to-date information. Much care planning was reactive, in that it was a response to a problem identified while care was given. The majority of these problems were not recorded on Care Plans although they might be persistent, for example, problems associated with the establishment of feeding. Care was also 'planned' by hospital routines and policies. For example, in the antenatal clinic, women were observed being directed to see the parentcraft sister when they had expressed no interest in attending classes, and on postnatal wards women were prevented from bathing their babies until the fourth day. These practices were commented on adversely by the case study women during the course of their interviews. On the wards the day was structured around the tasks to be done to the women and babies, for example observations, and routinized care was demonstrated by the giving of standardized information to women in the antenatal clinic, for example, on diet, regardless of their individual needs.

These data may usefully be considered in the context of the action framework (Figure 3.5). As far as action is concerned, then observation showed lack of individualized care. Comments on the questionnaires, however, indicated that midwifery staff did value the provision of such care. On the other hand, data from interviews showed that staff from other disciplines and women attending the hospital had little or no understanding of the nursing process and of the concept of individualized care. Observation showed that progress towards providing individualized care was inhibited by hierarchical systems of management and relationships with other professional groups that resulted, for example, in the development of hospital policies to be applied in the care of all women. Lack of development of the use of the nursing process in midwifery in general may also have contributed to the problems experienced in changing to a more individualized approach to care.

Figure 3.5 Use of the nursing process in midwifery

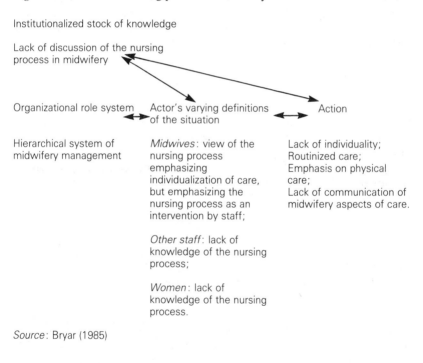

Institutionalized stock of knowledge

Lack of discussion of the nursing process in midwifery

Organizational role system Actor's varying definitions of the situation Action

Hierarchical system of midwifery management

Midwives: view of the nursing process emphasizing individualization of care, but emphasizing the nursing process as an intervention by staff;

Other staff: lack of knowledge of the nursing process;

Women: lack of knowledge of the nursing process.

Lack of individuality; Routinized care; Emphasis on physical care; Lack of communication of midwifery aspects of care.

Source: Bryar (1985)

CONCLUSION

By use of an action framework this project sought to examine the intro-duction of individualized care into midwifery practice. Examination of the literature focused the collection and analysis of data while also contributing to an understanding of the strengths and weaknesses of the different research methods used. The research design used methodological triangula-tion, on the grounds that examination of change in midwifery practice can not be considered adequately by use of a single method. By use of the action framework, midwifery practice was considered in the wider context of change within health care organizations and society in general. Findings from this project suggest the need for education and change in many areas. There is a need to develop the skills of individual midwives to enable them to provide individualized care as well as to provide midwives and midwifery managers with research skills to appreciate and undertake research. The effects of changes on other groups within the organization (childbearing women, doctors, physiotherapists, etc.) need to be considered, as do means for involving them in the changes. If the move towards individualized care is to be paid more than lip-service (Hayward, 1986) then consideration will have to be given to changes required in the wider society to alter the expect-ations that childbearing women have of care and that midwives have of midwifery.

ACKNOWLEDGEMENTS

This study would not have been possible without the hard work and interest of the midwifery staff at the study hospital and in the community. Their help is gratefully acknowledged, as is the advice of Sarah Whitfield and super-visors; Grace Owen and Pat Ashworth. The study was generously funded by the administrators of the endowment funds of the study hospital, and a bursary from the Edwina Mountbatten Trust allowed time for data analysis.

REFERENCES

Abdellah, F.G. and Levine, E. (1979) *Better Patient Care Through Nursing Research.* 2nd edn, McMillan Publishing Company, New York.

Adams, M., Armstrong-Esther, C., Bryar, R., Duberley, J., Strong, G. and Ward, E. (1981) The Nursing Process in Midwifery: Trial Run. *Nursing Mirror,* **153**(15), 32–5.

Arms, S. (1981) *Immaculate Deception.* Bantam Books, New York.

Ashworth, P. (1980) Nursing process: a way to better care. *Nursing Mirror,* **151**(9), 26–7.

Ashworth, P. (1982a) The Nursing Process: an International Perspective. In *Proceed-ings of International Critical Care Nursing Conference.* Organised by American Association of Critical Care Nurses and *Nursing Mirror,* **31**(8), 82–3; (9)82, 10–15.

Ashworth, P. (1982b) *Change from What?* A baseline descriptive study of clinical areas involved with the UK (Manchester) Collaborating Centre in research associated with the WHO Medium-Term Programme in Nursing/Midwifery in Europe, Unpublished report, World Health Organisation, Regional Office, Copenhagen.

Berger, P.L. and Luckmann, T. (1985) *The Social Construction of Reality. A treatise in the sociology of knowledge.* Pelican Books, Penguin, Harmondsworth, Middlesex.

Bryar, P. and Strong, G. (1983) Trial run – continued. *Nursing Mirror,* **157**(15), 45–8.

Bryar, R. (1985) A study of the introduction of the nursing process in a maternity unit. M.Phil (unpublished), South Bank Polytechnic, London.

Burns, T. and Stalker, G.M. (1961) *The Management of Innovation,* Tavistock Publications, London.

Chalmers, I. (1978) Perinatal epidemiology. *Midwife, Health Visitor and Community Nurse,* **14**(11), 380–2.

Chalmers, I. Oakley, A. and MacFarlane, A. (1980) Perinatal health services: an immodest proposal. *British Medical Journal,* **280**(6217), 842–5.

Chard, T. and Richards, M. (eds) (1977) *Benefits and Hazards of the New Obstetrics,* Spastics International Medical Publications, William Heinemann Medical Books, London.

Chin, R. and Benne, K.D. (1976) cited in: Hegyvary, S.T. (1982) *The Change to Primary Nursing,* C.V. Mosby Co, St. Louis.

Comaroff, J. (1977) Conflicting Paradigms of Pregnancy: Managing Ambiguity in Ante-Natal Encounters. In: Davis, A. and Horobin, G. (Eds) *Medical Encounters: The Experience of Illness and Treatment,* Croom Helm, London.

Cowell, B. and Wainwright, D. (1981) *Behind the Blue Door,* Balliere Tindall, London.

Davies, C. (1979) Organisation theory and the organisation of health care: a comment on the literature. *Social Science and Medicine* **13A**(4), 413–22.

Davies, C. and Francis, A. (1976) Perceptions of structure in National Health Service Hospitals. In Stacey, M. (Ed.) *The Sociology of the NHS. Sociological Review Monograph 22,* University of Keele.

Denzin, N.K. (1970) *The Research Act.* A Theoretical Introduction to Sociological Methods. Aldine Publishing Co, Chicago.

de la Cuesta, C. (1979) Nursing process: from theory to implementation. Unpublished MSc thesis. London University.

Dickinson, S. (1982) The Nursing Process and the Professional Status of Nursing. *Nursing Times Occasional Paper,* **78**(16), 61–4.

Dingwall, R. (1976) The Social Organisation of Health Visitor Training. 4. Method in Nursing Research. *Nursing Times Occasional Paper,* **72**(10), 37–40.

Duff, R. and Hollingshead, A.B. (1971) The organisation of hospital care. In Dreitzel, H.P. (ed.) *The Social Organization of Health.* Macmillan Co, New York.

Freidson, E. (1970) *Professional Dominance: the Social Structure of Medical Care,* Atherton, New York.

Garcia, J. (1982) Women's views of antenatal care. In: Enkin, M. and Chalmers, I. (Eds) *Effectiveness and Satisfaction in Antenatal Care.* Spastics International

Medical Publications, William Heinemann Medical Books Ltd., London.

Goss, M.E.W. (1963) Patterns of bureaucracy among hospital staff physicians. In Friedson, E. (Ed.) *The Hospital in Modern Society*, McMillan Publishing Co, New York.

Grant, N. (1979) *Time to Care*. Royal College of Nursing, London.

Hayward, J. (Ed.) (1986) Report of the Nursing Process Evaluation Working Group to the DHSS Nursing Research Liaison Group, NERU Report No. 5, Nursing Research Unit, King's College, University of London, London.

Hegyvary, S.T. (1982) *The Change to Primary Nursing: A Cross-Cultural View of Nursing Practice*, C.V. Mosby Co, St. Louis.

Holsti, O.R. (1968) Content analysis. In: Gardner, L. and Elliot A. (eds) *The Handbook of Social Psychology vol. 2 Research Methods* (2nd edn), Addison and Wesley Publishing Co, Reading, Massachusetts.

Hunt, J. (1979) *A comparative study to determine the most effective method of communicating nursing instructions.* The London Hospital, Whitechapel, London.

Jourard, S.M. (1971) *The Transparent Self* (2nd edn.) D. van Nostrand Co. New York.

Kitzinger, S. (1983) *The New Good Birth Guide.* Penguin Books, Harmandsworth, Middlesex.

Kratz, C.R. (Ed.) (1979) *The Nursing Process*, Bailliere Tindall, London.

Lofland, J. (1971) *Analyzing Social Settings*, Wadsworth Publishing Co. Belmont, California.

Marris, P. (1974) *Loss and Change.* Routledge and Kegan Paul, London.

Menzies, I.E.P. (1981) *The Functioning of Social Systems as a Defence against Anxiety.* Reprint of Tavistock Pamphlet No. 3, 1970. The Tavistock Institute of Human Relations, London.

Metcalf, C.A. (1982) A study of a change in the method of organising the delivery of nursing care in a ward of a maternity hospital. Unpublished PhD thesis, University of Manchester.

Methven, R.C. (1981) The Process of Childbirth. Nursing process related to midwifery care. A Dissertation for Diploma in Advanced Nursing Studies (unpublished), University of Manchester.

Moores, B. (1980) Towards rational midwifery service planning. *Journal of Advanced Nursing*, **5**(3), 301–11.

Newton, R.W., Webster, P.A.C., Binu, P.S., Maskrey, N. and Phillips, A.B. (1979) Psychosocial stress in pregnancy and its relation to the onset of premature labour. *British Medical Journal*, **2**(6187), 411–13.

Odent, M. (1984) *Entering the World. The De-Medicalisation of Childbirth*, Marion Boyars, London.

O'Neill, J. (1984) The use of nursing records in the evaluation of nursing care. MSc thesis (unpublished). University of Manchester.

Pembrey, B. (1980) *The Ward Sister – Key to Nursing.* Royal College of Nursing, London.

Phillips, D. (1981) *Do-It-Yourself Social Surveys. A Handbook for Beginners.* Research Report No. 4. The Polytechnic of North London.

Robinson, S. (1980) The vanishing midwife: are there enough midwives? *Nursing Times*, **76**(17), 726–30.

Robinson, S., Golden, J. and Bradley, S. (1983) *A Study of the Role and Responsi-*

bilities of the Midwife. Nursing Education Research Unit. Report Number 1, Chelsea College, University of London.

Roch, S. (1983) Is the midwife accountable? *Nursing Times* **79**(39), 38–9.

Schatzman, L. and Strauss, A.L. (1973) *Field Research. Strategies for a Natural Sociology,* Prentice-Hall Inc, Englewood Cliffs, New Jersey.

Silverman, D. (1972) *The Theory of Organisations.* Heinemann, London.

Strauss, A., Schatzman, L., Bucher, R., Ehrlich, D. and Sabshin, M. (1964) *Psychiatric Ideologies and Institutions.* The Free Press of Glencoe, Collier-Macmillan Ltd, London.

Thomson, A.M. (1980) Planned or unplanned? Are midwives ready for the 1980's? *Midwives Chronicle and Nursing Notes* **93**(1106), 68–72.

Towler, J. (1982) A dying species: survival and revival are up to us. *Midwives Chronicle* **95**(1136), 324–8.

Webb, C. (1981) Classification and framing: a sociological analysis of task-centred nursing and the nursing process. *Journal of Advanced Nursing* **6**(5), 369–76.

Weber, M. (1957) *The Theory of Social and Economic Organizations.* Collier-Macmillan, London.

Weitz, R. and Sullivan, D. (1985) Licensed lay midwifery and the medical model of childbirth. *Sociology of Health and Illness* **7**(1), 36–54.

World Health Organisation (1977) *The Nursing Process.* Report of the First Meeting of the Technical Advisory Group, Nottingham, December 1976. World Health Organisation, Regional Office, Copenhagen, ICP/HMDO49(1).

CHAPTER FOUR

Continuity of care provided by a team of midwives
- the Know Your Midwife scheme

Caroline Flint

INTRODUCTION

If we knew the person who was going to be with us in labour we wouldn't really need to come to these classes and ask you all these questions would we Caroline? We could just ask the person who is going to be there and get it all sorted out beforehand.

Time and again sentiments such as this were voiced to me in my sitting room where I held National Childbirth Trust antenatal classes every week from 1969. They reflect a maternity service in which care has become fragmented between an ever-increasing number of health professionals; women see a variety of care-givers throughout pregnancy, a different group of people during labour and yet another in the postnatal period.

By 1978 I was still hearing similar comments but by then I had completed my midwifery education and was working as a Community Midwife in South London, able to provide continuity of care for the 35 or so women I delivered as 'domino' deliveries and the 16 or so women I delivered at home every year. They loved having the same familiar face at every visit; equally I loved the closeness of the relationship I developed with each family. I learnt so much, especially when I delivered a woman of several babies. My husband and children enjoyed the christenings, but they were not so keen on this other family of mine when it intruded on holiday times – 'No not that month, Julie's due then', or 'I'm sorry we shall have to cancel coming this weekend, I've got someone who is overdue'.

Their complaints were always quite muted; it has always appeared to me that if the mother of the family is happy and fulfilled then it is likely that everyone else in that family will be satisfied also, but this may be me justifying my own selfish behaviour. Children seem able to adjust to many variations of parent; for example, our daughter as a very little girl showed a playgroup friend the pelvis I used for antenatal classes and which was kept in the sitting room. 'Haven't you got one in your sitting room?' she asked her friend, in an amazed tone obviously believing that a pelvis was 'de rigeur' equipment in any self respecting sitting room.

Not only was the practical application of the principle of 'continuity of carer' sometimes difficult for my immediate family, it also engendered hostility and jealousy amongst senior colleagues.

Sister Flint, do you think that you are a better midwife than any other midwife in the Health District? Do you have no respect for your colleagues on the labour ward? What are you doing here in the labour ward on your day off?

Of course I have respect for my colleagues on the labour ward, and obviously I know that I'm no better as a midwife than anyone else here but I do have one great and immeasurably important quality for this woman that none of the others has – she knows me. I am her friend on the inside.

Sometimes I shared provision of care with my friend and colleague, Sandra; her approach and mine were very similar, our philosophies were almost interchangeable. I began to experience the huge delight of sharing the responsibility and the experience of working with someone with whom I was close, and for the women the satisfaction of getting to know the two of us seemed as great as their satisfaction in getting to know just me. That awful worry that I might break a leg the day they were in labour, or have two women in labour at the same time was no longer so invasive – working in a pair was lovely and for the women they had the advantage of two people they were able to get to know and trust – two friends on the inside.

More and more I realized how important it was to and for women to be enabled to get to know their midwife. It was all very well for me to deliver 40–50 women a year who had been able to develop a relationship with me, but every year in England and Wales 60 000 women have a baby (Macfarlane and Mugford, 1984) and I wanted all those women to be enabled to get to know their midwife.

Others seemed to be expressing similar views: for example Micklethwaite, Beard and Shaw (1978) in a discussion document on a pregnant woman's expectations said:

she would like, if it were possible to have someone around during labour who had given her some antenatal care.

Based on the experience I had had working with Sandra, I wrote an article about, and worked out a rota for, a team of three midwives who would be able to give antenatal and labour care to 468 women every year. The rota took me the best part of a year to work out and I took it with me when I went to the Annual General Meetings of the Royal College of Midwives in Glasgow in 1979. There I heard a talk which moved me to tears

– a midwife called Ann Thomson gave a paper on exactly those thoughts I had in my heart. She led her audience through a vision of midwifery which took my breath away and described how the current midwife was either an antenatal clinic midwife, an antenatal ward midwife, a labour ward midwife, etc. She compared those midwives with assembly-line workers and suggested that this 'Division of Labour' reduced the size of the worker's contribution to the final product, and increased the meaninglessness of her work (Thomson, 1980).

Ann Thomson described her vision for the future in which teams of midwives looked after pregnant women from 'booking', through delivery, the puerperium, and right through to discharge from care, both at home and within hospital wherever the needs of that family dictated. The teams of midwives would be assisted by nursery nurses and auxiliaries who ran creches in the hospital for the pregnant and labouring woman and who helped out at home in the puerperium when necessary. I was breathless with delight and at the end of the session rushed up to Ann. I told her that I had a rota for such a scheme in my bag which I had been going to discuss with the editor of *Nursing Mirror* with a view to publication, but having heard her much wider vision I would tear mine up because it was not nearly as comprehensive as hers. Ann dissuaded me from destroying a year's work. She pointed out that her talk has been about the philosophy but she had not filled in the practical details, and I should carry on and do that. The article which arose from the meeting was called 'A continuing labour of love' (Flint, 1979). I ordered 40 copies of the journal to send to my old head-mistress, English teacher, parents and other poor unsuspecting friends. I waited for the postman to come to my door struggling under mountains of letters inviting me to come and set up this scheme in maternity units around the country. I waited in vain.

Finally, after three months I could wait no longer and took a copy of the article to the Head of Midwifery Services in the district in which I worked to ask if I could be allowed to set up such a scheme. The answer was to set up a working party to examine its feasibility. The working party brought up many disadvantages and concluded that women did not really mind who looked after them as long as they were kind. Women might not mind who looks after them so long as they are kind. There is, however, a growing body of evidence which indicates that continuity of care has positive physical and psychological effects. Before continuing with the history of how the Know Your Midwife scheme came to be set up, some of those studies are briefly reviewed.

RESEARCH ON THE EFFECTS OF CONTINUITY OF CARE

Continuity of care in health care is defined as the provision of care by one person or by a team of persons (Roos *et al.*, 1980). The concept of continuity of care has been examined in the specialities of paediatrics (Gordis and Markowitz, 1971; Becker, Drachman and Kirscht, 1974; Breslau and Haug, 1976), Ear, Nose and Throat (Roos, *et al.*, 1980) and Obstetrics (Carpenter, Aldrich and Boverman, 1968; Shear *et al.*, 1983). It has been demonstrated to have benefits for the recipients (Carpenter, Aldrich and Boverman, 1968; Becker, Drachman and Kirscht, 1974; Breslau and Haug, 1976; Shear *et al.*, 1983) and for the providers (Becker, Drachman and Kirscht, 1974).

In an attempt to evaluate the effectiveness of continuity of care in a paediatric clinic Becker, Drachman and Kirscht (1974) randomly allocated all patient families of a large Children and Youth project to either a clinic in which the patient was seen by the first available physician or to a panel clinic in which continuity of care was maintained by ensuring that the patient saw only his assigned physician on each return visit. The mothers of the children in the panel group reported a higher level of satisfaction with the service that they received and there was an increased incidence of child immunization in this group when compared with the group receiving conventionally organized care.

Breslau and Haug (1976) report a study in which the previously existing continuity of care was decreased following the move of a paediatric practice into a university setting. The number of paediatricians was increased from two to three and because of the different focus of a university setting the physicians were not able to provide the continuity of care that had existed in the original practice. There was an increase in the utilization of the clinic for acute illness without an increase in the incidence of illness in the rest of the community.

In an early study Carpenter, Aldrich and Boverman (1968) examined continuity of support during pregnancy. As part of their course at the Chicago Lying-In hospital, first year medical students were required to interview a woman six times at intervals during her pregnancy. These interviews were extra to consultations with obstetricians and were purely for the benefit of the medical students' education. In order to assess if these interviews affected more than the medical students' education Carpenter, Aldrich and Boverman (1968) compared 52 women who had had the benefit of the medical students' interviews with 50 who had not. The women were not randomly allocated to the two groups, they were allocated a medical student because they happened to be attending for antenatal care at the relevant time in the students' programme. Likewise, those who were not interviewed were attending for antenatal care when there were no students in the hospital. Those who had been interviewed by medical students reported feeling less nervous during pregnancy, were less worried and concerned during labour, and received less narcotic and tranquillizing medication in labour. The authors attribute these differences to the continuity of care the women received from the medical students.

In a retrospective assessment of the outcomes of care provided during pregnancy to women who attended either an obstetric clinic (OB) or a Family Practitioner (FP) clinic Shear *et al.* (1983) found that the babies born to the women attending the FP clinic were 220 grams heavier than those born to women attending the OB clinic. Although not statistically significant the women attending the FP clinic were more satisfied with the care they received. The babies born to women attending the OB clinic were four times more likely to be admitted to the Special Care Baby Unit (SCBU) but this was not statistically significant.

In other studies however, continuity of care has not been shown to have beneficial effects (eg. Gordis and Markowitz, 1971; Roos *et al.*, 1980). In the former study a randomized controlled trial of continuity of care for the babies of adolescents showed no difference in immunization take-up, utilization of medical resources, morbidity, mortality or compliance with medical recommendations. I felt sufficiently convinced however, from my own experience and from the findings of available literature, that continuity of care is important for childbearing women. I also felt that the person who can most easily provide continuity of care in maternity care in the United Kingdom (UK) is the midwife. It is the midwife who is most likely to be present during antenatal care even if the woman is seen by an obstetrician. The midwife is present throughout labour and for delivery, and if the delivery is complicated the midwife remains and assists the obstetrician. Moreover most of the care provided in the postnatal period is given by midwives.

GETTING CONTINUITY OF CARE INTO PRACTICE

After a short period licking my wounds and crying on my husband's shoulder, I approached all the hospitals within travelling distance of my home to ask if they would employ me to set up a scheme to provide continuity of care during childbirth. With one accord they all said no, because the suggested scheme was 'unnecessary' and because I had 'no experience of working within a hospital', therefore I could not possibly know what would work within a hospital.

I began to realize that I would have to get a job in a hospital to prove that I could work within a hospital setting and only then could I try and introduce the scheme I was proposing. I had the good fortune to meet Lynette Murray at a Royal College of Midwives meeting. She was the Director of Midwifery at St George's Hospital in Tooting and seemed dynamic and open. I felt I would like to work with her and was pleased to hear that she had a vacancy for an antenatal clinic sister. I applied and was appointed.

I have always been a good organizer. I knew that if this antenatal clinic was anything like my previous experience of antenatal clinics – long waiting times, impersonal care, sausage-machine type procedures – then I could only improve the situation. It would be hard to make it worse. With the friendly and talented midwives I was working with we were able to turn the Clinic into a more interesting place to receive antenatal care. We appeared in films about antenatal care and I wrote a series of nine articles about our clinic and how we ran it (Flint 1982a; 1982b; 1982c; 1982d; 1982e; 1983a; 1983b; 1983c; 1983d). Whenever women asked me if I would care for them personally in labour and deliver them I gave them my home phone number, and bought myself a radio bleep so that I could be available. I watched the midwives as they developed their skills while providing continuity of care. Each time a woman came to the clinic she saw 'her' midwife and the midwives involved developed from being obstetric nurses lacking in confidence who referred every other symptom to a doctor, to confident, professional midwives who made deep and caring relationships with the women they looked after.

I had published a series of articles which took the team concept a stage further (Flint, 1981a; 1981b; 1981c; 1981d) and asked one of the obstetricians to read them because I wanted to set up such a scheme at St George's. He read the articles and expressed an interest. I approached one of the other obstetricians who was also interested and then went to see Lynette Murray. She suggested setting up a working party to assess the feasibility of implementing the scheme.

The working party discussed the problems, the fears, the cost, and the implications of such a scheme and agreed it should go ahead. Finally, Giles, my husband, thought of the name the Know Your Midwife (KYM) scheme and we were scheduled to start in April 1983.

At that time very little in maternity care had been evaluated. For example Cochrane (1972) describes antenatal care as 'a multiphasic screening procedure which by some curious chance, has escaped the critical assessment to which most screening procedures have been subjected in the last few years ...'. The use of routine continuous fetal monitoring in labour has become policy in many maternity units (Chapter 2 in this volume) and yet in reviewing the available trials of this procedure Prentice and Lind (1987) could find no benefit from this practice.

If we were going to introduce a new style of care it seemed essential to scientifically evaluate the proposed scheme. I went to a Research and the Midwife conference in 1982 and heard Adrian Grant from the National Perinatal Epidemiology Unit give a talk on randomized controlled trials (Grant, 1983). I asked him if I could talk with him about undertaking such a trial with the KYM scheme. I had received help from Adrian before when he had introduced me to papers of which I would otherwise have had no knowledge (this was before the days of the Midwives Information and Resource Service, an organization that provides midwives in the UK with regular and up-to-date information about research and professional developments). He led a naive and totally inexperienced practical midwife through all that was involved in setting up a randomized controlled trial, and my gratitude is eternal to that unit which treats inexperienced researchers with such extreme kindness, gentleness, respect and patience. Sometimes through the turbulent years to follow the unit felt like a haven.

In the following section of this chapter I describe the KYM scheme and the way the team worked, and outline the associated evaluation, in order to place the rest of the chapter in context. Recruitment to the scheme and randomization into the trial are then discussed and this is followed by a description of the scheme in action. The next section provides details of the various methods used in the evaluation of the scheme, prior to a presentation of the main findings. The chapter is concluded with a discussion of the implications of the findings for midwifery.

THE SCHEME AND THE EVALUATION

The intention of the scheme was for a team of four midwives to provide continuity of care during pregnancy, labour and delivery, and the postnatal period for 250 women each year. The women would be deemed to be at low obstetric risk. Following the visit to the booking clinic those women at low obstetric risk who had been randomly allocated to the KYM group and who agreed to participate in the study would then be seen all the way through their pregnancy by the KYM team. Each woman would also be seen routinely by a consultant obstetrician at 36 weeks gestation and at any other time if this was requested by the midwife. During labour the women would be cared for by members of the KYM team whom they had got to know during pregnancy. The women would be transferred to the postnatal ward by a member of the team and visited twice daily thereafter, also by members of the team. On return home women who lived within a reasonable distance of the hospital would be visited by the KYM team for the required length of time.

How the team functioned

Except for Wednesdays there were two duty spans in the scheme:

1. The early shift from 8am to 4.30pm;
2. The 'on-call' shift where the midwife was 'on call' from 7.45am until 7.45am the following morning.

The early shift. The midwife working this shift visited the postnatal ward on arrival for work and provided postnatal care for those women in the KYM scheme (usually 4–5 women). She would also visit any KYM women who had been admitted to hospital during pregnancy (rarely more than one at a time). This midwife would then go into the community to provide postnatal care for KYM women who had been transferred home. The midwife returned to the hospital at lunchtime and in the afternoon provided antenatal care for 5–6 women.

The 'on-call' shift. The midwife working this shift had a long-range bleep and could be called upon to provide antenatal care, care in labour or postnatal care at any time during the 24 hours for one of the women in the KYM scheme. Her only fixed work during the 24 hours was to provide postnatal care between 4pm and 7pm for those postnatal KYM women who were still in hospital. If not called during the other hours the midwife was free to spend time at home, or go out so long as she was within range of her bleep functioning. If bleeped she responded as necessary. If the midwife was called to provide care she noted the length of time involved, if she was not called she just recorded the three hours she worked in the postnatal ward in the afternoon.

On Wednesdays one midwife would work from 1–9pm. She would provide antenatal care in the clinic from 1–4.30pm and from 6–9pm. Between 4.30pm and 6pm the KYM midwives held their weekly team meeting. Figure 4.1 shows a four-week on-duty rota span for four midwives. At the end of every month all the hours worked were totalled and all those who had worked more than 150 hours in a 28 day period were repaid their time.

Figure 4.1 The Know Your Midwife scheme rota

a) The rota repeated itself every three weeks and the basic line was as shown below.

Su	M	Tu	W	Th	F	Sa	Su	M	Tu	W	Th	F	Sa	Su	M	Tu	W	Th	F	Sa
OC	E	OC	E	D	D	OC	½	OC	E	1-9	OC	E	D	D	D	D	OC	E	OC	½

b) In practice the off-duty sheet was as shown below (the team leader (line 1) filled in for others on holiday and made up time for them).

Midwife	S	M	T	W	T	F	S	S	M	T	W	T	F	S	S	M	T	W	T	F	S	S	M	T	W	T	F	S
1	AL	AL	AL	AL	AL	AL	AL	D	D	D	OC	E	OC	½	OC	E	OC	E	D	D	OC	½	D	D	OC	E	X	OC
2	OC	E	OC	E	D	D	OC	½	OC	E	1-9	OC	E	D	D	D	D	OC	E	OC	½	OC	E	OC	E	D	D	X
3	½	OC	E	1-9	OC	E	D	AL	AL	AL	AL	AL	AL	AL	AL	AL	AL	AL	AL	AL	AL	X	OC	E	1-9	OC	E	D
4	D	D	D	OC	E	OC	½	OC	E	OC	E	D	D	OC	½	OC	E	1-9	OC	E	D	D	D	D	X	X	OC	½

OC = On-Call
E = Early Shift
½ = Early Shift which finishes early
D = Day off

AL = Annual Leave
1-9 = 1pm to 9pm shift
X = Day off when time is being paid back by the fourth midwife

The evaluation

In order to evaluate the scheme reliably we introduced it in the context of a randomized controlled trial. From its inception, women eligible for the scheme were randomized into two groups – the group who would be offered KYM care and a control group for comparison. The study had two main purposes. The first was to assess whether the provision of total perinatal care by a team of four midwives is feasible and does result in greater continuity of care. The second was to assess its acceptability to women at low obstetric risk. The differential effects of the two policies on the clinical management and outcome of perinatal care were also examined, but it was recognized in advance that a trial of the size envisaged would provide only imprecise estimates of these, particularly in respect of relatively uncommon adverse outcomes. An attempt was also made to assess some aspects of the comparative costs of care provided to the two groups. Funding for the study was provided first by the Wellington Nursing Research Bursary and then by the South West Thames Regional Health Authority.

RANDOMIZATION INTO THE TRIAL AND RECRUITMENT TO THE SCHEME

We debated how to randomize the two groups, and decided that women could be selected for the study if they were suitable for Midwife care, that is that they were of low obstetric risk and that they met the following criteria:

1. Over 5 feet tall;
2. No serious medical conditions;
3. No previous uterine surgery;
4. No more than two miscarriages or terminations of pregnancy;
5. No previous intrauterine growth retardation;
6. No previous stillborn babies or neonatal deaths;
7. No previous preterm labours;
8. No rhesus antibodies.

We decided that it would be best to select women for inclusion in the trial after their history had been taken and a physical examination carried out at the booking visit. We would then write to all the women eligible and ask them if they would be willing to be randomized into such a trial and then once affirmatory answers were received we could randomize them into the two groups. However, this did not appear to be practical, as it would take too long, we would lose a great number of eligible women because they would not reply to the question, and the women deprived of continuity of care by midwives might be resentful. We decided instead to randomize following the booking clinic with the knowledge that some women would opt out of KYM care and in fact receive ordinary hospital care. To comply with the theory of randomization (Meinart, 1986) we should have to include their findings with the women receiving total KYM care even though the 'refusers' as we came to call them had not actually received KYM care.

The subjects were drawn from women who booked for antenatal care and delivery at St George's Hospital, Tooting, London, between April 1983 and March 1985. The majority of the women booked for care when they were 12–20 weeks pregnant and so were expected to have between 12–14 antenatal clinic visits. The main sample were women who intended having full hospital care. A second sample of women who had booked for shared care between the hospital and their GP was also studied in response to a request from the Regional Research Committee.

The medical records of all the women who came within the listed criteria and who were intending to have full hospital antenatal care were then stamped Midwives Clinic and were randomized into two groups by pinning sealed envelopes containing either the motto Know Your Midwife or Control Group on their records.

The aim was to enrol about five women a week who were to be invited in to the KYM scheme and about five women who were to be in the control group. Some weeks there were less and some weeks there were more in each group, but over the year these differences equalled out. Five hundred and three women were randomized into the KYM group and 498 were randomized into the control group.

Those women randomized into the group to be offered KYM care were written to, given a new appointment and asked to return a tear-off slip giving their consent to take part in the scheme. The KYM care was described to the women as being care given by a team of four midwives who would look after the women throughout their pregnancy (with a check up by a consultant obstetrician at 36 weeks, and with a doctor at any other time if any illness or abnormality was detected). One of their team of midwives would be with them throughout their labour and delivery and would look after them postnatally. They were sent photographs and details of the four midwives. Four hundred and sixty women accepted KYM care and 43 (8.5%) refused KYM care.

The names of the women in the control group were noted together with their expected date of delivery. The date when they would be 36 weeks pregnant was also calculated so that a questionnaire would be ready to give to them when they attended the clinic at 37 weeks gestation. The women in the control group had normal hospital care; this was defined as being provided by an assortment of different doctors and midwives at various times during the childbirth continuum. Neither the women themselves nor the midwives were aware that they had been randomized into a control group.

The sample comprised both primigravid and multigravid women of all races. Overall, 15 KYM women (3%) and 19 controls (4%) moved away during pregnancy. The final size of the trial was dictated by the maximum length of time (two years) that recruitment could continue.

THE SCHEME IN ACTION

The first meeting of the Know Your Midwife Team was held on Thursday 7th April 1983. Wendy Pearce, Penny Church and I introduced ourselves, talked about ourselves and what we were doing and had done, and decided on dates for our clinics. I was writing to the women who had been randomized into the KYM scheme to give them new antenatal appointments and to invite them to join the scheme. I usually did this at the weekends as during the week I was still working as the Sister in the antenatal clinic. Penny was working on a postnatal ward and Wendy was in the labour ward obtaining her 'certificates of competency' in epidural 'topping-up', suturing perineums and 'scrubbing' for caesarean sections.

The first antenatal clinic for the KYM scheme took place on Tuesday 19th April 1983. Four women were seen by Penny Church and myself. They had been given appointments at twenty minute intervals – a pattern that was to continue throughout the period of the KYM scheme.

The women were welcomed to the scheme and it was explained to them that eventually they would be meeting all four midwives and that one of the four would be with them throughout their labour, and that the four midwives would be looking after them during the postnatal period. The philosophy behind the scheme was to try and develop a new type of midwife, neither a hospital midwife or a community midwife, but a woman-based midwife who would be available (and known) to the woman wherever she needed a midwife. At the time, approximately 75% of all women in Great Britain were delivered by midwives (Chamberlain *et al.*, 1978; Cartwright, 1979) and the other 25%, who were delivered by doctors because of complications, always had a midwife assisting and so it was envisaged that one of the four midwives would always be with the woman.

During April 1983 approximately five women were seen each week, during May the number grew to ten per week. By June the number of women seen was fifteen a week, by July twenty, and so the clinic was held on Monday and Tuesday afternoons as well. Claire Neil who was the fourth member of the team had been on night duty for many years while her children were small and came 'off nights' in order to join the rest of the team. The team was complete by June 1983 and in September 1983 began working to the rota described earlier in the chapter. Wendy and I were on call most of August for the women who were expected to deliver then but as there were only three this was not a problem.

We held a weekly team meeting. This involved all the midwives who were working that day unless the midwife on call was caring for a labouring woman (when the meeting took place outside the woman's labour room or in an adjoining labour room as appropriate). At the weekly meetings the midwives discussed women they were anxious about, and the wishes of women who would be delivering in the near future. The midwives also altered 'off-duties'; discussed any deficiences in their knowledge, and problems with other members of staff or with their children! The meetings were enormously supportive; in a safe environment it is easier to admit lack of knowledge and to learn from other members of the group. The team members grew very fond of each other and it is interesting to note that many of them spontaneously hugged and kissed each other on meeting, which is not usual amongst midwives working within a hospital setting.

Midwives working in the National Health Service are contracted to work 37 hours a week, this equates with 150 hours every four week period. The midwives in the KYM scheme kept very careful records of the hours they worked and meal-breaks they took and added this up at the end of every four weeks. When they had worked too many hours they were paid back as soon as possible, when they had worked too few hours they paid them back as time went by.

During the early days of the scheme we were amazed at how disorientated and depressed we felt. It was extremely difficult not having an office and it was very supportive and necessary to meet together every week. Once we had received the money from the Wellington Nursing Research Bursary Fund we set about advertising for a secretary. There was a hitch however. Following the glad news that the South West Regional Health Authority had agreed to give the Project a grant of £41 262 there was a moratorium on the filling of posts in Wandsworth Health District. It was only when the Medical School agreed to take on the administration of the project, under the direction of the Professor of Obstetrics, that we could appoint a secretary. Jane Sanderson started work in March 1984, and in the summer Carol Beth Cundy took over. The day before Jane came we were given an old ward nursery, complete with baby bath in the corner, as an office.

Having an office and secretary made many things much easier. I stopped staying up most of Saturday nights writing to the KYM women and also stopped carrying around all the documentation in my shopping bag which had now become two shopping bags. The midwives had somewhere to convene, we enjoyed our new-found freedom enormously. There was somewhere to put our midwifery bags, somewhere to hang coats, a cupboard to hold 'on call' clothes (a clean set of underwear and equipment for having a bath), desks were begged from the Deputy Head Porter who had a store of old furniture in the hospital basement, and a filing cabinet was ordered from medical school supplies. Polly Poulengeris, our Research Assistant, joined us in April 1984 and set about organizing and completing the questionnaires. It felt that everything was really underway.

During the spring, summer and autumn of 1984 the Know Your Midwife scheme flourished. The rota worked well except that about once every six weeks one of the midwives worked a very long stretch, when she had been 'on call' all the day before and had spent the night with someone in labour.

The midwives were aware of the lack of a second person on call which would have made life much easier and there were discussions that when the research stopped the team would be increased to five or six midwives in order to have a second person on call.

The smooth running of the scheme was shaken on 4th December 1984 when Wendy Pearce was suspended from midwifery practice pending investigation into her management of the first stage of labour of two women. This had a two-fold effect in that first, for a period of time, the team was understaffed and secondly the members experienced great anxiety, as their practice differed little from Wendy's. An additional midwife was appointed in March 1985 but until then it was necessary to write to all the women who were expected to have their baby in December 1984 and January and February 1985 explaining that they would not have a KYM midwife with them during labour. Altogether 66 women were not able to be delivered by the KYM team over this period.

While Wendy's disciplinary procedures progressed slowly another midwife, April Gloag, was appointed to join the KYM team and she started in March 1985 after the parameters for our practice had been discussed at a meeting with the Director of Midwifery Services and the Senior Midwifery Tutor. We started delivering women again as soon as April joined us, but it meant that for three months the KYM women were not delivered by midwives they knew and this had implications for the research, as well as being very upsetting for both the women and the midwives.

The researcher was instructed not to book for the scheme any women who were expected to have their baby after August 1985 as it was necessary to suspend the scheme while it was evaluated.

METHODS USED IN THE EVALUATION

Feasibility of the scheme

In order to assess whether the scheme was feasible we decided to examine the medical records of women having KYM care to see how many different care givers they saw during pregnancy, labour and the pueperium. This would then be compared with the numbers of care givers seen by women in the control group receiving standard care. In the end this proved to be too big a task, and so we only examined in detail the records of women who were expected to deliver in September and October 1984. We looked at and counted every signature on their records, and ascertained whether the signature was that of a midwife, an obstetric house officer or registrar, senior registrar or consultant.

Originally we decided to count all the different care givers who had signed the records antenatally, in labour/delivery and postnatally. However, in contrast to antenatal and labour/delivery care, postnatal care of the KYM group was relatively similar to that of the control group women. Postnatal care of the KYM women was shared between the KYM team who visited in the mornings and evenings, and ward staff who cared for the KYM women during the rest of the day and night. It was extremely difficult to ascertain who actually cared for the women in the postnatal ward because not everyone who provides care for a woman on the ward signs the Kardex. In fact only the midwife in charge of the ward did so. The Nursery Nurse who gave breast feeding advice, the Enrolled Nurse who gave encouragement and the Sister who gave analgesics for perineal pain would not necessarily write all this in the Kardex. It was therefore decided that we would only examine our subgroup in the antenatal and labour/delivery periods.

In total, the number of women who were due to deliver in September and October 1984 were 52 in the KYM group (one of whom had refused KYM care) and 49 in the control group. We compared the two groups in order to ascertain whether women in the KYM group had actually seen fewer care givers than women in the control group.

Women's satisfaction with care

We attempted to assess how women felt about their care by giving them questionnaires at three different periods – at 37 weeks of pregnancy, at two days following delivery and again at six weeks following delivery. They also received a General Health Questionnaire (Goldberg, 1978) with the six-week postnatal questionnaire.

The questionnaires were originally designed by the South London group of the Association for Improvements in the Maternity Services in 1982. I modified these in collaboration with a research midwife, psychiatrist and a social scientist. Further design and administration of the questionnaires were taken over by the research assistant and secretary and were approved by the Steering Group of the project. Questionnaire content and method of distribution were both piloted (see Flint and Poulengeris, 1987). The questionnaires were designed to:

1. Obtain information such as waiting time in clinic (37 week questionnaire), method of baby feeding (2 day questionnaire), discomfort after delivery (2 day questionnaire), problems experienced postnatally (6 week questionnaire);
2. Measure attitudes towards the care received, experiences of labour and feelings about motherhood.

The questionnaires were kept as simple as possible in order to avoid ambiguity. They were printed on different coloured paper as it has been suggested that this is more attractive to respondents and increases returns (Eastwood, 1940).

The questionnaires were not ready to be given out until after July 1984 which meant that some women delivered before they were ready (189 (38%) in the KYM group and 185 (37%) in the control group). We were able to collect obstetric data only for these women.

At 32 weeks of pregnancy a personally signed letter was given to all women asking them to participate in this research into maternity services. The letter emphasized the importance of the research and the confidentiality of any information given (these emphases have been shown to increase co-operation (Robins, 1963)). It was at this stage that it was discovered which women had moved away since booking.

Of the women available to receive questionnaires some were excluded because of language difficulties (three KYMs and nine controls) some refused to participate (three KYMs and three controls) and some women seemed to vanish mysteriously when the research assistant or secretary approached the antenatal clinic (six KYMs and 17 controls). Questionnaires were given to all the available women in the KYM scheme, those women who had declined the offer to be in the KYM scheme and the women in the control group. In practice it was easier to maintain contact with the KYM group who were being looked after by just four midwives than it was to maintain contact with the group receiving usual hospital care (i.e. the control group and KYM refusers).

37 week questionnaire. This was a 47 item self-administered questionnaire completed in the antenatal clinic and included questions on attitude to pregnancy, women's expectations and plans for labour, views on waiting time in the clinic, and an assessment of staff attitudes, care and helpfulness. Questions were designed to ascertain sample characteristics and these included social class based on husband's occupation, woman's education, drinking and smoking habits. The majority of questions were of a closed item format with two to four choices available in each. In addition, there were two open questions for comments. Women were approached in the antenatal clinic by either the research assistant or secretary; they were asked to fill in this first questionnaire and to apply the questions to the care that they were receiving (either KYM care or the normal hospital care for the control group and the women who had refused KYM care). Occasionally a woman would take the questionnaire home and return it at her following appointment. Women staying in the antenatal ward at this time were also given the questionnaire. At this stage women with language difficulties (three KYMs and nine controls) and those refusing to participate (three KYMs and three controls) were excluded from the questionnaire study. Of the women who were missed, it was possible to catch up with some in the puerperium and give them the 37 week questionnaire then. Twelve per cent of all 37 week questionnaires given out were given to women in the puerperium. In total 285 KYMs and 274 controls were given the 37 week questionnaire. The number returned was 277 (97%) from the KYMs and 268 (98%) from the controls.

Two day postnatal questionnaire. This was a 36 item self-administered questionnaire completed on the postnatal ward: it included questions on how the woman felt about her labour, how prepared she had felt, her satisfaction with her pain relief, whether she was experiencing any perineal discomfort or pain, her attitude towards her baby, and questions about the staff. As with the antenatal questionnaire, most questions were of closed item format with between three and five choices. There were also three open-ended questions for additional comments.

The two day postnatal questionnaire was handed out two to three days post delivery. The procedure was to give the questionnaire to the woman in the morning and then arrange a suitable time for collection. Questionnaires were sent on to any women who had left the ward early. Questionnaires were not given to women if it was felt that it would be distressing for them, as when their baby was in the Special Care Baby Unit (SCBU) and/or seriously ill.

In total, two day postnatal questionnaires were given to 279 KYMs and 267 controls. The number returned was 275 (99%) for the KYMs and 261 (98%) for the controls.

Six week postnatal questionnaire. This was a 28 item questionnaire with closed-item questions on how the woman felt about her labour, her satisfaction with her pain relief, whether she felt prepared for motherhood and to cope with her baby, her attitude towards the baby, her confidence, whether she had experienced problems and how she felt about her postnatal care. The questionnaire was printed on yellow paper, the colour found to yield the highest proportion of returns (Eastwood, 1940).

The six week postnatal questionnaire, together with a covering letter and the General Health Questionnaire were sent six weeks after the birth (the average age of the baby at this time as indicated on the returned forms was seven weeks (SD=3.1 days) for the KYM group and 7 weeks 5 days (SD=2.4 days) for the control group). Before sending the questionnaires we ascertained that the baby was still alive and well, especially if it had been in the SCBU. Any woman who had not returned the questionnaire within four weeks was either telephoned or sent a reminder letter. If she did not respond she was sent another questionnaire and letter, followed by another phone call if possible; it was stressed how important her contribution was and that returning the final form would complete the set of questionnaires.

In total, six week questionnaires were sent to 279 KYMs and 267 controls. Of these 249 (89%) were returned by KYMs and 227 (85%) returned by controls.

General Health Questionnaire. The 28 item General Health Questionnaire (GHQ) sent out with the six week questionnaire is a well-validated instrument for screening psychological health and wellbeing (Goldberg, 1978). The 28 item version with four sub-scales in addition to a total score was chosen in preference to the 30 item version which yields a single severity score. GHQs were sent to 279 KYMs and 267 controls. Of these 231 (83%) were returned by KYMs and 198 (74%) by controls. Unlike the 6 week postnatal questionnaire, GHQs were not sent out a second time to women who had not returned them within 4 weeks, and this accounts for the lower rate of GHQ returns compared with the return rate of the six week questionnaire.

Maternal and baby outcomes

Information was obtained on a wide range of aspects of clinical management of pregnancy, labour and delivery and of details of neonatal outcome. As already noted, it was recognized at the outset that a trial of the size envisaged would be too small to allow for a precise assessment of the differential effects of the two types of care on neonatal outcomes.

An obstetric record sheet was filled in for every woman randomized into the study (women offered KYM care whether they accepted or not, and the control group). The obstetric sheet covered all details of parity, age, marital status, race, labour, haemoglobin level at 36 weeks of pregnancy and two days postnatally, length of pregnancy, analgesia used during labour, the type of delivery, perineal trauma and estimated blood loss. Details of the baby included whether it was alive, stillborn, died neonatally or if the pregnancy had miscarried before 28 weeks gestation, birthweight, Apgar score at 1 and 5 minutes, whether any resuscitation was needed or if the baby had been admitted to SCBU. The length of the woman's postnatal stay, any antenatal admission and the reason for admission were also noted. All these details were taken from the medical records by the research assistant and secretary. If for any reason a set of records was persistently missing (very few) then as much information as possible was gleaned from the Birth Register in the labour ward and the index cards kept by the maternity secretary. We examined each woman's records following delivery and compared how the women and babies in the KYM group fared with those in the control group.

Costs

It proved impossible to ascertain the full cost of providing the KYM service and to compare it with the cost of providing the service to the control group. It also became apparent that within the National Health Service it is very difficult to find out the actual cost of procedures or use of facilities. We had to content ourselves with comparing the antenatal admissions in each group, the difference in costs as related to the use of epidural analgesia in each group and the different perceived costs of consultations with different personnel during the antenatal period.

Data processing and analysis

All the coded data from the obstetric sheet, the three questionnaires and the GHQ were put on to the London University Mainframe Computer (an Amdhal). The programme used for data input was Quip and Quote and the SPSSX programme was used for statistical analyses.

The sample size of approximately 250 women a year in each group was arrived at from a purely practical point of view. This was the number that it was decided a team of four midwives could look after in the way that the KYM team intended to function. This number was adequate for examining client satisfaction, feasibility and cost implications but as already noted was inadequate for assessing obstetric outcome. The findings could however be considered with those from similar studies undertaken in the future; they have already been considered (Robinson, 1989) in relation to the only two comparable randomized controlled trials (Runnerstrom, 1969; Slome *et al.*, 1976) identified from the Oxford Database of Perinatal Trials (Chalmers, 1988).

Chi square and Student's 't' statistical tests were used as appropriate. Confidence intervals of the relative risks were calculated using the method described by Katz *et al.* (1978), 99% rather than 95% intervals are presented because of the many comparisons made between the groups. If the 99% confidence interval does not include unity (i.e. 1) then the observed difference is significant at $p < 0.01$.

FINDINGS

A large data set was obtained in the course of the research, and the findings are available in full in Flint and Poulengeris (1987). The main findings are presented in this chapter and relate to:

1. Socio-demographic characteristics of the two study groups;
2. Continuity of care;
3. Women's views of the two systems of care;
4. Maternal outcome;
5. Neonatal outcome.

Individual items are missing for a few women in both the medical records and questionnaire data sets and this is why the denominators vary slightly.

Socio-demographic characteristics of the two study groups

The two groups derived by random allocation were similar at entry in age, parity, marital status, number in employment, and type of accommodation (Table 4.1). However, there were more Asian women in the control group and more smokers in the KYM group.

Table 4.1 Socio-demographic characteristics of the trial groups

	Know Your Midwife care	Standard hospital care
Data from case-notes	($n = 503$)	($n = 498$)
Mean (SD) maternal age	25.8 (5.1)	25.4 (5.0)
No. (%) primiparous	288 (57)	291 (58)
No. (%) married*	368 (76)	371 (78)
Ethnic group: No. (%)		
Caucasian	367 (73)	311 (63)
Asian	48 (10)	90 (18)
Afro-caribbean	74 (15)	74 (15)
Other	14 (3)	20 (4)
Data from questionnaires	($n = 274$)	($n = 264$)
No. (%) smokers	83 (30)	59 (22)
No. (%) in paid employment at 37 weeks' gestation	20 (7)	18 (7)
Housing: No. (%)		
Own home	142 (52)	136 (52)
Rented	88 (32)	87 (33)
Other	44 (16)	42 (16)

*Denominators for information on marital status were 483 for the KYM group and 473 for the controls.
Source: Flint *et al*. (1989).

Feasibility of providing continuity of care

It will be recollected that the first purpose of the study was to ascertain whether it is feasible for a team of four midwives to provide total perinatal care for a group of women at low obstetric risk and with a greater degree of continuity of care than is normally experienced. This was assessed by analysis of signatures on the medical records of a sub-group of KYM and control group women; the findings are shown in Table 4.2. It can be seen that women in the KYM group saw fewer care givers during pregnancy than did the women in the control group. The most striking finding in Table 4.2 is that KYM women were much more likely than control group women to have had someone with them in labour from whom they had also received antenatal care: 98% compared with 20%. The care giver known to the KYM women was almost always one of the midwives whom they had met antenatally, whereas for control group women this person was usually a junior doctor whom they had met in the antenatal clinic. Overall the findings in Table 4.2 show that the KYM scheme was associated with greater continuity of care.

Women's views of the two systems of care

The KYM scheme appeared to be more acceptable to the women in almost every aspect investigated, some of these findings are shown in Table 4.3. In the antenatal clinic the KYM women did not have to wait as long to be seen and found it easier to discuss their anxieties. Other findings, not shown in the table, indicate that although a majority of both groups expressed overall satisfaction with the experience of attending the antenatal clinic, this was more marked in the KYM group than in the control group. Both groups found midwives more approachable than doctors.

Two days after delivery women in the KYM group were more likely to feel that they had been well prepared for labour (Table 4.3). Other findings (Flint and Poulengeris, 1987), showed that KYM women were more able to take up a position of their choice during labour and to have been delivered in an alternative position (on a bean bag, a birthing chair, squatting or on 'all fours'). At two days post delivery the KYM group were more likely to rate those who had looked after them in labour as 'very caring'. Six weeks after delivery there were striking differences in the women's recollection of labour in that the KYM women looked back on it as a 'wonderful' or 'enjoyable' experience more often than did women in the control group (Table 4.3). Findings in Table 4.3 also show that KYM women were more likely to have felt in control during labour and to have been satisfied with pain relief. Moreover, KYM women were more likely than controls to have felt well prepared for child care and felt able to discuss problems postpartum. There were no statistically significant differences in the GHQ scores of the KYM and control group.

Table 4.2 Continuity of care

	Know Your Midwife care	Standard hospital care	Relative rate	99% CI
Fewer than 8 care givers seen during pregnancy	41/52 (79%)	24/49 (49%)	1.6	1.1–2.4
Fewer than 3 midwives seen during labour	34/49* (69%)	22/46* (48%)	1.5	0.9–2.3
Fewer than 3 doctors seen during labour	43/49* (88%)	35/46* (76%)	1.2	0.9–1.5
Met intrapartum care giver during pregnancy	48/49* (98%)	9/46* (20%)	5.0	2.3–11.0

Data from 2 month case-notes study.
*Three women in each group either miscarried or delivered elsewhere.
Source: Flint *et al.* (1989).

Table 4.3 Women's view of the two systems of care

	Know Your Midwife care		Standard hospital care		Relative rate	99% CI
Clinic waiting time <15 min[a]	169/275	(61%)	18/267	(7%)	9.1	5.0–16.6
Ability to discuss anxieties[a]	243/272	(89%)	200/261	(77%)	1.2	1.1–1.3
Well prepared for labour[b]	144/275	(52%)	102/254	(40%)	1.3	1.0–1.7
Enjoyment of labour[c]	104/246	(42%)	72/223	(32%)	1.3	1.0–1.8
Feeling of control during labour[c]	103/246	(42%)	54/225	(24%)	1.7	1.2–2.5
Satisfaction with pain relief[c]	121/209*	(58%)	104/205*	(51%)	1.1	0.9–1.4
Well prepared for child care[c]	104/242	(43%)	64/222	(29%)	1.5	1.1–2.1
Ability to discuss problems post-partum[c]	157/246	(64%)	112/220	(51%)	1.3	1.0–1.5

Data from [a]37-week; [b]2-day postnatal; and [c]6-week postnatal questionnaires.
*Based on women who had a normal delivery.
Source: Flint *et al*. (1989).

Maternal outcome

Women cared for by the KYM team were less likely to be admitted to the hospital antenatally than women in the control group. Clinically, the KYM scheme was characterized by less obstetric intervention during labour and delivery (Table 4.4). The KYM women received less analgesia despite being recorded as having longer labours. The differences in the rates of acceleration of labour, epidural and intramuscular analgesia, and episiotomy were statistically significant. However, the overall rates of perineal trauma were almost identical because of a corresponding rise in the incidence of vaginal tears in the KYM group. There were fewer instrumental deliveries in the KYM group when compared with the control group but the differences were not statistically different. The tendency for labours to be longer in the KYM group may be related to the difference in the rate of acceleration of labour, but could also be due to a different definition of the onset of labour by the known care givers.

Neonatal outcome

The outcome for the babies was generally similar in the two groups (Table 4.5). There were significantly more low five-minute Apgar scores in the KYM group but resuscitation was used significantly less often for the babies in this group and the final status on the delivery suite, as judged by the numbers of babies who were transferred to the SCBU, was similar. There were four stillbirths and four neonatal deaths in the KYM group compared with two stillbirths and two neonatal deaths in the standard care group. Review by an experienced obstetrician of the medical records of these 12 cases suggested that it is unlikely that any of the deaths could have been prevented by a change in care. With such a small number of events the confidence intervals are wide (Table 4.5) and include both a clinically important increase and a clinically important decrease in the risk of perinatal death associated with the KYM scheme.

Secondary analyses showed that adjustment for ethnicity and smoking makes no important difference to the findings. Women of European origin were more likely to have epidural analgesia and less likely to have pethidine in labour. Adjustment tended to accentuate the contrast between the groups in epidural use and slightly reduce the difference in pethidine use.

Costs

As noted in the methods section it proved impossible to obtain the information necessary to compare the full costs of the two systems of care. Some evidence was afforded by the study however. The KYM service cost less than the standard care service, in terms of fewer days spent in hospital

Table 4.4 Maternal outcome

	Know Your Midwife care	Standard hospital care	Relative rate	99% CI
Delivered at St George's Hospital	488	479		
Antenatal admission	123/484 (25%)	146/475 (31%)	0.8	0.6–1.1
Induction of labour*	51/465 (11%)	60/458 (13%)	0.8	0.5–1.3
Artificial rupture of membranes*	247/465 (53%)	270/454 (59%)	0.9	0.8–1.0
Augmentation of labour*	80/465 (17%)	114/458 (25%)	0.7	0.5–1.0
Length of first stage >6 hrs†	276/445 (62%)	229/439 (52%)	1.2	1.0–1.4
Epidural analgesia	88/479 (18%)	143/473 (30%)	0.6	0.4–0.8
Any analgesia other than Entonox	233/479 (49%)	293/473 (62%)	0.8	0.7–0.9
Operative vaginal delivery	56/479 (12%)	66/473 (14%)	0.8	0.5–1.3
Caesarean section	37/479 (8%)	35/473 (7%)	1.0	0.6–1.9
Episiotomy†	152/443 (34%)	185/438 (42%)	0.8	0.7–1.0
Vaginal tears†	184/443 (42%)	149/438 (34%)	1.2	1.0–1.5
Intact perineum†	107/443 (24%)	104/438 (24%)	1.0	0.7–1.4

* Elective caesareans excluded
† All caesareans excluded
Source: Flint et al. (1989).

Table 4.5 Neonatal outcome

	Know Your Midwife care	Standard hospital care	Relative rate	99% CI
Babies born at St George's Hospital*	478	471		
Birthweight <2500g	31/478 (6%)	38/471 (8%)	0.8	0.4–1.5
Apgar score				
<8 at one min	90/471 (19%)	91/467 (19%)	1.0	0.7–1.4
<8 at five min	17/470 (4%)	6/468 (1%)	2.8	0.8–9.5
Neonatal resuscitation	97/474 (20%)	128/465 (28%)	0.7	0.5–1.0
Admission to Special Care Nursery	23/475 (5%)	21/470 (4%)	1.1	0.5–2.3
Stillbirth or neonatal death	8/478 (2%)	4/471 (1%)	2.0	0.4–9.5

* 15 miscarriages and 3 terminations not included in this Table
Source: Flint et al. (1989).

antenatally, difference in the grade and number of personnel seen during antenatal consultations, less use of epidural and other analgesia and less frequent acceleration of labour. A fuller discussion of these differences and their associated costs can be found in Flint, Poulengeris and Grant (1989).

DISCUSSION

The main aims of this study were to assess the feasibility of providing total perinatal care by a team of four midwives, to assess whether this style of care did provide greater continuity of care and to assess the acceptability of such a scheme to women. The experiment has shown that a team of four midwives can successfully care for 500 women at low obstetric risk over a two year period. The trial has provided clear evidence that the KYM scheme as practised at St George's Hospital during 1983–1985 did improve continuity of care and was more acceptable to women at low obstetric risk than the standard hospital care. The KYM scheme was also associated with a reduction in obstetric intervention, particularly in respect of acceleration of labour and intrapartum analgesia. The lower rates of episiotomy and instrumental delivery are also similar to the findings of the only two comparable controlled trials (Runnerstrom, 1969 and Slome *et al.*, 1976) indentified from the Oxford Database of Perinatal Trials (Chalmers, 1988).

The difference in the 5 minute Apgar scores is likely to reflect the difference in the use of neonatal resuscitation; the rates of admission to the SCBU do not suggest a major adverse effect of the KYM scheme on pregnancy outcome. Although there were more baby deaths in the KYM group the total number is small and the confidence interval is very wide; as recognized at the outset, the trial was too small to assess with any precision the safety of the scheme in terms of perinatal mortality.

Women in the KYM group were significantly more likely to be able to discuss anxieties during pregnancy than the control group receiving standard care. Similarly, when comparing the views of women seeing few care givers during antenatal care with those of women who saw a different person at each antenatal visit, O'Brien and Smith (1981) found that those who saw few care givers were significantly 'more able to discuss things'; this advantage of seeing fewer care givers held for both the hospital and the GP's surgery.

The women in the KYM group wanted to be more active in labour that did those in the control group and were able to achieve this (Flint, Poulengeris and Grant, 1989). The KYM women found their care givers in labour to be 'more caring'. It is interesting to note that Kirke (1980) found a close association between the woman's reports of her treatment and attention by staff in labour and whether a woman would return to the same hospital for a subsequent birth. At six weeks post delivery the women in the KYM group had significantly more positive views of their labour and felt that they had been much more in control during labour. Oakley (1980) has shown that this latter finding is associated with a lower incidence of post-natal depression.

The popularity of the scheme with women is not in question. However, the scheme does demand extra responsibility from midwives than is usual in the current maternity services in the UK. This change in practice was sometimes stressful, particularly at first, for both those implementing the scheme and those administering it. The provision of continuity of care over a 24-hour period also meant that occasionally a midwife worked for long hours without formal back-up at nights or at weekends. Expansion of the team to 5 or 6 midwives would provide a second midwife 'on-call' and greater flexibility in the rota, although this might reduce continuity of care. The four midwives were very supportive of each other and worked closely together, to some extent independently of other staff in the hospital. This led to some problems in the working relationship between KYM midwives and other personnel (see Chapter 5, part 1 for a description of similar problems of working in an innovative scheme). All these difficulties should be taken into account when setting up similar schemes elsewhere.

In the time that has elapsed since I started my efforts to get the scheme into practice, concern about lack of continuity of care during pregnancy and childbirth has been expressed continually. In giving evidence to the Social Services Committee one witness said:

> I think this is what women complain about most: they do not have continuity of care which they want very much during their antenatal visits but certainly during labour and delivery.
>
> (Social Services Committee, 1980)

The Social Services Committee (1980) go on to state:

> We recognise the difficulties of providing continuity of care throughout pregnancy and labour but consider that a measure of it can be attained by better organisation.
>
> (Social Services Committee, 1980)

These sentiments were echoed by a National Childbirth Trust Working Party in 1981:

> there is an almost complete absence of continuity of care and each time she attends a woman sees different, anonymous faces.
>
> (NCT, 1981).

and again by the Maternity Services Advisory Committee in 1982:

> Continuity of care. It is important that the woman should be able to build up a relationship of trust with the staff she meets, and efforts should be made to involve the same group of staff at each visit.
>
> (MSAC, 1982)

The Royal College of Obstetricians added their voice in the same year:

> It has been suggested to us that women should have the same midwife to attend them in labour as in the antenatal period. We consider this continuity of care to be an ideal aim and it may be possible in some circumstances.
>
> (RCOG, 1982).

Three surveys, albeit not all methodologically ideal, of parents' views highlighted a desire for continuity of care. Comments made by respondents to Boyd and Sellers (1982) study included the following:

> I was more relaxed because my midwife was with me.

> By and large it is the midwife who makes or breaks a happy delivery.

> My labour was a truly delightful experience – attended by professional people that I regarded as friends.

The same themes emerged from a survey carried out for Parents Magazine in 1983 and again in 1986:

> Mothers would like antenatal, delivery and postnatal care to be provided as far as possible by the same people. Again and again, letters expressed the anxiety that arises when seeing a different doctor at each visit to the antenatal clinics, and at being delivered by total strangers – sometimes two different shifts of total strangers if a woman had a long labour.
>
> (Parents Magazine, 1983)

> Good communications between parents and the medical staff were helped where women saw the same doctor and midwife regularly ... most mothers saw different people at almost every antenatal visit and were delivered by total strangers. While full of praise for the care they received, many women wished they could have had more continuity of care through pregnancy and beyond.
>
> (Parents Magazine, 1986)

It is not known how much the observed effects of this style of provision of perinatal care were due to the enthusiasm, personality and efficiency of the midwives in the KYM team. There are still questions about whether the findings are generalizable to a similar scheme worked by other midwives in other settings. However, in view of the continuing demand for continuity of care and on the basis of the very encouraging findings presented here I believe that this scheme, or a modification of it, should be introduced widely elsewhere, in such a way that allows further evaluation of its effects on neonatal outcome.

At the time of writing attempts to provide such schemes are now taking place throughout the country – notably in the Rhondda, Oxford, Guildford and Riverside Health Authority (Flint, 1989). It is to be hoped that formal scientific evaluation of all the schemes will be undertaken.

ACKNOWLEDGEMENTS

This chapter could not have been written without the generous and unstinting help of Adrian Grant, Epidemiologist at the National Perinatal Epidemiology Unit, and Polly Poulengeris, research assistant to the KYM scheme. The research was generously funded by the South West Thames Regional Health Authority and the Wellington Foundation. I would like to acknowledge the help and support of the obstetricians at St Georges Hospital (Mr A. Amias, Professor G. Chamberlain, Mrs U. Lloyd, Mr M. Pearce, Mrs T.R. Varma). Commitment and help towards the scheme and the midwives in it were given by David Rosenberg, Debbie Moncrief, Jill Dixon, Jon Cresswell and Malcolm Stewart.

The midwives at St Georges Hospital gave us great help and support, and especial thanks are due to Mrs L. Murray, Director of Midwifery Services, who financed the four midwives and enabled the scheme to be started. It was a joy and privilege to work with Penny Church, Claire Neil, Wendy Pearce, April Gloag and Clover Dixon. Carol Beth Cundy was our stalwart support who found notes, typed the report and kept us all sane. Computing help was generously given by Valerie Dickenson, Tariq Rasheed and Andrew Tickle. Help with statistics and many other aspects of the report was given by Martin Bland.

The guidance of the steering group (Miss M. Arnold, Professor G. Chamberlain, Ms R. MacNair, Mrs L. Murray, Dr K. Poulton) was appreciated. Much support and guidance was generously given by colleagues at the National Perinatal Epidemiology Unit, which is supported by a grant from the Department of Health.

Giles Flint as ever, provided much love and support. The women who participated in the scheme allowed us the privilege of taking part in a chapter of their lives which we, and probably they, will never forget.

A full report of this study (plus the report of a study of women receiving 'shared' care with their GP) is available from The Midwives Information and Resource Service, Institute of Child Health, Royal Hospital for Sick Children, 65, St Michael's Hill, Bristol BS2 8BJ. Price: £8.50 plus £1.00 package and postage. Cheques with order made payable to MIDIRS please.

REFERENCES

Becker, M.H., Drachman, R.H., Kirscht, J.P. (1974) A field experiment to evaluate various outcomes of continuity of physician care. *American Journal of Public Health*, **64**, 1062–70.

Breslau, N. and Haug, M.R. (1976) Service delivery structure and continuity of care: a case study of a pediatric practice in process of reorganization. *Journal of Health and Social Behavior*, **17**, 339–52.

Boyd, C. and Sellers, L. (1982) *The British way of birth*. Pan Books Ltd, London.

Carpenter, J., Aldrich, C.K., Boverman, H. (1968) The effectiveness of patient interview. *Archives of General Psychiatry*, **19**, 110–12.

Cartwright, A. (1979) *The dignity of labour*. Tavistock, London.

Chalmers, I. (1988) (ed.) *The Oxford Database of Perinatal Trials*. Oxford University Press, Oxford.

Chamberlain, G., Phillip, E., Howlett, B., and Master, K. (1978) *British Births 1970*, Vol. 2, *Obstetric Care*. William Heinemann Medical Books, London.

Cochrane, A.L. (1972) *Effectiveness and Efficiency*. Nuffield Provincial Hospitals Trust, London.

Eastwood, R.P. (1940) *Sales control of quantitative methods*. Columbia University Press, New York.

Flint, C. (1979) A continuing labour of love. *Nursing Mirror*, **149**(20), 16–18.

Flint, C. (1981a) Our pregnant lady. *Nursing Mirror*, **153**(23), 22–3.

Flint, C. (1981b) Emma, Joan, Liz and A.N. Other. *Nursing Mirror*, **153**(24), 31–4.

Flint, C. (1981c) Crisis at night. *Nursing Mirror*, **153**(25), 26–7.

Flint, C. (1981d) Small is intimate. *Nursing Mirror*, **153**(26), 36.

Flint, C. (1982a) Where have we gone wrong? *Nursing Mirror*, **155**(21), 26–8.

Flint, C. (1982b) Get off the conveyor belt. *Nursing Mirror*, **155**(22), 37–8.

Flint, C. (1982c) Make it worth the wait. *Nursing Mirror*, **155**(23), 15–16.

Flint, C. (1982d) More than a laying on of hands. *Nursing Mirror*, **155**(24), 41–2.

Flint, C. (1982e) Continuity of care. *Nursing Mirror*, **155**(25), 67.

Flint, C. (1983a) Using the midwifery process. *Nursing Mirror*, **156**(1), 16–17.

Flint, C. (1983b) Involving the community. *Nursing Mirror*, **156**(2), 35–6.

Flint, C. (1983c) Growing in confidence. *Nursing Mirror*, **156**(3), 22.

Flint, C. (1983d) Encouraging feedback. *Nursing Mirror*, **156**(4), 49–50.

Flint, C. (1986) The Know Your Midwife Scheme. *Midwife, Health Visitor and Community Nurse*, **22**, 168–9.

Flint, C. and Poulengeris, P. (1987) *The Know Your Midwife Report*, 49, Peckarmans Wood, Sydenham Hill, London.

Flint, C. (1989) Riverside Midwife Teams. *Midwife, Health Visitor and Community Nurse*, **25**(3), 102–4.

Flint, C., Poulengeris, P., Grant, A. (1989) The Know Your Midwife scheme – a randomised trial of continuity of care by a team of midwives. *Midwifery* **5**(1), 11–16.

Goldberg, D. (1978) *Manual of the General Health Questionnaire*. NFER Publishing Co., Slough.

Gordis L. and Markowitz, M. (1971) Evaluation of the effectiveness of comprehensive and continuous pediatric care. *Pediatrics*, **48**(5), 766–76.

Grant, A. (1983) Evaluating midwifery practice: the role of the randomised controlled trial. In Thomson, A.M. and Robinson, S. (eds) *Research and the Midwife Conference Proceedings*, Department of Nursing, University of Manchester, Manchester.

Grant, A. and Chalmers, I. (1985) Epidemiology in Obstetrics and Gynaecology: Some research strategies for investigating aetiology and assessing the effects of clinical practice, in Macdonald, R.R. (ed.) *Scientific Basis of Obstetrics and Gynaecology*, 3rd edn Churchill Livingstone, Edinburgh.

Huggins, C. (1985) *A comparative study of two antenatal care systems in terms of waiting time and staff encounters.* Unpublished BSc dissertation, Department of Nursing, Chelsea College, University of London, London.

Katz, D., Baptista, J., Azen, S.P., Pike M.C. (1978) Obtaining confidence limits for the risk ratio in cohort studies. *Biometrics*, **34**, 469–74.

Kirke, P.N. (1980) Mother's views of care in labour. *British Journal of Obstetrics and Gynaecology*, **87**, 1034–7.

Macfarlane, A. and Mugford, M. (1984) *Birth Counts. Statistics of pregnancy and childbirth.* HMSO, London.

Maternity Services Advisory Committee (1982) *Maternity Care in Action. Part 1, Antenatal Care.* HMSO, London.

Meinart, C.L. (1986) *Clinical Trials. Design, conduct and analysis.* Oxford University Press, Oxford.

Micklethwaite, P., Beard R., Shaw, K. (1978) Expectations of a pregnant woman in relation to her treatment. *British Medical Journal* **2**, 188–91.

National Childbirth Trust (1981) *Change in antenatal care, a report of a working party.* NCT, London.

Oakley, A. (1980) *Women Confined: towards a sociology of childbirth.* Martin Robertson, Oxford.

O'Brien, M. and Smith, C. (1981) Women's views and experiences of antenatal care. *Practitioner*, **25**, 123–5.

Parents Magazine (1983) Birth in Britain, A Parents special report. *Parents Magazine*, **92**, November.

Parents Magazine (1986) Birth, 9000 mothers speak out, Birth survey 1986 – results. *Parents Magazine*, **128**, November.

Prentice and Lind, T. (1987) Fetal heart rate monitoring during labour – too frequent intervention, too little benefit. *Lancet*, **ii**(8572), 1375–7.

Robins, L.N. (1963) The reluctant respondent. *Public Opinion Quarterly*, **27**, 276–86.

Robinson, S. (1989) The role of the midwife, opportunities and constraints. In Chalmers, I., Enkin, M., Keirse, M.J.N.C. (eds) *Effective care in pregnancy and childbirth.* Oxford University Press, Oxford.

Roos, L.L., Roos, N.P., Gilbert, P., Nicol, J.P. (1980) Continuity of care: does it contribute to quality of care? *Medical Care*, **18**(2), 174–84.

Royal College of Obstetricians and Gynaecologists (1982) *Report of the RCOG working party on antenatal and intrapartum care.* RCOG, London.

Runnerstrom, L. (1969) The effectiveness of nurse-midwifery in a supervised hospital environment. *Bulletin of College of Nurse-Midwives*, **14**, 40–52.

Shear, C.L., Gipe, B.T., Mattheis, J.K., Levy, M.R. (1983) Provider continuity and quality of medical care. *Medical Care*, **21**(12), 1204–10.

Slome, C., Wetherbee, H., Daly, M., Christensen, K., Meglen, M., Theide, H. (1976)

Effectiveness of certified nurse-midwives. A prospective evaluation study. *American Journal of Obstetrics and Gynecology*, **124**, 177–82.

Social Services Committee (1980) *Perinatal and Neonatal Mortality, second report (Short Report)*, HMSO, London.

Thomson, A.M. (1980) Planned or unplanned? Are midwives ready for the 1980s? *Midwives Chronicle and Nursing Notes*, **93**(1), 1016,68–72.

CHAPTER FIVE

The Newcastle Community Midwifery Care Project

Part 1 The project in action
Jean Davies
Part 2 The evaluation of the project
Frances Evans

Part 1 The project in action

BACKGROUND TO THE STUDY

Although perinatal mortality rates in England and Wales have been falling since the late 1930s (Macfarlane and Mugford, 1984) public concern was expressed in the 1970s that these rates were not falling as fast as in other countries (DHSS, 1977). In response to this concern the UK government set up a parliamentary sub-committee to enquire into perinatal and neonatal mortality; its findings and recommendations were subsequently published in a report, commonly referred to as the Short Report (Social Services Committee, 1980). The major direct causes of perinatal mortality are low birth weight, congenital abnormality, antepartum haemorrhage, birth trauma and maternal disease (McIlwaine *et al.*, 1979). However, there are also underlying causes, as indicated by the fact that perinatal mortality is significantly higher amongst those who come from the lower socio-economic groups and there are wide regional variations in mortality rates throughout the UK (Macfarlane and Mugford, 1984). Armand-Smith (1980) has also demonstrated that there are wide variations in perinatal mortality rates within one city. By comparing rates between local authority wards in 1971–73 he demonstrated that perinatal mortality in Edinburgh, for example, varied between 8.5 and 37.9 per thousand. The Social Services Committee drew attention to lack of education, poverty, poor housing, unplanned pregnancy, smoking and the drinking of alcohol during pregnancy as contributory factors to perinatal mortality (Social Services Committee, 1980). The report also stated that the perinatal and neonatal mortality rates among those in the lowest socio-economic classes were twice as high as in the highest groups, a fact that the committee felt was totally unacceptable.

It has long been suggested that one of the ways to reduce perinatal mortality is to provide each woman with a good standard of antenatal care (Butler and Bonham, 1963). However, the Short Report (Social Services Committee, 1980) states that 'While we unhesitatingly accept the often reiterated aim of antenatal care as a means of reducing perinatal and neo-natal mortality, what exactly antenatal care consists of and how it works has been less clear to us'. Despite this lack of understanding of what antenatal care does or how antenatal care achieves success, the report recommends that provision of antenatal care should be improved, in particular to those most 'at risk' of a perinatal death. Those seen to be most at risk are 'single mothers, teenagers at school, mothers of families living on social security, wives of low-wage earners, and those with large families in poor circum-stances' (Social Services Committee, 1980). The committee recommended that a 'commando group' composed of members of the primary care team should target the services to those in the 'at risk' groups within each District. The community midwife was seen as a key member of this 'commando group'.

This chapter describes the response of one Health Authority to the Committee's recommendations. I was a member of a team of community midwives that provided care in two inner-city areas of social and economic deprivation, and in the first part of the chapter I describe the setting up and running of the scheme. From the outset it was agreed that the project should be evaluated, and this is described in the second section of the chapter by Frances Evans, the research officer to the project. (see p. 115).

The situation in Newcastle

The perinatal mortality rates in Newcastle for the years 1978–80 were 14.7, 17.1 and 14.1 per thousand births respectively. This should be compared with national rates of 15.5, 14.7 and 13.4 per thousand births for the same years. Newcastle Health Authority was particularly interested in the rela-tionship between socio-economic disadvantage and poor pregnancy outcome. In examining the mortality rates within Newcastle it was noted that some of the perinatal deaths were clustering in five areas of the city. Two of these areas, Cowgate and Newbiggin Hall, did not have existing additional preventive health initiatives – schemes to promote health through preventive education and group work where broad health issues could be raised and discussed. A report of consumer views of health and health services in Newcastle (Newcastle Inner City Forum, 1983) demonstrated that women in Cowgate were not attending the hospital as frequently as the health pro-fessionals would appear to have liked. The reasons for this were that the women could not always see the relevance of the hospital visits, they found it extremely difficult to travel to the hospital – one woman describing a long walk – and the women did not like being 'poked'.

There were no comments in this report from women in Cowgate about antenatal care provided by a community midwife, but women in other comparable areas of Newcastle described situations suggesting that the community midwife was more a doctor's assistant than an independent professional. The midwives did not seem to be functioning as experts in normal childbirth and did not seem to have a community identity (Newcastle Inner City Forum, 1983).

In response to the Short Report, the Health Authority drew up a list of six recommendations. The first five were to improve ultra-sound, laboratory, neonatal surgical and clinical genetics services, and to set up a perinatal/ neonatal pathology unit. The sixth was for a community-based antenatal care project which had two aims:

1. To provide enhanced support by midwives to childbearing women in their own home in an area of the city defined as having a concentration of high risk factors;
2. To measure the effects of this intervention on maternal, fetal and infant well-being; consumer satisfaction; and relationships between hospital and community services.

In 1982 the Director of Midwifery Services put forward a proposal for extra midwifery care to be provided within the community to those women considered to be 'at risk' of a perinatal death. The women would continue to have the usual package of antenatal care, either total hospital or 'shared care', as provided in Newcastle. Although the emphasis of this extra care was to be during pregnancy, continuity was to be provided throughout the childbearing experience into the postnatal period. The extra resources were to be focused in the two areas of the city identified as having an existing high rate of perinatal mortality and as being without health initiatives. Evaluation was to be an integral part of the project as it was recognized that benefits of the extra care, if they existed, needed to be demonstrated if their subsequent continuation was to be justified.

It was suggested that funding for the project might come from the Department of the Environment's Inner City Partnership funds. This money, provided by central government, is specifically for initiatives in areas of economic need and includes initiatives in health care provision. Allocation of the funds is through a process of consultation, culminating in a bid made by a sponsor to the relevant partnership committee within the local authority.

There was initial resistance to the proposed project from the consultant obstetric staff who were under the impression that the women would be denied the assumed benefits of antenatal care provided by the hospital. However, this resistance was overcome and the Department of the Environment allocated funds for four midwives to provide the extra care for three years, and a social scientist to evaluate the project. The project began in August 1983.

The project areas

The four midwives were to work in the two previously identified inner city areas, both council estates with very close-knit communities. These estates were characterized by poor-quality housing, high levels of unemployment, a high proportion of single mothers, high rates of vandalism, and those who were in work were concentrated in social classes 4 and 5. Despite these similarities there were distinct differences between the two areas.

Newbiggin Hall is on the outskirts of the city, but had been classified as an 'inner' area of stress by Newcastle City's Priority Area Planning Team in the light of the estate's economic standing. It consists of flats, houses and bungalows built in the 1960s to re-house those made homeless by slum clearances. The estate is not popular with its residents due to the quality of the housing. The houses were built on a steep slope and several streets have been seriously affected by subsidence. Frequently the houses have had to be vacated for structural and maintenance work. The tenants feel that their homes are unsafe and the building work inconveniences them. Condensation is a recurrent problem. Most of the houses have a convector heating system which is expensive to run, does not provide the residents with radiators on which they can dry clothes and many residents say that the dry heat which is generated gives them bronchial problems, itchiness and sore throats.

Another factor contributing to the unpopularity of this estate is the high level of crime and vandalism. Petty crime and vandalism in the flats means that clothes are stolen from washing lines, the contents of bins are strewn across the stairways, and gangs of youths shout and fight late into the night. Burglaries are so frequent that residents in parts of the estate have been unable to obtain household insurance. Rapid house moves are a feature of the estate. Strangers in Newbiggin Hall attract both interest and suspicion, but midwives and general practitioners are, in general, welcome visitors.

Initially, only half of the estate was going to be included in the project. However, it was felt by the midwives who had worked in the area and knew it well that the whole estate was an entity, and that if the neighbourhood aspects of community midwifery were to be examined, then the estate should not be divided. This has meant that there have been more women and babies cared for in this estate than in the other area chosen. There are two antenatal clinics in Newbiggin Hall, one in the Welfare Clinic and the other at a general practitioner's surgery.

Cowgate is an older area having been built in the 1930s and 40s, and has a more stable population in that there are third and fourth generations living there. The houses are stone-built and each has its own garden. The layout of the estate is in an attractive 'garden city' style giving a feeling of space, but there is a lot of litter and a large number of the houses are boarded up. Dogs and small children roam around all day. Cowgate is known as the city's most problematic area, due mostly to the high levels of crime and vandalism.

House break-ins are extremely common and as in Newbiggin Hall, residents in some parts of the estate cannot obtain insurance cover. Although most of the crime is of a relatively petty nature, vandalism reaches more serious proportions at times. Male unemployment is very high and the number of single-parent households is twice that of the average for the city of Newcastle. There is strong suspicion of strangers but midwives are one of the few groups of professionals who are made welcome. There is no clinic or general practitioner's surgery in Cowgate.

Project midwives' working patterns in action

Two midwives worked in each area, covering their own off duty and holidays. They also covered the other area for holidays and off duty. Initially, the project midwives were included in the rotas of the established community midwives for the city, but it was realised that the project could only be evaluated if the project midwives were autonomous. However, they remained in the same administrative structure as all the city community midwives, receiving information about childbearing women, attending meetings with them and taking their share of the night, city wide, on-call rota.

There was daily contact between the pair of midwives working in each area. All four project midwives met once a week, in order to discuss problems as they arose. This meeting was invaluable as inevitably there are problems that arise from working in an innovative way. Through the meetings the midwives were able to give each other support. The social scientist appointed to evaluate the project started work in May 1984 by which time some of the early difficulties had been ironed out, and attended the weekly meetings.

The project's location in the community

The two teams functioned differently. The main difference was that in Cowgate the midwives were responsible for a concurrent project that was run alongside social workers. The midwifery and social work projects were sited in a converted Local Authority house on the estate. The house was named the Cowgate Neighbourhood Centre, although it became known in the community as 'the midwives' house'. The Centre was next door to another house used by the Housing Department's local management team, with whom there is close liaison. It was hoped that by basing both the midwifery and social work projects in defined accommodation within the community a neighbourhood base would be provided for preventive health care. The philosophy of the Centre was to increase self esteem through friendly contact with workers in an unthreatening place.

The Cowgate Neighbourhood Centre had financial support from both Local and Health Authorities through the Joint Care Planning Team's support of the scheme. The Centre is managed by the two midwives and social workers. It is open in the morning for a drop-in coffee session and the midwives are easily accessible at this time. In the afternoons, various groups meet at the Centre, the group relevant to childbirth meeting on a Tuesday. These sessions are run jointly by the midwives and a health education worker, the first part of each session being for both pregnant and postnatal women. During the second half the midwife would work with the pregnant women while the health education worker would focus on those who had already had their baby. The traditional formal approach of parentcraft education whereby women were required to sit and listen in a classroom-like environment proved impossible to establish, even if it had been desired. The sessions have dealt with a range of topics and use more varied teaching techniques than in traditional courses on preparation for parenthood. As poor nutrition was recognized as being a major problem for women in this area, sessions on how to eat nutritiously and relatively cheaply were started early in the project. For safety and insurance reasons the professionals working in the Cowgate Centre were not allowed to teach women to cook on the premises. However, the professionals would partially overcome this problem by preparing a nutritious item of food, take it to the childbirth session, share it with the women who attended, provide them with a copy of the recipe and discuss with them how the dish had been cooked. Education about nutrition, smoking and fitness were high priorities. Other sessions have included teaching assertiveness strategies, and help with gaining the relevant social security entitlements. Taking the group swimming was one of the activities that was very popular, many of the women not having been since they were at school. They enjoyed coming to the Centre and did not want to stop when they had had their baby, so this class developed into a mothers' group, known as the Pregnant in Cowgate group.

In Newbiggin Hall the midwives work from a health centre as do midwives not working within this project. Preparation for parenthood sessions are held within the health centre and the content of the classes is very similar to the content in other classes throughout the city. However, because the project midwives know the women better due to the extra antenatal contact, the midwives are able to adapt the classes to meet the needs of the women.

NATURE OF CARE PROVIDED BY THE PROJECT MIDWIVES

Initially, referral of women to the project midwives came through the usual hospital maternity service channel. However as the project progressed and as the midwives came to be recognized within the communities the women began to refer themselves and each other for midwifery care. It was possible, and appropriate, for the midwife to initiate care at this point of contact. This development could only occur because the work was geographically defined.

The midwives were responsible for all the women within their areas. At each initial contact a history was taken, potential and actual problems were identified and care planned to meet individual needs. Each woman would be visited in her home at least four times during pregnancy, she would be encouraged to attend the parentcraft classes run by the midwives, and would be visited in hospital during any hospital admission – antenatally, during labour (when appropriate) and postnatally. It was hoped that it would be possible to begin providing a Domino service but unfortunately this did not come to fruition.

Each woman was seen mainly by one midwife, but through parentcraft classes, during postnatal care and because of the geographical organization of the work, the other midwives became familiar figures. The midwife kept a profile for each woman; this provided a guideline for the midwives and was a reminder about what was to be discussed. Initially the first page of the profile was filed in the woman's hospital records; this contained a birth plan in which the woman might express any preferences about her care. Unfor-tunately, the consultant obstetricians objected to the profiles being filed in the notes, so they had to be removed.

Different areas have different needs. The inhabitants of the Cowgate estate have special needs because of the effects of long-term unemployment. It was hoped that the Centre would provide a facility through which the residents would become more confident and self-reliant. The combination of midwifery with social work proved to be effective in creating an accessible and accepted service. Midwives are usually trusted and accepted, perhaps more than social workers whose work is not always understood; together, the midwives and the social workers provided care that was welcomed, both professions learning and benefiting from each other. Many residents have been helped and are increasingly helping themselves, not least in taking responsibility for the Centre. Initially there was a lot of vandalism, but this has improved as local residents have become involved in the management and running of the building.

In Newbiggin Hall there are two antenatal clinics, one based in the Welfare Clinic and one at a surgery. The majority of women who had 'shared care' given by the general practitioner were seen at these clinics, and the midwives attended them. In Cowgate there is no clinic or general prac-titioner. The midwives attended the antenatal clinic of the nearest doctor. A lot of general practitioners from across the city provided care for only one or two pregnant women on the estate and the benefits of working in a neigh-bourhood would be lost if midwives were attached to these practices. The travelling would be time consuming and expensive, and giving continuity of care within the community would be difficult if several different midwives were all visiting the estate. The work in Cowgate gave substance to the view that primary health care should be neighbourhood based.

As already stated parentcraft classes were established by the project midwives in both areas. Women from these estates had not previously attended parentcraft classes, but once the midwives became known, and the bases from which they worked were established as part of the community the number attending the classes increased.

One advantage of early contact with the women was the possibility to visit them during antenatal hospitalization. Women would sometimes ask questions of the project midwives, admitting that they did not wish to bother the staff. This indicated that meeting a woman in her own environment enabled her to feel that her unique identity was understood. A history taken in hospital may not reflect the reality of a woman's life (see Methven in Volume 1 of this series). Make-up and clothes can disguise and cover up and may have been used to do so. Adverse domestic situations may come to light only at a second or a subsequent home visit, when trust in the community midwife has developed. Some problems may, of course, never come to light. Some women go through pregnancy lonely and afraid; one girl, for example, was visited three times and she had been seen several times at her cousin's house, before she confided that her electricity had been cut off for a year. It had not been obvious as she had run an extension cable from her neighbour's house, for which she paid. The baby was due in four weeks and it took almost that time for the problem to be sorted out, with the help of the Citizens Advice Bureau, the social worker, the DHSS and the Electricity Board. The baby came home to a lit house.

Another advantage of working geographically was hearing about a threatened miscarriage. It was often not possible to do anything 'medical', but it was possible to give counsel and support. As the project progressed, women informed the midwives of such an event and after appropriate medical aid had been sought and given there was still a lot of support needed. The network of information was useful and the midwives usually heard very quickly when a woman was having a problem or if someone had been admitted to hospital.

This networking is a very fascinating phenomenon whereby news is transmitted. It could be discounted as gossip, but it serves a useful social purpose. It only exists where there is familiarity, and it takes some time to establish the credentials of being a recipient. It developed as part of the work tools of the project midwives. If a woman was out, for example, her whereabouts were often established by neighbours. Women also used the clinic and the Centre to meet or leave messages for the midwives, but there was also a lot of street communication. Many a time the midwives' cars were hailed. It is not a 'sentimental notion' that professional care can utilize neighbourhood communication. For example a recently delivered woman was abandoned by her sometimes violent husband. She had a history of in-patient care at the local psychiatric hospital. She was seen in a distressed state in the street by a woman who came and told the midwife at the Centre. It took time to calm her down, the health visitor joined forces, so by the time the children

returned home from school the woman was able to cope. This woman subsequently used the Cowgate Neighbourhood Centre frequently, without
whose support she says she could not have managed. The social workers
became involved with the family and gave the mother some help. The
woman came to see that her problems were caused by feeling she could not
cope without the support of her husband, who was unable to offer any. She
felt that realizing this made her 'grow up' and her frequent visits to the
general practitioner reduced as she discovered that she could in fact cope
quite well. This was not an isolated case of co-operation and showed that
neighbourhood-based work can be effective and should be developed as an
efficient way of providing care that is relevant to people's lives.

THE EXPERIENCE OF WORKING IN A RESEARCH PROJECT

It was exciting having the opportunity to develop community midwifery with
a geographical base and to see how quickly the midwives become an identifi-
able part of the community. Students undertaking part of their community
experience with the project midwives commented on how everyone seemed
to know and acknowledge the midwives. This close professional contact
within the community provided a lot of job satisfaction. All the midwives
working on the project commented on enjoying this aspect of the work; of
knowing and being known to the women, and talking to them not only about
childbirth, but about menstruation, the menopause, men, contraception,
conception, the weather, the state of the nation, in particular its economy –
exemplified by the frequently perceived failure of the DHSS to do as
expected.

The professional profile of midwifery was raised with the users of the
service, but also with other professionals. The geographical base enabled
others to know exactly who was responsible for which aspect of care and
advice and this was particularly beneficial to the liaison between midwives,
health visitors and general practitioners. Giving antenatal care in areas of
economic stress will inevitably involve contact with others – the housing
department, social services, environmental health, citizens' advice bureaux,
the police, the schools, as well as various voluntary agencies. Providing care
for all the women who had a baby enabled the midwives to know a lot about
the families living in these areas.

Childbirth is a time of particular needs and vulnerability and midwives
are in a very privileged position; their expertise is not only needed but
usually welcomed. Meetings, case conferences and discussions held in multi-
disciplinary fora confirmed the project midwives' knowledge that 'Midwives
hold the key to healthy families' (International Confederation of Midwives,
1987). The evaluation of the project described in the second part of this
chapter showed that not only did the midwives hold the key but by working
geographically, with a manageable caseload, effective preventive health care

could be given and doors could be opened.

The opportunity to do this work was made possible because it was also a research project. The job satisfaction was, however, balanced by some of the disadvantages of working in a project that provided care different from that given by the majority of community midwives. There were two levels of care, with very different caseloads. When the existing community midwives were overladen their resentment was felt by all the project midwives. Although the project workload was different, close contact with unremitting poverty has its own inherent stresses. The fact that the project did so much extra antenatal visiting did not seem to be fully appreciated by the other midwives; nor was the hope that the outcome could eventually benefit community midwifery across the city. One project midwife said that she had never felt so isolated in all the time that she had been a midwife.

The isolation could have been reduced if the project midwives had had more opportunity to discuss the innovative work with their midwifery and obstetric colleagues. The latter would then perhaps have understood better what was being attempted and more importantly, why it was being attempted. It meant that the project was in the curious situation of not being understood by colleagues, yet being strongly supported within the community.

Initiatives are a new beginning, and most established systems have an inbuilt inertia and resistance to change. Attempts to look at work analytically, as in the course of the associated evaluation, are not always welcomed. Work was being studied and compared with that normally carried out by the other midwives working in comparable parts of the city. There was a lack of understanding that this was not comparing like with like, but rather an exercise to establish a base for good midwifery practice, that could be used as a tool for measuring establishment needs. A baseline of staffing and consumer needs did not as yet exist, with the consequence that too often the service was understaffed and very often undervalued.

Lack of appreciation about the potential of the evaluation led the project midwives to feel resented; not only for having a smaller case load (in terms of the number of women for whom they were responsible), but some of the other midwives seemed to think that the evaluation report showed their own work as being less effective. What it actually showed was the need to have more midwives if the potential for preventive health care within the 'inner city' was to be realized. For effective care to be provided realistic case loads are essential. Moreover a geographical base increases the efficacy of the work. Far from showing midwives to be wanting, the evaluative aspect of the project demonstrated the potential of midwifery care in improving maternal and infant wellbeing.

Tensions could have been reduced if the project midwives had discussed not only the work but also the evaluation with their colleagues. When the report was published the project midwives did not make themselves party to the presentation about the work, and some of them felt that the innovative midwifery had come to be secondary to the evaluation.

This aspect of the project midwives' experience is important, because it illustrates how midwifery may inhibit its own development by its lack of confidence about innovation and development. If the outcome of research shows that there is a better way of working, then the findings of the research should be used to argue for consolidation and development. The Department of the Environment gave a fourth year's full funding for the midwives and the Health Authority's Annual Programme stated:

> The evaluation of the work undertaken in the Project Area of Cowgate and Newbiggin Hall will be completed in 1987. It is the intention to review the allocation and style of midwifery services in the light of the report.

However, at the end of the fourth year it was decided that funding for the Community Midwifery Project should be discontinued. The Know Your Midwife (KYM) scheme in London (see Chapter 4 in this volume), which has the same philosophical base as the Community Midwifery Care Project, met with the same assumption that once the project was over 'normal work' would resume as usual; as if no benefit, including cost, could be gained from implementation. However, unlike the termination of the KYM scheme the termination of the Newcastle Community Midwifery Project met with stiff opposition from community workers and from the women that the project served. The Cowgate Task Group protested; the women collected a petition and presented it to the Health Authority. The project was re-instated and at the time of writing is still in existence.

REFERENCES

Armand-Smith, N.G. (1980) Perinatal health in the Lothians. *Edinburgh Med.*, 10–11.

Butler, N.R. and Bonham, D.G. (1963) *Perinatal Mortality. The first report of the British perinatal mortality survey*, E & S Livingstone, Edinburgh.

DHSS (1977) *Prevention and Health, reducing the risk: safer pregnancy and childbirth*, HMSO, London.

ICM (1987) *Midwives hold the key to healthy families*, title of triennial Congress. International Confederation of Midwives, The Hague.

Macfarlane, A., and Mugford, M. (1984) *Birth Counts: Statistics of pregnancy and childbirth*, HMSO, London.

McIlwaine, G.M., Howat, R.C.L., Dunn, F., and MacNaughton, M.C. (1979) Scotland 1977 *Perinatal Mortality Survey* Dept of Obstetrics and Gynaecology, University of Glasgow.

Newcastle Inner City Forum (1983) *What we need is*, Newcastle upon Tyne Inner City Forum, MEA House, Ellison Place, Newcastle upon Tyne.

Social Services Committee (1980) *Perinatal and Neonatal Mortality Report: Follow-up* (Short Report), HMSO, London.

Part 2 The evaluation of the project

The Newcastle Community Midwifery Care Project (CMC) described in the first part of this chapter had two aims:

1. To provide enhanced support by midwives to childbearing women in their own homes in an area of the city defined as having a concentration of high risk factors;
2. To ensure the effects of this intervention on maternal, fetal and infant well-being; consumer satisfaction; and relationships between hospital and community services.

I am a sociologist, and was employed for three years to carry out the second of these two aims. In this part of the chapter 1 discuss the methodology of the study, present some of its findings, and suggest some of the implications of these for midwifery practice and education.

METHODS

Studies of the maternity services tend to have one of three perspectives. The first focuses on the medical outcome of pregnancy (Butler and Bonham, 1963; Davie, Butler and Goldstein, 1972). This approach typically relies on quantitative methods, and studies the epidemiology of pregnancy and childbirth. A second perspective looks at the role of the consumer in the service (Cartwright, 1979; Graham and McKee, 1980; Oakley, 1979). This uses qualitative methods insofar as it focuses on consumer opinion, but it has also used large data sets as, for instance, in one mass study that was administered through a popular TV programme (Boyd and Sellars, 1982). A third perspective analyses the process of maternity care. Such work is typically 'desk' research, often using archive material relating to the development of the professions involved in maternity care (Ehrenreich and English, 1973; Oakley, 1984).

Researching the Newcastle CMC Project presented a particular challenge because of the need to draw from each of these perspectives. The underlying hypothesis of the project is that social intervention may affect health outcomes (although specific health outcomes were not identified). Therefore, it was necessary to design a quantitatively based outcome study in order to test this hypothesis. A second hypothesis was that the project would increase consumer satisfaction with the service and this demanded a more qualitative approach. At the same time, some of the implications of the project style of work could only be understood with reference to the changing process and structure of care.

In seeking to unravel these complexities I chose to use a variety of research techniques and these are described below.

Case note survey

The first major method of data collection was a case note survey. This was a quantitative measurement of health outcome, based on extractions from hospital medical records. Data recorded included maternal weight, height, social history at booking, obstetric history, complications of pregnancy and labour, clinic attendance, and clinical investigations. Data relating to the baby included weight, gestational age, and any malformation or mortality.

It was felt that clinical outcome measures should be analysed, even though the limitations of the quantitative approach with respect to a small study were recognized. The strength of research into clinical outcome (Butler and Bonham, 1963; Davie, Butler and Goldstein, 1972) has been to analyse large data sets in order to chart and seek to explain changes in indices such as birthweight, gestational age, and perinatal mortality. In this study, it was understood that the smallness of the data set and the restricted timescale of the research limited the validity of results insofar as they could not be claimed to completely support or refute the particular impact of the midwifery intervention. However, it was felt that the analysis of certain clinical outcomes could reveal trends and patterns of change, which might be significant indicators of the effect of midwifery work. An increasing number of studies have tested the effectiveness of social intervention strategies aimed to improve clinical outcome (Donovan, 1976; Sokol, 1980; Oakley, 1985 and in preparation in Volume 3 of this series) and it was felt that the CMC Project offered the opportunity to make a contribution to this literature.

In identifying a study population for evaluation, it was agreed that it would be preferable to restrict the numbers of cases rather than the detail in which they were studied. It was therefore decided that the main study population should consist of all women resident in the project area who booked in for antenatal care between October 1984 and October 1985. In all, there were 263 subjects.

The quantitative method typically relies on the comparison of cases with controls and the identification of a control group for evaluative purposes proved to be a difficult task. There were three options. First, a randomized controlled trial (RCT). This would have randomly allocated some women to the study group for midwifery intervention and others to a control group having no intervention. Although the advantages of the RCT have been widely recognized in the literature on the evaluation of maternity services (Cochrane, 1972) it was unfortunately an unworkable option in a study that focuses on developing a neighbourhood service, and in which women are encouraged to report their suspected pregnancy straight to a midwife. Project midwives needed to be able to respond directly to women's needs, rather than to the complex randomization procedures of the researcher. Secondly, evaluation could have been based on a before and after study, comparing the women in the project with a group of women who gave birth in the same part of the city before the project started. This option was rejected because it was felt that consumer satisfaction with a current service could not be reliably compared with a service that had been provided at least a year previously. Thirdly, project women could have been compared with women in an area of the city that is as similar to the Community Midwifery Care Project area as possible, but which does not have a project. Pursuing this option was not possible precisely because the project area is so distinctive in terms of its concentration of socio-economic disadvantage. There are very few areas of the city that have similar disadvantage, and these were unsuitable as control areas because special health initiatives were already in operation there.

It was decided that these problems could be overcome by drawing control women from an area of the city which is as similar to the project area in terms of socio-economic factors as possible, but which is larger. Certain women could then be selected from within it, if they match the project women in key respects. To select possible control areas, ward census data were used. These were the percentage of the economically active male population in social classes 1, 2 and 3, and the percentage of households in council rented accommodation. In addition to this, travelling proximity to the hospitals and existing levels of health intervention were taken into account.

Key matching variables were identified, in order to select women for the study from within this geographical area. Research into the clinical outcome of pregnancy (Adelstein and Fedrick, 1978; Baird and Thompson, 1969; Brennan and Lancashire, 1978; Butler and Alberman, 1969; Cullinan and Treuherz, 1982; MacVicar, 1976; Meechan, 1980) has found that age, parity, social class and marital status are highly significant indicators of outcome, and these were therefore selected as the first four matching variables. In addition to these, two variables relating to the management of pregnancy were used – place of booked delivery and type of antenatal care.

Matched group, rather than matched pair, analysis was used. Matching women in pairs could be done either retrospectively or prospectively. Retrospective matching pairs would necessitate the construction of a control group after the case group was complete, and this would precipitate a time lag that was felt to be unacceptable. Prospective matching would be based on partnering women with controls, as they entered the project. It was decided that it was extremely unlikely in practice that women with identical matching characteristics would book in for maternity care simultaneously. Using matched group analysis was therefore a preferable option, and debate on this method in the statistical literature suggests that results achieved by it are no less valid than those achieved by matched pair analysis and may even be preferable (Billewicz, 1964).

Each of the matching characteristics was split into categories for matching as follows:

Age	19 and under; 20–30; 31+
Parity	0; 1 and 2; 3+
Social class	1; 2; 3; 4; 5; unemployed
Marital status	Married; other
Hospital of booking	Newcastle General Hospital; Princess Mary Maternity Hospital
Type of maternity care	Hospital only; shared care

Using these categories, women were used as controls so long as their addition to the matching frame did not mean that the numbers in each category varied between cases and controls by more than a difference of six.

The second study population in the case note survey was therefore a control group of women identified by the method described above. A before and after dimension to the study was also developed, and data were collected from two additional control groups. The first was made up of all women who lived in the project areas and who delivered during the year preceding the onset of any midwifery intervention (1982–83). The second consisted of women who matched these women (according to the matching method described above), who were resident in the control areas, and who also delivered between 1982 and 1983. The reason for having a prospective and a retrospective group in the project area and in the control areas was to ascertain whether changes occurred over time, and if so, whether they differed in the two areas.

In total, 862 case notes were reviewed in this survey. There was rather more difficulty in tracing some notes than had been anticipated, and the main problem was that notes were removed from the shelves, with no insertion of a tracer card, so that the coder simply had to keep checking the shelves until they were returned. Eventually, the time available for this study ran out. However, by then 88% of the notes for the four groups had been traced and reviewed.

Client opinion survey

The second method used in the study was a questionnaire based survey of client opinion. Women in the project group and in the control group were interviewed twice, once antenatally and once postnatally. The two questionnaires used in these interviews focused on four areas: women's behaviour and their explanations of it; their opinions of the maternity service; and their socio-economic environment. Questions about behaviour related to clinic attendance (including general practitioner, hospital, child-health, and postnatal clinics); smoking, drinking, and eating practices; and contraceptive use. At the antenatal interview, women who had had children before were asked about their behaviour in the pregnancy immediately preceding the study pregnancy. Considerable detail about the socio-economic environment was recorded, including both characteristics (such as employment status and income) and behaviour (such as spending patterns, and use of support networks).

Throughout the questionnaires, there was an emphasis on explanation, and a series of open-ended questions was used to ask women why they behaved as they did. Answers to these were recorded in full, and coded manually after all the interviews were finished. Open-ended questions about opinions of all aspects of the maternity services were asked. Again, the answers to these were post-coded, but at the same time women were asked to rate their satisfaction on a scale of one to five.

It was decided that only the two prospective study groups would be included in this survey because of the time constraints, and because of the validity difficulties associated with retrospective data. Of the 263 women in the project group, 222 were interviewed in the antenatal period, 198 of whom were also interviewed in the postnatal period (non response was due to women moving, refusing to take part, having a miscarriage or being untraceable). The corresponding numbers in the prospective control group were 208 and 184, making a total of 812 maternal interviews in all. I carried out all these interviews myself, and all except three took place in the woman's own home.

The refusal rate in this client opinion survey was low; this was perhaps unexpected in an area in which middle-class professionals are often treated with suspicion. However, in general women were keen to participate in a study that was concerned with improving the maternity services and many expressed pleasure that their opinions on possible changes were being sought. The researcher was usually welcomed into the women's homes and there seemed to be very few barriers of hostility to be overcome.

The consumer survey was accorded a high degree of research priority for three main reasons. First, the possibility of disparate views between those who determine policy concerning the delivery of care, usually male medical staff, and the users of the service who are female. Secondly, although there have been several substantial studies of consumer opinion, much of the published work has been carried out with middle-class samples. For example, the percentage of the study population in social classes one, two and three was 93% in Oakley's study (Oakley, 1979); 88% in Graham and McKee's (Graham and McKee, 1980); 82% of Boyd and Sellars' (Boyd and Sellars, 1982); and 81% of Cartwright's study (Cartwright, 1979). In the Newcastle study population, the corresponding figure was 22%. Since social class is known to be an important variable in structuring access to and experience of the health service, it cannot be assumed that the findings from studies of middle-class women will be applicable to a working-class popu-lation. Drawing on his own research and on findings from other studies, McIntosh (1989 in Volume 1 of this series) has in fact shown that working-class women often hold expectations and priorities in relation to pregnancy and childbirth that differ from those of middle-class women. Thirdly, there is a new emphasis on consumer orientation as part of the strategic planning process of the National Health Service, and it was therefore felt important that consumer views of working-class women should be collated. This new orientation was highlighted in the *Griffiths Report* which states:

> It is central to the approach of management in planning and delivering services for the population as a whole, to:
>
> −ascertain how well the service is being delivered at local level by obtaining the experience and perceptions of patients and the community. These can be delivered from CHC's and by other methods, including market research and from the experience of general practice and the community health services;
> −respond directly to this information;
> −act on it in formulating policy (DHSS, 1983).

In short, the consumer survey was seen as central to the whole research exercise because it gave voice to a group of women whose views have previously not been well-researched, despite their centrality to the whole service.

Time budget study

The aim of this part of the research was to quantify the use of midwives' time in order to provide an accurate description of how project midwives' time is spent, and to demonstrate how this is different from the work of other community midwives. Typically, studies on time use rely on either continuous observation or work sampling (Abdellah and Levine, 1954; Burke, Chall and Abdella, 1956). Neither method was felt to be practical here, firstly, because of the non-routinized nature of the working day in the community and secondly, because of the need for observation to take place in women's own homes rather than in the wards. It was felt that the intrusion of an observer into the home, in addition to the visits of the researcher to complete questionnaires, would have been unreasonable. Instead, a diary study was carried out. The four project midwives and nine midwives working in the control areas were asked to keep a very detailed diary for a week, of how their time was spent. I spent four days accompanying the midwives, and this observation period served as a pilot for the diary study.

Staff survey

Time limitations meant that it was not possible to carry out a fully comprehensive survey of all the staff whose work might have been affected by the midwifery intervention. However, certain outcome measures related specifically to staff and it was therefore necessary to collate staff opinion about this. Four main areas were considered. First, whether or not community midwives' job satisfaction was enhanced by working on the project. Secondly, whether or not the existence of the project affected other members of the primary health care teams in the project areas. Thirdly, the response of midwives other than project midwives to the initiatives. Fourthly, the response of hospital midwifery and medical staff to the project. These areas were explored by means of a series of semi-structured interviews held with a number of staff that included all the hospital consultants and project midwives, a small number of general practitioners and midwifery managers, and by a postal survey of general practitioners and non-project midwives. This part of the study dealt only with qualitative issues, and it was recognised that the evidence collected by it would be individual and subjective.

The project in total

The Community Midwifery Care Project was set up in response to a call for research and policy initiatives relating to the health needs of women living in areas of multiple socio-economic deprivation (Social Services Committee, 1980). It aimed to provide enhanced midwifery care to women in particularly disadvantaged parts of the inner city and to measure the effects of the intervention. The evaluation study was based on four methods: a case note survey, a client opinion survey, a time budget study, and a staff survey. The data enabled the measurement of a range of outcomes from quantitative indices such as birth weight to more qualitative indices relating to opinion. The chi-square test was used to assess the extent to which views and experiences of the project and control groups of women differed. The evaluation study made a particular contribution to literature about maternity services because of its focus on working-class women who have tended to be underrepresented in published studies of consumer opinion about maternity care.

FINDINGS

The research produced an extensive data set, and only a small part of it is presented in this chapter. The findings included are concerned with the provision of care, consumer satisfaction, client behaviour, perinatal outcome and staff issues. The findings are available in full in Evans (1987).

Provision of enhanced care

The project's primary aim was 'to provide enhanced midwifery care to childbearing women in their own homes'. Quantitative and qualitative data obtained in the course of the evaluation demonstrated that the midwifery intervention did provide enhanced care and that this did not duplicate that already available. First, antenatal home visiting was substantially increased: the majority of project group women (55%) received between 4 and 10 antenatal home visits, whereas the majority of control group women (62%) received only one ($p < 0.001$). Similarly the amount of postnatal home visiting was increased in the project area; 90% of project women compared with 44% of control group women had been visited more often than the statutory norm of daily, up until the 10th day ($p < 0.001$). Project women were more likely than control group women to have telephoned the midwife antenatally ($p < 0.001$) and postnatally – (this difference did not reach a level of statistical significance) – and to have met her informally outside the home ($p < 0.001$).

Project group women were more likely than control women to have been visited at home during the first trimester of pregnancy (53% compared to 16%, $p < 0.001$). Continuity of care between the antenatal and postnatal period was greater in the project group, in that 63% had previously met all the midwives who visited them postnatally compared with 20% of the control group of women ($p < 0.001$). Data from interviews with women in the two groups showed that project women were significantly more likely than control group women to report that their midwives had discussed the following issues with them in the home: infant feeding, contraception, eating, drinking, smoking and baby care.

It could, of course, be argued that enhanced midwifery care was unnecessary as it duplicated care that was already available from existing midwifery services or from other agencies. Consequently, the possibility of duplication of care was investigated as part of the evaluation, but was found not to occur (full details can be found in Evans, 1987).

Consumer satisfaction

Findings from interviews with women show that those in the project group were significantly more likely than those in the control group to say that they were very satisfied with their community midwifery care (Table 5.1). This was most marked during the antenatal period ($p < 0.001$).

In interpreting these data, it should be noted that the opinions of control group women were artificially high, because their expectations of community midwifery care were often extremely low. Women did not expect a particularly close relationship with their midwife, and neither did they expect to receive several visits. They were therefore relatively easily satisfied: 'I was satisfied. None of them was stuck up. They were nice, I didn't mind them coming at all'.

Although the majority of control group women did not express dissatisfaction with the community midwifery service, there was evidence of a

Table 5.1 Rating of community midwifery care

| Satisfaction rating | Antenatal care | | | | Postnatal care | | | |
| | project women | | control women | | project women | | control women | |
	%	No.	%	No.	%	No.	%	No.
Very satisfied	72	143	35	65	77	153	55	102
Satisfied	19	38	41	76	14	28	22	40
Indifferent	4	7	12	22	7	14	15	27
Dissatisfied	4	7	6	12	1	1	6	12
Very dissatisfied	1	1	1	2	1	2	2	3
Don't know/No answer	1	2	4	7	–	–	–	–
Total	100	198	100	184	100	198	100	184

Source: Compiled by the author.

majority wish to have had different care. In total 63% of control group women said that they would like to have been included in the project. Many of those who did not say this commented that, although they themselves had not wanted the extra care, they felt it would be an excellent service for particular groups with special needs, such as first-time mothers.

This complicating factor of different expectations of care between the project and control groups is eliminated in a comparison between women who have previously had children (Table 5.2). These data show again that project group women were significantly more likely than were control group women to feel that their midwifery care had improved since their most recent pregnancy ($p < 0.001$).

The project was thus clearly an extremely popular intervention among women. In some respects this finding was counter-intuitive, since the project was located in an area where middle-class professional input can be met with hostility. Indeed, early interviews with non-project staff had indicated some anticipation that women might complain about the possible intrusion, and that they might feel that they were being rather too energetically 'policed' by the health service.

Analysis of the qualitative data relating to consumer satisfaction showed that women gave two main reasons for such very high satisfaction rates.

Table 5.2 Comparison of current midwifery care with that of the most recent pregnancy

| Rating of care | Antenatal care | | | | Postnatal care | | | |
| | project women | | control women | | project women | | control women | |
	%	No.	%	No.	%	No.	%	No.
Better	90	96	28	29	92	98	32	34
The same	9	10	70	73	8	9	61	64
Worse	1	1	3	3	–	–	7	7
Total	100	107	100	105	100	107	100	105

Source: Compiled by the author.

First, they felt that their care was appropriate to their needs. Second, they particularly valued the quality of their one-to-one relationship with the midwife.

Comments about the appropriateness of project care were usually made in the context of a feeling that care in previous pregnancies or during previous encounters with the medical profession had been inappropriate. Most typically, this was because there had not been an adequate recognition of the poverty in which women were living. This woman, describing her failure to attend parentcraft during her previous pregnancy, made the point clearly:

> It was awful. I really couldn't afford it. The travelling, and you had to buy raffle tickets and coffee, and you just felt daft. You couldn't spend – I couldn't. I didn't have the money to. They were all sitting there talking about new prams and clothes. I could have died. I had no money at all. I thought, will I even get a pram off the social? I couldn't stand it. So I stopped going. I was only 20 as well – you take it all in then.

By contrast, project group women felt that the midwives were able to give them appropriate advice:

> I was very satisfied. They weren't too prim and proper at all. Really nice and down-to-earth. They know the problems that single parents face and were just dead sensible.

It was clear that midwives were able to give appropriate advice because of the extra time they had to get to know the woman and her family circumstances during the pregnancy. Continuity of care meant that this knowledge could be used to good effect in the postnatal period too:

> I was very satisfied. You can really get to know who is coming, so that afterwards it's not a stranger who's coming. It's someone who knows your problems, and they can give you the right sort of advice. For me, it was advice on ex-husbands that I needed.

Comments about the quality of the one-to-one relationship with the project midwife were usually made in the context of women having very few supportive relationships in their lives. This qualitative evidence challenged the frequently-held assumption that working-class women are well protected by a network of supportive family relationships:

> I was very satisfied. It's an important time in your life. You want to feel important, and the midwives I saw did that for me, they made me feel really important.

> I wouldn't have pulled through the postnatal depression if it hadn't been for her. She used to come and sit with me, every day, for the first few weeks.

Women commented on several aspects of the one-to-one relationship with the midwife which they particularly appreciated. The most frequently mentioned of these was trust. The interview data repeatedly showed that women trusted the midwives not only during the pregnancy, but in the longer term too:

> They still come to see us. I've got their phone numbers now in case anything happens. It's nice to know they care for you. I would have been dead worried without them.

Other aspects of the one-to-one relationship that were mentioned by women included friendliness, openness, patience, and ease of communication.

It is clear that the project significantly improved client opinion of the community midwifery service. Interestingly, client opinion of certain parts of the hospital service was also significantly improved among the project group. In particular, the midwifery intervention had an effect on client opinion of the hospital antenatal service, labour care, and the length of postpartum stay. The following series of tables shows improved client opinions in all these respects (the difference between ratings of project group and control group women shown in Tables 5.5, 5.6 and 5.7 did not reach the 0.05 level of significance but conforms to a pattern of greater satisfaction with hospital services among the former).

Table 5.3 Rating of hospital antenatal service

Satisfaction rating	project women		control women	
	%	No.	%	No.
Very satisfied	34	153	29	114
Satisfied	43 `77`		33 `62`	
Indifferent	10	20	19	35
Dissatisfied	9	17	12	22
Very dissatisfied	4	7	7	12
Don't know	1	1	1	1
Total	100	198	100	184

Source: Compiled by the author.

Table 5.4 Opinion of frequency of antenatal visits to hospital

Opinion of frequency	project women		control women	
	%	No.	%	No.
Too many	8	17	17	31
Right number	85	169	75	137
Too few	6	12	8	16
Total	100	198	100	184

Source: Compiled by the author.

The findings show that project group women rated their opinion of nearly all hospital care higher than did the control group women. This could have been a consequence of project group women being given preferential treatment in the hospitals, but interviews with hospital staff confirmed that there was no such policy. The findings, therefore, demonstrate that the midwifery intervention improved client satisfaction with hospital maternity services.

Table 5.5 Opinion of labour care as compared with most recent previous pregnancy

Opinion of care	project women		control women	
	%	No.	%	No.
Better	53	56	44	46
The same	23	24	32	34
Worse	24	26	24	25
Don't know/No answer	1	1	–	–
Total	100	107	100	105

Source: Compiled by the author.

Table 5.6 Adequacy of explanations given during labour

Views on adequacy	project women		control women	
	%	No.	%	No.
Adequate	74	147	65	119
Inadequate	25	49	34	62
Don't know	2	2	2	3
Total	100	198	100	184

Source: Compiled by the author.

Qualitative data from maternal interviews suggest that the reason for this perhaps unexpected spin-off effect was that the midwifery intervention improved women's confidence and understanding so that they were able to make informed use of the hospital services, and this, in turn, improved their satisfaction with them. For example, many women said that they had used the midwife to role-play forthcoming appointments at the hospital and this

Table 5.7 Opinion of length of postpartum hospital stay

Opinion	project women		control women	
	%	No.	%	No.
Too long	25	50	36	67
About right	67	132	56	104
Not long enough	8	16	7	13
Total	100	198	100	184

Source: Compiled by the author.

had improved their subsequent experience:

> You get used to the same person and can talk to them. That's how I managed to get my tubes tied; they really helped me to learn how to ask for my tubes tied. I talked it all out with them, how to ask for what I wanted.

Women in the control group did not have this opportunity and they consequently experienced considerable frustration during their hospital visits:

> A lot of the doctors use big words and everything, and, well, I can't understand that language at all. I didn't like it, seeing different doctors each time. You can't explain how you feel if you haven't seen them before.

A further reason for the higher ratings of hospital care among project women as compared with control group women was that the former turned to project midwives after a visit to hospital if they had not been satisfied with it. This may have made the memory of dissatisfaction shorter, and reduced its impact. It is also likely that using the midwife in this way lowered project women's expectations of the hospital, so that they could more easily be met.

More generally, project midwives had enough time to prepare women for what was likely to happen at the hospital in terms of waiting time and feelings of being rushed. Interview data from the midwives confirmed that they felt it was important to give women a realistic preparation for the clinics. They told them they would have to wait, but they also made sure that they explained why this was, so that women did not feel it was because staff devalued them as individuals. They explained how busy the clinics were, but they also made it clear that staff were there to help, and that the feeling of being on a conveyor belt could be challenged if women made a planned interruption at an appropriate point.

Similarly, project women's improved satisfaction with labour care was related to their enhanced preparations for labour. Qualitative data showed clearly that project women felt they had been well-prepared for labour and that meant they were more satisfied with the experience:

> It was better than last time – I knew what to expect. With the first one I didn't know nothing. With the midwife coming and talking to us and explaining it beforehand, I had a much better time. It definitely made a difference.

> You could talk to them more. [The community midwife] told me that if I didn't want something to happen when I was having him, I could say no. No-one had said that to me before, that I could say what I wanted. I did that. I told them at the hospital. In fact, it made it much better when I was having him.

Client behaviour

Findings relating to four aspects of client behaviour are discussed in this section: attendance at antenatal and postnatal clinics; attendance at parent-craft classes; smoking and diet. At the outset, one of the key hypotheses in the project protocol was that the intervention would increase low attendance at hospital antenatal clinics. The study showed firstly, that there was little impact on attendance and secondly, that chronic defaulting (missing three or more appointments) was not so great a problem as had been assumed. These findings are shown in Table 5.8 for the present pregnancy and, by way of comparison, those relating to the most recent previous pregnancy.

Thus, the findings show clearly that the level of chronic defaulting is not as high as local anecdote stated. They also show that the level of chronic defaulting is extremely stable. The similarity of attendance rates between this and previous pregnancies suggests an established pattern of clinic use that would be very hard to change. The changed working practice of the project midwives gave women every encouragement to attend clinics. For example, they gave women regular reminders about appointments, offered to arrange child-care, and even offered transport. The fact that the level of chronic defaulting remained so constant demonstrated the difficulties in changing the behaviour of this particular group of women. However, the project resources enabled midwives to identify defaulters, drawing on their extensive local knowledge, and to take care to them in their own community.

This pattern of little project impact on attendance rates was repeated in the data relating to attendance at child-health clinics (Table 5.9). There was

Table 5.8 Antenatal hospital clinic attendance

Frequency with which appointments kept	Study pregnancy				Previous pregnancy			
	project women		control women		project women		control women	
	%	No.	%	No.	%	No.	%	No.
Kept every appointment	78	154	83	153	77	98	83	98
Missed one or two appointments	15	30	12	22	11	14	9	11
Missed three or more	7	14	5	9	11	14	8	9
Don't know	–	–	–	–	1	1	–	–
Total	100	198	100	184	100	127	100	118

Source: Compiled by the author.

Table 5.9 Postnatal child-health clinic attendance

Attendance at clinic	Study pregnancy				Previous pregnancy			
	project women		control women		project women		control women	
	%	No.	%	No.	%	No.	%	No.
Yes	96	190	97	179	90	114	89	105
No	2	5	3	5	9	12	11	13
Not known	2	3	–	–	1	1	–	–
Total	100	198	100	184	100	127	100	118

Source: Compiled by the author.

also repetition of the finding that, contrary to the assumptions of those working in the field, defaulting was not a widespread problem.

These findings disprove one further early hypothesis about the project that was raised by several staff during individual interviews. This was that the intervention would instil dependence in women, so that they would become passive and fail to attend antenatal or child-health clinics. There is no evidence from the study to support this view.

By contrast, the intervention has had a significant effect on attendance at local parentcraft classes (Table 5.10) with project women significantly more likely to attend some classes than control group women ($p < 0.001$).

This effect is particularly marked when comparisons are made between attendance during the most recent previous pregnancy and attendance during the study pregnancy.

Analysis by age showed that younger women were more likely than older women to attend parentcraft classes. Indeed, in the project group, 38% of teenage mothers attended classes. These were women who were shown by analysis of hospital attendance data to be most likely to default from hospital clinics. Their high attendance at parentcraft confirms the earlier suggestion that the project facilitated the provision of care in the community for women who defaulted from the hospital.

This significant and successful impact on attendance at parentcraft classes can be attributed to four aspects of the classes, all of which are different from classes held elsewhere in the city. First, project midwives had enough time to actively recruit for the classes. They would remind women about the

Table 5.10 Attendance at local parentcraft classes

Attendance at classes	Study pregnancy				Previous pregnancy			
	project women		control women		project women		control women	
	%	No.	%	No.	%	No.	%	No.
Attended some classes	31	61	6	12	4	5	3	4
Attended no classes	69	137	94	172	96	122	97	114
Total	100	198	100	184	100	127	100	118

Source: Compiled by the author.

class whenever they saw them, including when they met them informally in the street. They also put reminder notes through women's doors. Secondly, the classes were more informal than is usual, and they had a curriculum that was wider than usual. For example, cooking lessons and practice opportunities were given, and visits were made to the local swimming pool. Thirdly, because the classes had a small catchment community, the women came from a homogenous socio-economic background. This meant that education could be focused on their particular needs. For example, advice on which new pushchair to buy would be superseded by advice on how to make a sterilizing unit out of an old ice-cream tub. Finally, a wider group of women than simply the pregnant were encouraged to attend. Women were invited to bring relatives and friends as well as partners. They were also welcomed as part of the group after the birth of the baby, as well as before it.

Clearly, improved attendance rates alone do not ensure the improved health of the mother and baby. It is, therefore, important to investigate whether or not there was a change in the health-related behaviour of project women. Analysis of data relating to smoking and eating patterns shows that the intervention did have an impact in terms of encouraging both reduced smoking and a healthier way of eating.

The impact of smoking advice was particularly marked when the data were analysed by the social class of the head of household. In the project group, 47% of women whose head of household was unemployed either stopped or cut down smoking during pregnancy, compared with only 25% in the control group. It is known that women whose head of household is unemployed and who rely on a supplementary benefit income are likely to be living in poverty and that this would be particularly stressful during pregnancy. This would increase the likelihood that this group of women would smoke more cigarettes than usual, as a response to stress. The reverse held, and this shows that antenatal education about smoking was successfully targeted by project midwives at women who were under particularly strong socio-economic disadvantage.

The intervention affected diet in several ways. A higher proportion of project women changed their diet during the study pregnancy than they had in their most recent previous pregnancy. This was not true in the control group.

Project women were more likely than were control group women to modify their diet in order to improve their health during pregnancy, rather than simply in order to satisfy hunger cravings or relieve nausea. One instance of this is that project women were more likely than were control group women to make an effort to reduce their intake of sweet foods, such as cakes, biscuits and sweets. Project women were also more likely than were control group women to continue this modification into the postnatal period.

Analysis by age showed that a higher proportion of teenage mothers in

Table 5.11 Changes in diet

Changes in diet	Study pregnancy				Previous pregnancy			
	project women		control women		project women		control women	
	%	No.	%	No.	%	No.	%	No.
Changes made to diet	64	126	67	123	48	61	65	77
No changes made to diet	36	72	33	61	52	66	35	40
No answer	–	–	–	–	–	–	1	1
Total	100	198	100	184	100	127	100	118

Source: Compiled by the author.

the project group as compared with the control group improved their diet during the pregnancy. Since this was also the group with the highest attendance rates at parentcraft classes, there seems to be an association between attendance at parentcraft classes and modification of diet.

Perinatal outcome

Data from the case note survey provided information on some aspects of obstetric history, the management of pregnancy and perinatal outcome. Findings in relation to the latter are considered in this section. The intervention had no effect on perinatal mortality, nor on the incidence of abnormalities in the baby. As already discussed, it was not expected that the intervention would affect these outcomes and the numbers involved are so small that statistical tests could not be carried out on these data.

However, the intervention may have had an impact on two perinatal outcomes. First, there is evidence of a reduced incidence of low birth weight babies among the project women. This is most clearly seen in an analysis of those women who have previously had a low birth weight baby, and who are therefore at risk of having another during the study pregnancy. The numbers involved are small, and should thus be treated with caution. Twenty one per cent of project group women who had a previous low birth weight baby had another at the end of the study pregnancy. Among control group women this figure was 46%. There is a slight difference too among women who had not had a previous low birth weight baby: 9% of project women in this group had a low birth weight baby at the end of the study pregnancy, compared with 14% of controls. Secondly, the intervention may have had a small effect on the percentage of pre-term deliveries. In the prospective project group, 6% of all women had pre-term deliveries, compared with 11% in the retrospective project group. Among the controls, 8% in the prospective study had pre-term deliveries, compared with 6% in the retrospective group. Thus, a downward trend in pre-term deliveries could be identified among women in the project area, but not among women in the control group areas.

The data also suggest that the pattern of pain relief during labour may have been affected by the intervention. Although there were only very small differences between the groups in terms of method of delivery, project women were more likely than control group women to use no pain relief or self-administered inhalation only (40% of project women, compared with 32% of control group women). The retrospective data show that there has been a change over time in the project group, but not among the controls. Eighteen per cent of the retrospective project group used no pain relief or self-administered inhalation only, whereas 33% of the retrospective control group did so.

These three findings suggest that the midwifery intervention may have affected clinical health outcome. Such findings replicate those of other studies that have linked social interventions with health outcome. For example, social interventions such as home visits by midwives (Spira *et al.*, 1981); nurse-midwife antenatal care (Runnerstrom, 1969); anti-smoking programmes (Sexton and Hebel, 1984); dietary supplementation (Mora *et al.*, 1979); income maintenance (Kehrer and Wohin, 1979); and intensive education (Sokol, 1980) have all been shown to have the capacity to affect outcomes such as birth weight and neonatal health. The pilot study for a major DHSS-funded project (Oakley, 1985) found a significantly increased mean birth weight in a group of babies whose mothers received socially supportive interviewing during pregnancy. (The findings from the main study are reported in Volume 3 of this series [Oakley, in preparation]). Observational studies documenting pregnant women's social support networks have suggested that a combination of high stress and low social support are accurate predictors of pregnancy complications (Nuckolls, Cassel and Kaplan, 1972; Norbeck and Tilden, 1983; Berkowitz and Kasl, 1983; Smilkstein *et al.*, 1984).

It should be noted that a reduced incidence of low birth weight babies has significant implications for cost savings, since low birth weight is associated with short- and long-term mortality and morbidity. Although neonatal intensive care has reduced mortality in low birth weight babies, there is no evidence that the long-term morbidity of such babies has fallen to the same extent (Kitchen *et al.*, 1982).

Effect on staff: job satisfaction and inter-professional collaboration

Interviews held with project midwives indicated that the project enhanced their job satisfaction in several ways. The main source of increased job satisfaction was an improved relationship with women: this had five main strands:

1. Opportunity to give women all the time they needed to be fully reassured and educated;
2. Ability to provide women with continuity of care;
3. Offering women individualized care;
4. Becoming known and recognized in a defined geographical area;
5. Opportunity to get to know all the members of the woman's family and to help them become as involved as possible with the birth.

Other aspects of improved job satisfaction included the extra time for teaching both on a one-to-one basis and in groups, and the opportunity to offer domino deliveries.

Although there was this significant improvement in job satisfaction among community midwives, they felt that this would have been further enhanced were it not for the opposition that they felt they encountered from some of the hospital medical staff. Two of the project midwives said their main source of job dissatisfaction was that they felt some of the hospital medical staff were antagonistic towards the project and others mentioned a feeling that hospital medical staff were disinterested in the project and this, too, was a source of regret.

Data from staff interviews indicated that the project enhanced relations between midwives and those general practitioners and health visitors who were based in the project areas. However, there was evidence of some weaknesses in communication and general practitioners and midwives outside the two estates knew little about the project. Although the project improved communication between hospital midwifery staff and community midwives, there was no impact on relations with the hospital medical team. (Full details of these findings can be found in Evans, 1987.)

DISCUSSION OF FINDINGS

The findings show that the midwifery intervention improved client satisfaction with the midwifery and hospital services, increased attendance at parentcraft classes, encouraged reduced smoking and improved diet. These findings make it clear that the project style of midwifery enables the development of a service that is in line with that proscribed in all the recent DHSS thinking about community health services. Thus, the project has played an important role in enabling the Newcastle Health Authority to move towards meeting the recommendations of the Black Report (Townsend and Davidson, 1982); the Short Report (ocial Services Committee, 1980); the Cumberlege Report (DHSS, 1986); the Griffiths Report (DHSS, 1983); and the DHSS publication *Prevention and Health* (DHSS, 1976). All these outline a general strategy for health that forms the broader context of the community midwifery service. The two main themes of this strategy are prevention and consumer orientation, and the study shows the project has made a significant contribution in the development of each of these.

The study has wide implications for the midwifery profession. In general terms, it highlights the need for an increase in the numbers of community midwives. It is recognized that increasing the number of midwives requires additional resources at a time of economic stringency. However, this expansion is a priority because, in the longer term, it can become a cost-saving measure. For example, the easier identification of clinic defaulters, and caring for them in the community ensures that there can be early diagnosis among this 'at risk' population. The increased take-up of antenatal education about preventive health issues may promote a longer-term improvement in health, and this will bring a reduction in the demands made on the NHS. Similarly, project midwives have helped women to become more confident and articulate users of the health services, and this saves expensive professional time, both in clinics and in following up potential defaulters in the community.

More specifically, the study highlights the need to identify the primary focus of midwifery as the woman in her own community, rather than in the hospital clinic or labour ward. Focusing midwifery in this way has implications for both education and practice. Currently, midwifery education relates mainly to the physiology of pregnancy, and practical work is disproportionately concentrated in the hospital rather than the community. However, the evidence from the Newcastle Project, shows that the educational emphasis should be shifted to include an understanding of social issues, counselling, and group development work. A basic grounding in theories of social policy and social structure would enable midwives to make analytical sense of the links between social issues and health outcome. This, in turn, would encourage an understanding of the value of 'community work' with relation to the practice of community midwifery. Counselling and group work skills do not form part of the usual midwifery curriculum, and yet the intensive community midwifery approach outlined here is based on such skills.

Turning now to practice, the focus on women in the context of their own communities requires that midwives become involved in community development work. This involves taking an active part in community initiatives such as the Cowgate Neighbourhood Centre, and building relationships with people other than the pregnant woman.

It might be thought that the argument presented in this chapter is close to re-inventing the wheel! Indeed, one of the more experienced of the project midwives made exactly this point, and often commented that she was now working more closely than ever before to the model of midwifery in which she had been trained. This point should perhaps be emphasized and stated in a more political way. For some time the role of the midwife has been declining (Towler, 1982; Robinson, Golden and Bradley, 1983; Robinson, 1985, 1989). As the percentage of births taking place in hospital has risen to almost a hundred, so the task of the community midwife has become increasingly restricted to that of providing postnatal care. The project made resources available for community midwives to take back some of the areas of work that have been taken from them, and so regain some of the expertise that they have more recently been denied.

Thus, it is clear that the main implications of this study can only be fully acted upon if there is a significant increase in staff resources. As described in the first part of this chapter, there are considerable difficulties in achieving this, and Newcastle Health Authority was involved in fraught negotiation with the Local Authority about the future of the CMC Project. Despite the strength of the research evidence, and widespread agreement with its findings, there was considerable difficulty in securing funding to protect and extend this particular style of community midwifery. However, it is likely that, as a result of this study there will be some modification of midwifery practice in the city. For example, there is already a commitment to increase the midwifery establishment from 21 to 25. Although progress towards a fully resourced community midwifery service focusing on the needs of the mother in her own community has been slow, it is clear that projects such as the Newcastle CMC Project speed this progress and make an important contribution to the development of a more professional and pertinent community midwifery service.

REFERENCES

Abdellah, F.G. and Levine, E. (1954) Work sampling applied to the study of nursing personnel. *Nursing Research*, **3**(1), p. 11–16.

Adelstein, P. and Fedrick, J. (1978) Antenatal identification of women at increased risk of being delivered of a low birthweight infant at term. *British Journal of Obstetrics and Gynaecology,* **85**(1), 8–11.

Baird, D. and Thomson, A.M. (1969) General factors underlying perinatal mortality rates. In Butler, N.R. and Alberman, E.D. *Perinatal Problems,* Churchill Livingstone, Edinburgh.

Berkowitz, G.S. and Kasl, S.V. (1983) The role of psychosocial factors in spontaneous pre-term delivery. *Journal of Psychosomatic Research*, **27**(4), 283–90.

Billewicz, W.Z. (1964) Matched samples in medical investigations. *British Journal of Preventive and Social Medicine,* **18**(4), 167–73.

Boyd, C. and Sellars, L. (1982) *The British Way of Birth.* Pan, London.

Brennan, M.E. and Lancashire, R. (1978) Association of childhood mortality with housing status and unemployment. *Journal of Epidemiology and Community Health*, **32**(1), 28–33.

Burke, C., Chall, C.L. and Abdellah, F.G. (1956) A time study of nursing activities in a psychiatric hospital. A first step in improving patient care. *Nursing Research* **5**(1), 27–35.

Butler, N.R. and Alberman, E.D. (1969) *Perinatal Problems*. Churchill Livingstone, Edinburgh.

Butler, N.R. and Bonham, D. (1963) *Perinatal Mortality*. E. and S. Livingstone, Edinburgh.

Cartwright, A. (1979) *The Dignity of Labour?* Tavistock, London.

Cochrane, A. (1972) *Effectiveness and efficiency. Random reflections on Health Services* Nuffield Provincial Hospitals Trust, Oxford.

Cullinan, T. and Trenherz, J. (1982) *Ill in East London 1979–1981*

Davie, R., Butler, N., and Goldstein, H. (1972) *From Birth to Seven*. Longmans, London.

DHSS (1976) *Prevention and Health: Everybody's Business*, HMSO, London.

DHSS (1983) NHS Management Enquiry, *The Griffiths Report*, HMSO, London.

DHSS (1986) Neighbourhood Nursing – A focus for Care, *The Cumberlege Report*, HMSO, London.

Donovan, J.W. (1977) Randomized controlled trial of anti-smoking advice in pregnancy. *British Journal of Preventive and Social Medicine* **31**(1), 6–12.

Ehrenreich, B. and English, D. (1973) *Witches, Midwives and Nurses*, Glass Mountain Pamphlets, The Feminist Press, New York.

Evans, F. (1987) *The Newcastle Community Midwifery Care Project. An Evaluation Report*. Newcastle Health Authority, Newcastle upon Tyne.

Graham, H. and McKee, L. (1980) *The First Months of Motherhood*, HEC Monograph No. 3, Health Education Council, London.

Kehrer, B.H. and Wohin, C.M. (1979) Impact of income maintenance on low birthweight. *Journal of Human Resources*, **14**(4), 434–62.

Kitchen, W.H., Yu, V.Y.H., Lissenden, J.V. and Basuk. B. (1982) Collaborative study of very low birthweight infants: techniques of perinatal care and mortality. *Lancet*, **1371**, 1454–7.

McIntosh, J. (1989) Models of childbirth and social class: a study of 80 working class primigravidae. In Robinson, S. and Thomson, A.M. (eds) *Midwives, Research and Childbirth Vol. 1*. Chapman and Hall, London.

MacVicar, J. (1976) *Perinatal Mortality in Leicestershire*, Leicestershire Health Authority, Leicestershire.

Meechan, D.F. (1980) *Perinatal Mortality in Humberside*. Unpublished MSc Thesis. University of Hull, Hull.

Mora, J.O., de Paredes B., Wagner, M., de Navarro, G., Suescur, J., Christiansen N. and Herrera, M.G. (1979) Nutritional supplementation and the outcome of pregnancy 1: Birthweight. *American Journal of Clinical Nutrition*, **32**, 455–62.

Norbeck, J.S. and Tilden, V.P. (1983) Life stress, social support and emotional disequilibrium in complications of pregnancy: a prospective multivariate study. *Journal of Health and Social Behaviour*, **24**(1), 30–46.

Nuckolls, K.B., Cassel, J. and Kaplan, J.H. (1972) Psychosocial assets, life crises and the prognosis of pregnancy. *American Journal of Epidemiology*, **95**(5), 431–41.

Oakley, A. (1979) *Becoming a Mother.* Martin Robertson, Oxford.

Oakley, A. (1984) *The Captured Womb.* Basil Blackwell, Oxford.

Oakley, A. (1985) *Social Support and Pregnancy Outcome.* Unpublished research proposal. Thomas Coram Research Unit, Institute of Education, London University.

Robinson, S. (1985) Midwives, obstetricians and general practitioners: The need for role clarification. *Midwifery,* 1(2), 102–13.

Robinson, S. (1989) Caring for childbearing women: the interrelationship between midwifery and medical responsibilities. In Robinson, S. and Thomson, A.M. (eds.) *Midwives, Research and Childbirth. Volume 1.* Chapman and Hall, London.

Robinson, S., Golden, J. and Bradley, S. (1983) A study of the role and responsibilities of the midwife. *NERU Report, No. 1.* Nursing Research Unit, Kings College, London University, London.

Runnerstrom, L.R. (1969) The effectiveness of nurse-midwifery in a supervised hospital environment. *Bulletin of the American College of Nurse-Midwives,* 14(2), 40–52.

Sexton, M. and Hebel, J.R. (1984) A clinical trial of change in maternal smoking and its effects on birthweight. *Journal of the American Medical Association,* 251(7), 911–15.

Smilkstein, G., Helsper-Lucas, A., Ashworth, C. *et al.* (1984) Prediction of pregnancy complications: an application of the biopsychosocial model. *Social Science and Medicine,* 18(4), 315–21.

Social Services Committee (1980), Perinatal and neonatal mortality, *The Short Report.* HMSO, London.

Sokol, R.J. (1980) Risk, ante-partum care and outcome: impact of a maternity and infant care project. *Obstetrics and Gynecology,* 56(2), 150–6.

Spira, N., Audras, F., Chapel, A. *et al.* (1981) Surveillance à domicile des grosses pathologiques par les sages-femmes. Essai comparatif contrôle sur 996 femmes. *Journal of Gynaecology, Obstetrics and Biological Reproduction (Paris)* 10(6), 543–8 (Eng.Abst.)

Towler, J. (1982) A dying species: survival and revival are up to us. *Midwives Chronicle,* 95(1136), 324–8.

Townsend, P. and Davidson, N. (1982) *Inequalities in Health.* Penguin, London.

CHAPTER SIX

Providing care at a midwives' antenatal clinic

Ann M. Thomson

INTRODUCTION

In defining the Sphere of Practice of the midwife the World Health Organisation (WHO, 1966) states that the midwife 'must be able to give the necessary supervision, care and advice to women during pregnancy, labour and the postpartum period ...'. The care includes preventive care, the detection of abnormalities and referral for medical care where appropriate. The WHO also states that the midwife may 'practise in hospitals, clinics, health units, domiciliary conditions or in any other service'. In the United Kingdom (UK), however, medical involvement in the provision of care for normal childbearing women has been increasing since the beginning of this century, eroding the extent to which midwives have been able to practise in accordance with the WHO definition (Walker, 1976; Robinson, Golden and Bradley, 1983; Robinson, 1985; Robinson, 1989). By the 1970s the midwife had come to be seen, and was only allowed to act, as little more than a maternity nurse. In the provision of antenatal care in particular midwives were not allowed to take the degree of responsibility for which they were qualified (Robinson, Golden and Bradley, 1983).

In the early 1980s in the UK there appeared to be some attempts to alter the way in which care was provided, particularly in the antenatal period, so that midwifery practice was fulfilling the role as defined by the WHO. There were many personal communications and some reports (Morrin, 1982; Callis, 1983; Stuart and Judge, 1984) that midwives had begun to provide their own antenatal clinics. One of the continuing complaints about antenatal care has been of the lack of continuity of the professionals providing the care (Fleury, 1967; Chamberlain and Cave, 1977; King's Community Health Council, 1978; Oakley, 1979: Kitzinger, 1981; Boyd and Sellars, 1982; Turnball, 1984). Before the provision of facilities for childbirth moved wholesale into the hospital, continuity of care during pregnancy was provided by midwives in hospital and in local authority clinics. Recently midwives have advocated the reinstatement of midwives' antenatal clinics, stating that this is one way to provide continuity of care (Callis, 1983; Stuart and Judge, 1984). No research had been undertaken, however, to record for whom the midwives in these clinics were providing care, how the care was provided and most importantly to evaluate the outcomes of such care.

As well as the re-establishment of midwives' clinics there have been other initiatives in the provision of maternity care of women during pregnancy. These included a scheme in which midwives provided antenatal care as part of a package of care for the whole childbirth continuum (Flint and Poulengeris, 1987 and Chapter 4, this volume), and a scheme in which extra community midwifery care was provided in addition to the standard hospital antenatal care, to women living in an area of socio-economic deprivation (Evans, 1987 and Chapter 5, this volume). Both these initiatives have been the subject of evaluation studies.

The purpose of the study reported here was to document the social and obstetric profile of women who attended a midwives' clinic, to describe some aspects of the care received, and to relate the outcomes of care in terms of the problems identified in the antenatal period. A further intention was to compare the findings from this study of women attending a hospital midwives' clinic with the findings of a study of women attending a community midwives' clinic and a study of women attending an obstetrician's clinic. The data for the study was obtained from medical records; the use of these as a source of data are considered in terms of their availability and reliability.

In order to place the re-emergence of midwives' clinics in context some aspects of the history of midwives involvement in antenatal care are described.

DEVELOPMENTS IN MIDWIFE-PROVIDED ANTENATAL CARE

Recognition of the need for antenatal care in the UK occurred at the beginning of this century when it was felt that antenatal care could make a contribution to the reduction of the unacceptably high maternal and infant mortality rates (Oakley, 1984). The midwifery profession recognized the need to include teaching about antenatal care in midwifery training early in its development. The Midwives' Institute's (later the College of Midwives) first course of lectures in 1915 were devoted to various aspects of antenatal care (Cowell and Wainwright, 1981) and some instruction in antenatal care was included in the revised and extended syllabus for midwives in 1917 (Central Midwives Board, 1917). Midwives and general practitioners (GPs) were encouraged to provide antenatal care, and pregnant women were urged to attend local-authority antenatal clinics which had been set up in existing maternal and child welfare centres (Lewis, 1980; Robinson, Golden and Bradley, 1983). Take-up of the available service increased and most antenatal care was provided in these local-authority clinics. Although women would usually be examined twice during pregnancy by the Medical Officer of Health, most of the care at these clinics was provided by midwives who were responsible for assessing whether pregnancy was progressing satisfactorily (Wood, 1963).

Following the introduction of the National Health Service, and the facility for the GP to be given financial remuneration for providing antenatal care, GP involvement in antenatal care increased. The extent of this increased involvement led to complaints being made to a government Working Party on Midwives (Ministry of Health *et al.*, 1949). The complaints stated that GPs were taking over all the care provided by the local-authority clinics and were 'relegating midwives to the status of maternity nurses' (Ministry of Health *et al.*, 1949). Midwives did in fact continue to provide antenatal care in women's homes and in local-authority clinics but they worked more closely with GPs than they had before 1948 (Wood, 1963; Robinson, Golden and Bradley, 1982; Robinson, 1990).

In 1970 the government report on the facilities needed for the provision of a satisfactory maternity service (DHSS, 1970) recommended that there was a need to make provision for 100% hospital confinement on the grounds that delivery at home was unsafe (see Campbell and Macfarlane, 1987 for a discussion of the latter assumption). In the years that followed an increasing proportion of women who were 'booked' for hospital confinement had their antenatal care provided at the hospital antenatal clinic. The vast proportion of this care was given by obstetricians, although much of the routine work was undertaken by midwives. Midwives' clinics which had existed in many hospitals were closed down (Robinson, Golden and Bradley, 1983). However, as the number of women 'booked' for hospital confinement increased it became impossible for the obstetricians to cope with the pressure of work. In order to ease the workload a system of shared care was introduced whereby the provision of care to women at low obstetric risk was divided between hospital and community. However the provider of care in the community was not the health professional qualified to provide care during normal pregnancy, the midwife, but the GP.

The midwifery profession expressed concern about this both as individuals and collectively through the Royal College of Midwives. In their evidence to the Royal Commission on the National Health Service the Royal College of Midwives stated, 'The midwife is trained and capable of giving prenatal care on her own responsibility, but in practice the medical staff do not fully utilise this valuable resource', and again; 'For example in some hospital prenatal clinics and family group practices, the total prenatal care is given by medical staff' (Royal College of Midwives, 1977). Barnett (1979) stated that 'many midwifery skills have been ignored or abandoned in the need to give sophisticated care in the electronic age' and Brain (1979) said 'I believe we are not using her (the midwife's) skills today in the community or in the hospitals'. This situation was still in existence nationally in the late 1970s (Robinson, Golden and Bradley, 1983).

As a result of the comments from individual midwives (Walker, 1976; Barnett, 1979; Brain, 1979; Flint, 1979; Thomson, 1980) the writings of the Royal College of Midwives (1977) and the national research study on the role and responsibilities of the midwife (Robinson, Golden and Bradley, 1983) midwives began to question their role in general but in the provision of antenatal care in particular (Flint, 1982a,b). The statutory bodies felt sufficiently concerned about the erosion of the role of the midwife to issue a document re-affirming the WHO definition of the midwife (Central Midwives Board for Scotland *et al.*, 1983). As noted at the beginning of this chapter there were a number of initiatives to re-establish midwives' clinics for women at low obstetric risk (Callis, 1983; Stuart and Judge, 1984).

RESEARCH INTO ANTENATAL CARE

Antenatal care, like Topsy, has 'just growed'. Oakley (1984) in tracing its history has shown that as medical knowledge increased more was included in the antenatal assessment and treatment. Because the maternal and perinatal mortality rates have fallen since the turn of the century (Social Services Committee, 1980; DHSS, 1989) the success of antenatal care was presumed without assessing the effect of general improvements in socio-economic status and the environment. Antenatal care is assumed to do good, to do no harm, that the earlier it starts the better, the more that is given the better and is better when provided by highly specialized people (Hall, 1984). In the national study of all births occurring in one week in 1958 (Butler and Bonham, 1963) it was found that perinatal mortality was lowest among those who had the greatest number of visits for antenatal care. The authors therefore recommended an increase in antenatal supervision. However, it is women from socio-economic classes 1 and 2 who have the lowest perinatal mortality rates (OPCS, 1987) and as these women book earliest for ante-natal care, they therefore have more chance to attend for a greater number of visits. Conversely women from the lower socio-economic groups who have the highest perinatal mortality have higher rates of spontaneous pre-term delivery or develop problems which necessitate induction of labour. Their chances of attending for a large number of antenatal appointments are therefore reduced.

Cochrane (1972) describes antenatal care as a:

multiphasic screening procedure which by some curious chance, has escaped the critical assessment to which most screening procedures have been subjected in the last few years and there seems no reason why the same approach that has proved so useful elsewhere should not be used here.

Chng, Hall and MacGillivray (1980) and Hall, Chng and MacGillivray (1980) took up this challenge and carried out a retrospective analysis of antenatal records in order to conduct an audit of antenatal care. They found that doctors failed to note relevant previous medical and/or obstetric histories which might have a bearing on the outcome of antenatal care (Chng, Hall and MacGillivray, 1980). They also found that when these relevant histories were missed the women were not booked for specialist antenatal and intrapartum care. For example a woman who has given birth to an intra-uterine growth retarded (IUGR) baby has a 27% chance of delivering a subsequent IUGR baby (Thomson, Billewicz and Hytten, 1968). It is therefore particularly important that the woman who has delivered a previous IUGR baby receives continuity of care in her antenatal care and is delivered in a unit with specialist paediatric facilities in case they are required by the baby. This woman should not have shared care nor be delivered in a maternity home with no Special Care Baby Unit (SCBU). In Aberdeen Chng, Hall and MacGillivray (1980) found that 68% of women who had delivered a previous IUGR baby were not identified and they were booked inappropriately for style of antenatal care and for place of confinement.

As a result of their research, Hall, Chng and MacGillivray (1980) state that the obstetric profession has an unrealistic expectation of the productivity of antenatal care. They found that there was an over and an under-diagnosis of IUGR in the pregnancies under study, in that although 189 women delivered an IUGR baby only 89 were suspected antenatally. However, 289 women were suspected during pregnancy of having an IUGR fetus but only 83 delivered an IUGR baby. Although 190 women developed pre-eclampsia only 70% of women developed signs in pregnancy, the remaining women developed it in labour. They also found that a significant proportion of emergency antenatal admissions occured despite good antenatal care. As a result of this study the authors suggest a much reduced programme of antenatal examinations and subsequently introduced and evaluated such a programme (Hall, Macintyre and Porter, 1985). Although there were various difficulties in instigating the new regime, no adverse effects were demonstrated for the women who did receive fewer antenatal examinations.

Several studies have been undertaken asking women their views of antenatal care. Complaints have been about long and difficult journeys to the antenatal clinic, long waiting times, lack of privacy, poor communications from health professionals, and conveyor belt systems in which care is not individualized (Fleury, 1967; Richards, Donald and Hamilton, 1970; Chamberlain and Cave, 1977; King's Community Health Council, 1978; Oakley, 1979; Graham and McKee, 1980; Hogg and Hague, 1980; Kirke, 1980; O'Brien and Smith, 1981; Boyd and Sellers, 1982; Perfrement, 1982; Rajan and Oakley, 1990). In reviewing the literature on women's views of antenatal care Garcia shows that sadly the complaints in the 1980s are the same as those recorded in the 1940s (Garcia, 1982).

There have, however, been some initiatives in taking antenatal care out of the hospital into the community. In Lambeth (Zander *et al.*, 1978; Zander, 1982; Taylor, 1984) and at Sighthill in Edinburgh (McKee, 1984) antenatal care is provided in the Health Centre as integrated care between the GP, community midwife and consultant obstetrician. In Glasgow (Reid, Gutteridge and McIlwaine, 1983), however, the antenatal care is provided by obstetricians in local authority premises. The thinking behind these moves into the community was to try to reduce the number of complaints about antenatal care and to reduce the defaulting from care rate which was seen to be a contributor to perinatal mortality (Reid, Gutteridge and McIlwaine, 1983; Taylor, 1984). All these clinics have shown that community antenatal care does no harm, that the defaulting rate is lowered and that the women are more satisfied with the care they receive. At Sighthill there has been a dramatic reduction in the perinatal mortality rate from 25/1000 in 1975 to 8/1000 for the period 1976–80, whereas perinatal mortality for women living in Sighthill and not attending this antenatal scheme is 21/1000 (McKee, 1984).

Research has been undertaken assessing antenatal care provided by obstetricians (for example, Chng, Hall and MacGillivray, 1980; Hall, Chng and MacGillivray, 1980; Reid, Gutteridge and McIlwaine, 1983; Taylor, 1984), and by midwives in initiatives such as the Know Your Midwife scheme (Flint and Poulengeris and Chapter 4, this volume) and the Newcastle Community Midwifery scheme (Evans, 1987 and Chapter 5, this volume). However, at the time that the research described in this chapter was undertaken there had been no studies of care provided at midwives' clinics.

METHODS

The research described in this chapter was undertaken at a Maternity Unit in a District General Hospital serving an inner city area in the North of England, which undertook 2500 deliveries a year. Antenatal care was provided by the obstetricians in the hospital clinic but in order to provide student midwives with the opportunity to observe midwife-provided antenatal care a Teaching Midwives clinic had been in existence for some years. The clinic was run, and care was provided, by the Midwife Teachers who taught in the maternity unit's school of midwifery. Student midwives attended the Teaching Midwives Clinic (TMC) when they were gaining clinical experience in the antenatal clinic. The TMC was held on one afternoon a week and the women who attended it were referred by one of the three consultant obstetricians. There was no facility for systematically referring all women suitable for midwifery-provided care to the clinic. The obstetricians would be told when the clinic was 'short of women' and be asked to refer a few more from the next 'booking' clinic.

The aims of the study were:

1. To describe the characteristics of the women referred to this clinic and compare them with those of women who attended the obstetrician's clinic and a clinic run by community midwives at a satellite clinic;
2. To assess whether those who attended the TMC and community midwives' clinic come within the groups identified as being at low obstetric risk. If not, were they noted as being at high obstetric risk and was appropriate care targeted to them?
3. Did the Midwife Teachers and community midwives provide continuity of care?
4. Were problems which occurred in labour, the early puerperium and the perinatal period identified antenatally?

Source of data

Due to time and financial constraints it was decided to undertake a retrospective analysis of the records of the women who had attended the clinics during one calendar year. Hockey (personal communication) has stated that medical records are a vast untapped store of readily available data. The data are relatively easy to extract, they do not change over time, and because they are always there it is possible to go back to them. However, medical records are a secondary source of data which 'were collected by someone other than the researcher with some other purpose in mind' (Bulmer and Atkinson, 1979). In this case the data were collected for medico-legal reasons so that subsequent care providers would know of previous findings and treatment. A large number of people may be involved in recording this information and they may not always record the same information or record in the same way. This can affect the validity and reliability of the data. In their study comparing the reliability of medical records with the recall of women of the medical events of their childbearing experience Cartwright, Jacoby and Martin (1987) have also shown that errors can be made in extracting data from the records. They describe the task as a 'difficult and tedious job demanding some medical knowledge and much patience and persistence' (Cartwright, Jacoby and Martin, 1987).

Obtaining the data to undertake an analysis of medical records has proved a problem in obstetrics. Simpson and Walker (1980), and Evans (Chapter 5, this volume) have only had success rates in finding records varying between 72% and 90%. Non-availability of records affects the validity and reliability of the data. However, Chng, Hall and MacGillivray (1980) and Hall, Chng and MacGillivray (1980) used medical records in their audit of antenatal care in Aberdeen and found that a retrospective examination of the records produced adequate data for their study. It was therefore decided that this method would be suitable for the study described in this chapter.

Access to the study site was gained by application to the Division of Obstetrics and Gynaecology. The author was not required to gain permission from the District Ethical committee. A proforma was designed to collect information on demographic data, information about previous pregnancies, the antenatal period under study, the outcome of the pregnancy and postnatal and perinatal morbidity.

Information obtained

Ethnic origin. Although concern has been expressed at the high incidence of perinatal mortality among women who were not themselves born in this country (Social Services Committee, 1980), ethnic origin and place of birth of women attending the hospital for antenatal care were not noted in the medical records. In a crude attempt to ascertain the ethnic origin of the women a subjective assessment of the origin of the woman's surname (e.g. British, African, Chinese) was made and cross tabulated with the religion noted in the records.

Area of residence. Armand-Smith (1980) reported that perinatal mortality varied widely within the city wards of Edinburgh, and Davies (Chapter 5, part 1 in this volume) reports similar findings from Newcastle. Roland (1981) demonstrated that the area in which the woman lived had a bearing on the incidence of low birth weight in Manchester. In an attempt to discover if place of residence was a relevant factor in the outcome of pregnancy in this study the women's addresses were grouped according to electoral ward.

Continuity of care. As noted earlier one of the continuing complaints about antenatal care has been of the lack of continuity of professionals providing the care. During informal discussions with the Teaching Midwives in the early days of this study the impression was gained that they thought they were able to provide a greater degree of continuity of care than was available in the obstetrician's clinic. Certainly, with the small number of Midwife Teachers it seemed a feasible supposition. In an attempt to discover how many health professionals the women had seen for their antenatal care at the TMC a simple count of the number of different types of writing and initials/signatures on the records was made. These signatures/initials included those of the obstetrician seen at the first visit to the hospital clinic. In the antenatal record there were columns in which weight and urinalysis were recorded and a section in which blood pressure, period of gestation, fundal height, fetal presentation etc. were recorded. It was obvious that the writing recording weight and urinalysis in each set of records was different from that recording blood pressure, period of gestation etc. There were no signatures or initials beside the recording of weight and urinalysis but there were signatures or initials beside the other information recorded.

Outcomes. Data on labour and delivery were extracted from the labour summary sheet and, when this was deficient, from the partogram and written labour records. Data on the woman's postnatal period were obtained from the medical notes made during the puerperium and from the ward Kardex.

At birth all babies were given a medical record chart separate from that of their mother. This chart was filed in the mother's medical records unless the babies were admitted to the Special Care Baby Unit (SBCU) or were to be 'followed-up' by the paediatricians when they were given a new file of their own and the chart given them at birth was incorporated in this file. In spite of the valiant efforts of the ward clerk on the SCBU, who even managed to find the records of a baby whose first and second names had changed, five sets of baby records were not found. In order to assess the health and perinatal problems of the babies the medical records (when available) and Kardex were examined.

Data collection and analysis

The proforma was piloted and minor adjustments made. Facilities for the punching of data were available within the University. Data were analysed using the Statistical Package for the Social Sciences (Nie *et al.*, 1975). Differences between values were assessed using the chi square test.

In order to use available time most efficiently it was decided to code the data directly from the medical records on to the proforma. Anonymity was guaranteed by the use of 'study numbers' only, not names, on the proforma. Because of the pressure of work experienced by the medical records clerks in the antenatal clinic the author undertook to 'pull' and put back all the relevant medical records. A list of all the women who had attended the clinic during the study year, 1982, was provided by the medical records clerks.

It had been intended to complete the data collection in June and July of 1983 but unexpected problems were encountered. Two hundred and eighteen names were obtained from the appointment sheets for the Teaching Midwives' Clinic for 1982. However, medical records were found for only 76% (165) of these women. Twenty-four per cent of the records of the women listed in the antenatal appointment sheet could not be found despite extending the projected data collection period of two months to nine months. The problem did not lie in the author's inexperience in tracing records because as a last resort the records clerks did assist and look for missing records, but to no avail. The difficulties encountered were due to several factors. The medical records of pregnant women and those delivered within the last five years were kept in the antenatal clinic, not in the main hospital medical records department. In the antenatal clinic these records were kept in five different places depending on whether the woman was pregnant, recently delivered or had delivered in the last two years. In two of these record stacks the records were not in alphabetical or numerical order. As found by Evans (Chapter 5, part 2 in this volume) tracer cards were not used and there was no central record of where a set of records for a child-bearing woman might be at any one time. The data collection was discontinued in January 1984 because the productivity of records searches was so poor at that time. Because of the difficulties in obtaining medical records it was decided not to pursue that part of the study which would have compared outcomes of women attending the Teaching Midwives clinic with those of women who attended the community midwives' clinic and the obstetrician's clinic. The findings presented here therefore relate only to antenatal care provided by Midwife Teachers at an antenatal clinic designed to demonstrate midwife-provided antenatal care to student midwives. However these findings can usefully be compared with the findings from other studies on the provision of antenatal care.

FINDINGS

Examination of the 165 records that were found showed that only 86% (142) of the women had actually attended the Teaching Midwives' Clinic (TMC). The findings reported relate to:

1. Socio-demographic characteristics of the sample;
2. Antenatal attendance and care;
3. Referral back to the obstetrician during pregnancy;
4. Labour and delivery outcomes;
5. Postnatal outcomes.

Social and demographic characteristics

Information on factors such as age, socio-economic status, support from partner and nationality was collected to determine if the women came within the low risk categories discussed earlier.

Age. The ages of the women who attended this clinic ranged between 16 and 38 years (Table 6.1). A fifth of the sample were aged 19 or younger. This is a slightly higher proportion than Reid, Gutteridge and McIlwaine (1983) found in their study of women attending Glasgow Royal Maternity Hospital (13%) and women attending for antenatal care in the Greater Glasgow Health Board area (13%) or than McKee (1984) found in relation to the Sighthill Clinic in Edinburgh (12%). The proportion of teenagers attending the Easterhouse Clinic in Glasgow was 23% however (Reid,

Table 6.1 Ages of women attending clinic

Age in years	No.	%
<19	28	20
20–24	65	46
25–29	31	22
30–34	12	8
35+	6	4
Total	142	100

Source: Compiled by the author.

Gutteridge and McIlwaine, 1983), higher than that reported for other studies.

Marital status. The women's marital status was recorded at booking and at delivery. At the time of booking 67% (95) of the women were married with a further 12% (17) living in a common law relationship. Seven women who were single at the time of booking had married before the baby was born. There was no indication in the records of whether any of the women were supported, either financially or emotionally.

Social class. This was assessed on both the woman's and partner's occupation using the Registrar General's Classification of Occupations (OPCS, 1970) (Table 6.2). Over half of the women had stated that they were housewives and 18% of the partners were unemployed. Only 16% of the women came from social classes 1, 2 and 3N when classified by their partner's occupation. Although the greater proportion came from the lower socio-economic groups the proportion in groups 4 and 5 was considerably lower than the 46% at Glasgow Royal Maternity Hospital, 40% at the Easterhouse clinic (Reid, Gutteridge and McIlwaine, 1983) and the 26% at the Sighthill clinic (McKee, 1984).

Women's place of birth. Using the assessment described above, 73% (104) of the women had a surname considered to be British and had a Christian religion. Twenty per cent (29) of the women had a surname which was considered to be Asian in origin and were noted to be of the Sikh, Moslem or Hindu religion. Two 'British' named women had 'other' religions, one woman with a 'South American' name was recorded as having a Christian religion and one 'Asian' and four British women were not noted to have a religion.

Parity. Forty-nine per cent (70) of these women were having their first baby (Table 6.3). The parity of the other 72 women ranged between 1 and 7.

Table 6.2 Social class by own and partner's occupation

Social class	Own		Partner	
	No.	%	No.	%
1	–	–	1	1
2	6	4	6	4
3N	16	11	15	11
3M	18	13	46	32
4	3	2	11	8
5	–		1	1
Unemployed	11	8	26	18
Housewife	81	57	–	
No information available	7	5	36	25
Total	142	100	142	100

Source: Compiled by the author.

Table 6.3 Parity of women attending clinic

Parity	No.	%
Primipara	70	49
Para 1	40	28
Para 2	18	13
Para 3	10	7
Para 4	1	1
Para 6	1	1
Para 7	2	1
Total	142	100

Source: Compiled by the author.

Place of residence. It was not possible, from the information given in the records, to group the addresses of five women. Although women were more likely to live in the immediate vicinity of the hospital than further afield, the geographical spread was large and no pattern emerged.

The teaching midwives were therefore providing care for a group of relatively young women in that a fifth of them were teenagers, a high proportion were primiparous and came predominantly from the socio-economic groups 3M, 4 and 5. The Short Report (Social Services Committee, 1980) recognized that it was these women who were at greater risk of perinatal mortality and who should therefore be identified early in pregnancy as being 'high risk'. Care should then be targeted very specifically to these women. However, there did not appear to be an indication in the records that these women were potentially at high obstetric risk, neither did there appear to be any particular targeting of services. This targeting could have taken the form of provision of antenatal education, support from community midwives such as that described in chapter 5, or an attempt to discover if those who were unsupported financially were claiming all the Social Security benefits to which they were entitled.

The third report from the Social Services Committee (1984) on perinatal and neonatal mortality made particular comment on the high perinatal mortality and morbidity of babies born to women who were not themselves born in this country. They stated that there is a need to ensure better antenatal care delivery to these women and it is, therefore, a cause for concern that there was no indication in the records of the women in this study of their country of birth. The crude attempt made to assess the ethnic origin suggested that up to 20% of these women might have come into this potentially high risk category.

Antenatal attendance and care

The records were examined for information about the following aspects of antenatal care: gestational age at booking, number of clinic visits, the rate of defaulting, continuity of carer, detection of complications and referral back to the obstetrician.

Gestation at booking. 'Booking' was taken to be the first date of attendance at the hospital antenatal clinic when the women would have seen the obstetrician. It was not possible to assess from the medical records the gestational age at booking of two women. The range of gestational ages at booking of the other 140 women was from 8 to 35 weeks. These are shown in Table 6.4 grouped into the three trimesters of pregnancy. Advocates of antenatal care recommend that it should start as early as possible and definitely within the first trimester of pregnancy (McClure Brown and Dixon, 1978). It is a cause for concern therefore that 40% of these women

Table 6.4 Attendance for antenatal care

a) Trimester of pregnancy at first visit	No.	%
1st	83	59
2nd	51	36
3rd	6	4
Total	140*	100
b) Number of visits to antenatal clinic		
1 and 2	–	
3 and 4	3	2
5–9	42	30
10–14	90	64
15+	6	4
Total	141†	100
c) Number of appointments missed		
None	85	60
1	27	19
2	14	10
3	7	5
4	3	2
5	3	2
6	2	1
8	1	1
Total	142	100

* It was not possible to assess the gestation at booking of two women.
† Data on one set of records not collected.
Source: Compiled by the author.

had not attended the clinic for the first time before the end of the fourteenth week of pregnancy. It was not possible in the retrospective analysis of the records to determine why so many women had attended for their first visit to the hospital at such a late time in pregnancy.

Referral to the teaching midwives clinic. Ninety one per cent (127) of the women had been referred to the TMC by the obstetrician. In six sets of records there were statements such as 'wants to go to midwives' clinics'. These women were deemed to have referred themselves. In seven sets of records no note had been made of the referral.

Number of clinic visits. The women made between 3 and 17 visits to the antenatal clinic with a mean of 10.3 (Table 6.4). This is comparable with the findings of other studies (Reid, Gutteridge and McIlwaine, 1983; Flint and Poulengeris, 1987 and Chapter 4 in this volume); although very much more than considered necessary by Hall, Chng and MacGillivray (1980) on the basis of their study of the provision of antenatal care.

Obstetricians claim that one of the limitations placed on antenatal care is that women do not attend for care (Butler and Bonham, 1963). In order to assess whether the women attended for their appointments, the number of times DNA (did not attend) was written in the records was counted. As shown in Table 6.4, 60% (85) of the women did not have DNA written in their records. It would seem reasonable that a woman might miss one appointment during her pregnancy so for the purpose of this study a woman with an unacceptable level of defaulting was defined as a woman who had DNA written on her records two or more times. A total of 21% (30) of these women had DNA recorded on two or more occasions. Reid, Gutteridge and McIlwaine (1983) found that 9% of those attending the antenatal clinic at Glasgow Royal Maternity Hospital and 14% of those attending the Easter-house clinic missed two or more visits. The defaulting rate in Sighthill has fallen from 16% to 1% since the new antenatal care scheme was instituted (McKee, 1984). However, McKee (1984) does not give a definition of a 'defaulter'. In the Newcastle Community Midwifery project Evans (1987 and Chapter 5) found that 15% of women missed one or two antenatal appointments and 7% missed three or more. It would appear that the women attending this clinic had a higher defaulters rate.

The defaulters. The characteristics of the defaulting and non-defaulting women are shown in Table 6.5. There was a statistically significant difference between the women in the two groups in terms of the numbers who described themselves as housewives and the numbers who were multiparous. Ninety per cent of the defaulters but only 48% of the non-defaulters were housewives ($p < 0.0002$). Seventy-three per cent of the defaulters but only 45% of the non-defaulters were multiparous ($p < 0.01$). It is possible that women who already have one baby have ceased wage-earning employment and that these two factors are linked. There may be several explanations for the high proportion of multiparous women in the defaulting group. It could be that these women felt they were the 'competent childbearers' identified by Parsons and Perkins (1980), i.e. because they had already had a successful outcome to at least one pregnancy they felt less need to attend for antenatal care. It is also possible that these women did not have care

Table 6.5 Characteristics of defaulters compared with those of non-defaulters

Characteristics	Defaulters (n = 30)	Non-defaulters (n = 112)
Mean age in years	23.4	23.5
Married at booking	22 (73%)	73 (65%) NS
Married at delivery	23 (77%)	80 (71%) NS
Housewives	27 (90%)	54 (48%)
	$x^2 = 15.1$, 1df, $p < 0.0002$	
Partner unemployed	8 (27%)	18 (16%) NS
Asian name	9 (30%)	20 (18%) NS
Multiparous	22 (73%)	50 (45%)
	$x^2 = 6.687$, 1df, $p < 0.01$	
Booked within 1st trimester	14 (47%)	69 (62%) NS
Mean no. antenatal visits	9.2	10.6
Range of antenatal visits	4–13	3–17
Referral back to obstetrician	14 (47%)	60 (54%) NS

Source: Compiled by the author.

facilities for existing children and that to bring them to the hospital on public transport was too difficult. There was no statistical difference between mean age, proportion married at booking and at delivery, the proportion who had an unemployed partner, those born outside the UK and the number who booked for antenatal care in the first trimester of pregnancy. Although the defaulters had missed at least two appointments there was very little difference in the mean number of visits attended by the two groups of women; the defaulters having a mean of 9.2 visits and the non-defaulters having a mean of 10.6..

Continuity of care. Continuity was assessed by counting the number of different types of writing and the number of signatures on the antenatal record. However, the number of different types of writing in the first two columns made it impossible to distinguish between and count them separately. In the section recording blood pressure, period of gestation etc. the number of different signatures ranged between 3 and 10 with a mean of 5.3 (Table 6.6) These figures are a little worse than those for women in the experimental group of the only other known study (Flint and Poulengeris, 1987 and Chapter 4 in this volume) of antenatal care provided by midwives (not Teaching Midwives) which examined this aspect of the provision of care.

Table 6.6 Number of signatures on antenatal record

No. of signatures	Women	
	No.	%
3	8	6
4	29	20
5	54	38
6	31	22
7	11	8
8	8	6
9	–	–
10	1	1
	142	100

Source: Compiled by the author.

The figures are comparable with those of the obstetrician-provided care at Glasgow Royal Maternity Hospital (Reid, Gutteridge and McIlwaine, 1983) a little worse than those in Aberdeen (Hall and Chng, 1982) and do not compare favourably with those of the Easterhouse Clinic where 53% saw one or two doctors and 45% saw three or four (Reid, Gutteridge and McIlwaine, 1983).

Complications during pregnancy. Only 12% (17) of the women in this study did not have a complication noted in their records during this pregnancy. Of those who did have a complication, 'inadequate weight gain' and 'oedema' were the two noted most frequently (Table 6.7). Apart from investigations ordered, treatment for the various complications was not recorded.

Referral back to the obstetrician. Flint (Chapter 4) reports that all women in the KYM group in her study had to routinely see an obstetrician at 36 weeks gestation as well as whenever the midwife thought it necessary in pregnancy. There was no such ruling for the women in this study who attended the TMC; after the visit to the booking clinic they only saw the obstetrician if the midwife thought this necessary. Fifty-five per cent (78) of the women were in fact referred back to the obstetrician at some stage during pregnancy. Unfortunately this high referral rate was not identified during the pilot stage of the study. As it was not recognized initially as a problem the data collection proforma did not accommodate the collection of

Table 6.7 Antenatal complications noted in records

Antenatal complications	*(n = 142)*	
	No.	*%*
Inadequate weight gain	40	28
Oedema	35	25
Raised B/P	29	20
Vaginal discharge	19	13
Suspected IUGR	19	13
Malpresentation or position	16	11
Proteinuria	16	11
Excessive weight gain	13	9
Glycosuria	10	7
Urinary tract infection	9	6
Unsure of dates	5	4
Nausea	5	4
Anaemia	4	3
Large for dates	3	2
Polyhydramnios	2	1
Accidental APH	1	1
Incidental APH	1	1
Nausea and vomiting	1	1
Dysuria	1	1
Reduced fetal movements	1	1

Source: Compiled by the author.

information about the referral and inadequate information was extracted from the records. In particular the period of gestation at which the referral occurred, the reason for the referral and the outcome of the referral are not available. However it is possible to compare the group of women who were referred with those who were not in terms of social and demographic details, information about attendance for care and aspects of the care received (Table 6.8).

The referred women did not differ in terms of mean age and social class from those women who were not referred back. The two groups were also similar in relation to gestational age at booking and although 56% (44) of the women in the group referred back to the obstetrician were primiparae compared with 41% (26) in the non-referred group this difference was not statistically significant. However there was a statistically significant difference between the number who were single in the two groups both at booking

Table 6.8 Women referred back to the obstetrician: characteristics compared with those women not referred back

Characteristics	Referred back to obstetrician (n = 78)	Not referred back to obstetrician (n = 64)
Mean age in years	23.3	24.1
Single at booking	25 (32%)	5 (8%)
	$x^2 = 10.983$, 1df, $p < 0.001$	
Single at delivery	18 (23%)	3 (5%)
	$x^2 = 8.03112$, 1df, $p < 0.005$	
Housewives	44 (56%)	37 (58%) NS
Partner unemployed	15 (19%)	11 (17%) NS
Primiparous	44 (56%)	26 (41%) NS
Booked within 1st trimester	48 (62%)	31 (48%) NS

Source: Compiled by the author.

and at delivery. Thirty-two per cent (25) of the referred women compared with 8% (5) of the non-referred women were single at booking ($p < 0.002$), similarly 23% (18) of the referred and 5% (3) of the non-referred were single at delivery ($p < 0.005$). There was no difference between the groups in the number of health professionals seen during pregnancy (Table 6.9). In both groups, inadequate weight gain was the complication noted most frequently in pregnancy, but whereas the second most frequently occurring complication among women referred back to the obstetrician was raised blood pressure (18 women (23%)); the corresponding item for the non-referred group was oedema (18 women (28%)).

Table 6.9 Cross-tabulation of whether referred back to the obstetrician by number of health professionals' signatures on the antenatal record

	Number of health professionals' signatures							
	3	4	5	6	7	8	10	Total
Referred to obstetrician	2	13	30	21	6	5	1	78
Not referred to obstetrician	6	16	24	10	5	3	–	64

Source: Compiled by the author.

The Social Services Committee (1980) recognized that those who were unsupported were at high obstetric risk, and it is therefore not surprising that the group of women referred back to the obstetrician contained a statistically significantly higher number of single women than did the group which had midwife care only. As women having their first baby are also at greater obstetric risk, the higher, though not statistically significant, number of primiparae in the referred group could be expected.

Labour, delivery and the puerperium

The women who had received care from the Midwife Teachers during pregnancy were cared for by hospital midwives during labour and the hospital postnatal period. No attempt was made to provide care by the Midwife Teachers beyond the antenatal period. However if one of the women who had attended the TMC was in part of the Maternity Unit (e.g. one of the postnatal wards) when one of the Midwife Teachers was supervising the clinical experience of a student midwife, then the teacher might provide care if appropriate.

Seventy-two per cent (102) of these women went into labour spontaneously. The labours of 9% (13) were augmented and 18% (25) women had their labour induced. As 78 women had been referred back to the obstetrician, a decision for induction of labour had obviously not been the reason for referral for the greater proportion of the referred women. Information on gestation at delivery was obtained from the labour and delivery summary sheet; it was not calculated from the information on the antenatal care sheets. Eighty-seven per cent (124) of the women were noted to be between 37 and 42 weeks gestation when labour commenced, and 9% (13) were noted to have a gestation of less than 37 weeks. It was not possible to assess, from the labour records, the gestation at delivery of five of the women. As could be expected from a group of women in which 75% did not appear to be at high obstetric risk 79% of the total sample had a normal vaginal delivery, 7% (10) women were delivered by a simple forceps delivery and 3% (4) by rotational forceps. One woman had an elective caesarean section, 8% (11) women had an emergency caesarean section and three had a vaginal breech delivery.

Just over two-thirds (68%) of the women were not noted to have experienced a postnatal complication. The complications experienced by the other 54 are shown in Table 6.10. However, the validity of the data from the postnatal period has to be questioned on two points. First, 53% (69/130) of the women had an episiotomy, a second-degree or a third-degree tear, and yet only one woman is noted to have a 'sore perineum'. This seems strange especially as the women in Logue's study (Chapter 9) reported that this type of trauma was painful. Secondly, while searching through one set of records a letter from the physiotherapist to the obstetrician was found. The letter

Table 6.10 Postnatal complications noted in records

Postnatal complication	(n = 142)	
	No.	%
Pyrexia	16	11
Engorged breasts	10	7
Sore nipples	9	6
Anaemia	6	4
Infected lochia	3	2
Haemorrhoids	2	1
Postpartum haemorrhage	2	1
Subinvolution of uterus	1	1
Urinary tract infection	1	1
Relaxed uterus	1	1
Dysuria	1	1
Sore perineum	1	1

Source: Compiled by the author.

was referring the woman back to the obstetrician and stated that the physiotherapist's treatment had done nothing to alleviate the woman's urinary incontinence. There was no note in the medical records or the Kardex that this woman had urinary incontinence. It was obvious that there was an under-recording of information on perineal pain and one woman's incontinence. It is not know if other relevant information was omitted from the records.

Of the recorded complications experienced by the women during the postnatal period the only ones which might have been influenced by antenatal care were the ones relating to engorged breasts and sore nipples. Antenatal teaching on these two problems might have prevented their occurrence, but there was no information in the records as to whether or not such teaching had been given.

The babies

There were 72 boys and 70 girls born to the women who attended the TMC for antenatal care during 1982. One baby was stillborn.

Gestational age at delivery. Gestational assessment by a paediatrician was only noted in three sets of records. However, gestational length was recorded by the midwife admitting the woman in labour in 137 sets of labour records. Thirteen labours were reported to be ending before the thirty-seventh week of gestation, one each at 28, 32 and 35 weeks, and the remaining 10 at 36 weeks gestation. This latter data did not always appear to coincide with the antenatal records but unfortunately this was not detected during the pilot work and the proforma had not been altered to accommodate this difference.

Perinatal complications. Sixty per cent (85) of the babies had no noted perinatal complications, but 53 of the 141 babies born alive had been discharged home on the second day after birth and the Community Midwife's records were not available for this study. Thirty-six babies who had not been admitted to the SCBU were noted to have had the perinatal problems shown in Table 6.11. Jaundice not requiring phototherapy was the most frequently recorded perinatal problem. The only complications which some authorities claim are amenable to good antenatal care were prematurity and 'small for dates' (Butler and Bonham, 1963).

Intra-uterine growth retardation. Using the charts produced by Milner and Richards (1974) twelve (8.5%) of the babies had a birth weight

Table 6.11 Noted perinatal complications of babies not admitted to the SCBU

Perinatal problems	(n = 36) No. of babies
Jaundice	18
Jaundice requiring phototherapy	5
Sticky eyes	3
Spots	2
Vomiting	2
Bowels not open	2
Talipes	2
Prematurity	1
Small for dates	1
Cephalhaematoma	1
Sutures and fontanelles wide	1
Undescended testicle	1
Cardiac murmur	1
Hydrocoele	1

NB, some babies had more than one noted perinatal complication
Source: Compiled by the author.

which was below the 10th centile for gestational age. The numbers in this study are small but an intra-uterine growth retardation (IUGR) rate of 8.5% is higher than the IUGR rate at the Sighthill clinic where it was 6.9% (McKee, 1984). Only four of these IUGR babies had been suspected antenatally, and yet 19 (13%) women had been suspected of having an IUGR fetus during the antenatal period (Table 6.7). Hall, Chng and MacGillivray (1980) noted a similar under- and over-diagnosis of intra-uterine growth retardation when antenatal care was provided by obstetricians. However the antenatal detection rate of 33% in this study is lower than the antenatal detection rate (44%) by obstetricians in Aberdeen (Hall, Chng and MacGillivray, 1980). The over-diagnosis of 15 in this study gives a false positive rate of 3.75, very much higher than the rate of 2.5 found by Hall, Chng and MacGillivray (1980).

As already stated the number of babies born in this study with a birth weight below the 10th centile for gestational age is small, and the data should therefore be treated with caution. However, a profile of the mothers of these babies born small for gestational age is given in Table 6.12 and is compared with the rest of the women in the sample. The two groups were similar in terms of maternal age and marital and occupational status. Equal numbers appeared to be Asian as indicated by the name on their records. Women who delivered an IUGR baby had attended the clinic as frequently as those women whose baby's birth weight was within normal limits, but they

Table 6.12 Comparison of women who delivered an IUGR baby with women who did not

Characteristics	Women who delivered IUGR baby (n = 12)	Women who did not deliver IUGR baby (n = 130)
Mean age in years	22.3	23.5
Married	7 (58%)	88 (68%)
Housewives	6 (50%)	75 (58%)
Partner unemployed	1 (8%)	25 (19%)
Asian name	3 (25%)	26 (20%)
Primiparous	6 (50%)	64 (49%)
Booked within 1st trimester	5 (42%)	78 (60%)
Mean no. antenatal visits	8.9	9.7
No. who were defaulters	2 (17%)	28 (22%)

Source: Compiled by the author.

were less likely to have booked for care within the first trimester of pregnancy, although this difference was not statistically significant. The number of health professionals seen by these women was less than for those who did not deliver an IUGR baby (Table 6.13). Two women who had delivered an IUGR baby had no noted antenatal complication and this included one woman who had been referred back to the obstetrician. The complications experienced by the remaining 10 women that were noted in their records are listed in Table 6.14. As can be seen suspected IUGR and vaginal discharge were the most frequently reported complications. Although only four of these women who delivered an IUGR baby were suspected to have an IUGR fetus, eight of the 12 had been referred back to the obstetrician during the antenatal period. The gestation at delivery of these babies, as assessed from the labour records, ranged between 37 and 42 weeks. Hall, Chng and MacGillivray (1980) noted that a small-for-gestational-age fetus should be delivered in a maternity unit which had adequate obstetric and paediatric facilities should they be required.

It is of interest that there were relatively few complications in labour, at delivery and in the postnatal period in this group of babies. Seven of the labours were spontaneous in onset, two were accelerated and three were induced. Ten of the deliveries were normal, one was a vaginal breech delivery and the remaining baby was delivered by caesarean section. There were six boys and six girls. None of these IUGR babies was admitted to

Table 6.13 Number of health professionals seen by women who delivered an IUGR baby compared with those whose baby was the correct weight for gestational age

No. of health professionals	Women who delivered IUGR baby	Women who delivered a 'normal weight' baby
3	–	8
4	6	23
5	5	49
6	1	30
7	–	11
8	–	8
10	–	1
Total	12	130

Source: Compiled by the author.

Table 6.14 Recorded antenatal complications of women who delivered an IUGR baby

Complication	(n = 10) No. of women
Vaginal discharge	4
Suspected IUGR	4
Proteinuria	3
Oedema	2
Malpresentation/position	2
Urinary tract infection	1
Inadequate weight gain	1
Blood pressure raised	1
Nausea	1

n = 10

Source: Compiled by the author.

SCBU. Eight of the babies had no noted perinatal problem. Of the remaining four babies, two had jaundice, one had jaundice requiring phototherapy, one was noted to be 'small for dates', one was noted to be 'preterm' and one had sticky eyes.

Baby feeding. Although it has been shown that the decision on how a baby will be fed has usually been made before a pregnant woman comes into contact with a midwife (Thomson, 1989) it is recognized within the midwifery profession that antenatal teaching about breast feeding contributes to its success (Towler and Butler-Manuel, 1973; Myles, 1981; Helsing and Savage King, 1982; Fisher, 1989). As the purpose of the TMC was to demonstrate midwife-provided antenatal care to student midwives it could be presumed that in providing an example to the students the Midwife Teachers would discuss baby feeding with the women. There was no information in the antenatal records on teaching about any aspect of child care let alone baby feeding although this does not necessarily mean that it was not given.

In order to discover the rates of breast and bottle feeding the mothers' records and Kardex and the babies' records and Kardex were examined for this information. Forty-two per cent of the babies were breast fed on discharge from hospital. This is lower than the national rate of 51% for 1975 (Martin, 1978) and the national rate of 67% in 1980 (Martin and Monk, 1982). However Martin (1978) and Martin and Monk (1982) defined their incidence of breast feeding as 'the proportion of babies put to the breast at all, even if this had been on one occasion only'. In this study 53% (75) of babies had been put to the breast on at least one occasion, comparing favourably with the national rate for 1975 but not so favourably with the national rate for 1980. However, Martin (1978) and Martin and Monk (1982) showed that breast-feeding rates were lower in the north of England when compared with the south. In 1975 the breast feeding rate in the north was 41% and in 1980 it was 59% whereas in London and the South East the rates were 62% and 76% respectively (Martin, 1978; Martin and Monk, 1982). A prospective study of baby feeding practices in Newcastle upon Tyne in the period 1978–80 (Hally *et al.* 1981) found that 58% of all women began to breast feed their baby, but that only 45% were wholly or partially breast feeding on discharge from hospital. The study reported in this chapter was undertaken in the north of England and relates to all women who had attended the TMC in 1982. Although the breast-feeding rate compares favourably with the rate for the north for 1975, it would appear that there is still room for improvement when compared with the findings of Hally *et al.*, (1981) and the breast-feeding rate for the north in 1980 (Martin and Monk, 1982). The DHSS (1974) recommend that all women should be encouraged to breast feed their baby for a minimum of two weeks and preferably for 3 to 4 months. The proportion breast feeding in this sample is not surprising considering that the study was undertaken in the north of England and considering the high proportion of women who were in the lower socio-economic groups. The proportion of women giving up breast feeding gives cause for concern and it is hoped that the Breast Feeding Initiative which was launched in the UK in 1988 will give health professionals information on how to assist women to succeed with breast feeding.

Admission to SCBU. Within the midwifery and obstetric professions it is recognized that the aim of antenatal care is to produce a live, healthy mother and baby. For this to happen the baby must be born at term and not require any medical care in the first weeks of life, the baby should not need to go to the SCBU. It is recognized that one of the primary reasons for admission to a SCBU is prematurity although the major underlying cause is poor socio-economic status (OPCS, 1987). The prevention of premature delivery has been the concern of obstetricians for some time, but unfortunately they have had very little success in reducing the incidence. However, in two studies (McKee, 1984; Evans, 1987 and Chapter 5) women who were given a different style of midwifery provided antenatal care in the community had a lower incidence of preterm delivery.

The records of the babies born to women who had attended the TMC were examined to discover the number of admissions to SCBU, the reasons for the admissions and the length of time in days spent in a SCBU. Fourteen per cent (20) of the 141 babies born alive were admitted to the SCBU for a period ranging from 1–67 days. The reasons for admission as noted in the records and the number of days that the babies stayed in the SCBU are shown in Table 6.15. Although 9% of the babies born alive were born preterm, 'prematurity' as a reason for admission to the SCBU was only recorded in four sets of records. In this study, as in those of McKee (1984) and Evans (1987 and Chapter 5), the numbers are small and so comparisons have to be made with caution. However, in both the McKee (1984) and Evans (1987) studies the incidence of prematurity was 6%, somewhat lower than in this study. Seven of the babies spent over one week in either a medical or surgical special care unit. Seven of the babies admitted to the SCBU did not appear to have a medical reason for admission.

The stillborn baby. This baby was born to a woman who had been a poor attender at the antenatal clinic in the pregnancy under study and in previous pregnancies. The midwives suspected IUGR, and when the woman

Table 6.15 Reasons for admission to special care baby unit

No. of babies	Reason for admission	No. of days
2	? for adoption — no complications	3
5	Post caesarean section — no complications	1
1	Vomiting and pyrexia	2
1	Hypothermia	2
1	Meconium aspiration	1
1	Bruising from delivery	1
1	Grunting respirations	1
1	Abdominal pathology → regional SU	1
1	Laparotomy and ileostomy ×2	54
1	Prematurity (28/52), RDS' apnoea	67
1	Hirschprungs disease → regional SU colostomy	18
1	Prematurity (35/52)	26
1	Prematurity (35/52), ? neurological problems	26
1	Apnoea RDS → regional SCBU	48
1	Hypothermia, subcostal recession	8

RDS = respiratory distress syndrome
SCBU = special care baby unit
SU = surgical unit
Source: Compiled by the author.

was seen at 38 weeks gestation were of the opinion that the fetus was of a size compatible with a 34 week gestation. The woman was admitted to the antenatal ward immediately where she was seen by the obstetrician the next day. It was noted in the records that the woman was 'four weeks out on her dates' and she was discharged home to return to the clinic in one week's time. She did not, and was next seen two and a half weeks later when she appeared in labour with a fetal death *in utero*. The baby's birthweight was just above the 10th centile for 38 weeks gestation (the gestation recorded on the labour record) but was below the 10th centile for 40 weeks gestation (the gestation as assessed by the midwives in the TMC). There was no clinical or post mortem assessment of the gestational age of the baby at delivery. During the data collection period for this study this woman was again pregnant. She was receiving her antenatal care from the obstetrician 'because of the previous stillbirth'.

DISCUSSION

In this section the findings from this study are considered in relationship to the following issues:

1. Availability, validity and reliability of the data;
2. The style of antenatal care at the Teaching Midwives' Clinic;
3. Continuity of care;
4. Detection of intra-uterine growth retardation;
5. Evaluation of care.

Availability, validity and reliability of the data

In carrying out this research it was hoped to study the antenatal care provided by midwives to a group of women experiencing a normal pregnancy and to compare this with antenatal care received by women attending a community midwives' clinic and an obstetrician's clinic. To obtain the data medical records were examined because it had been suggested that this was a source of data which was always available and which did not change over time (Hockey, personal communication). However, as was shown in this study, the data are not always available. Murray and Topley (1974), Lovell *et al.* (1986) and Elbourne *et al.* (1987) have demonstrated that it is practical and feasible for a woman to retain her own records during pregnancy. It was very obvious during the data collection period for this study that the records clerks were spending a lot of time 'pulling' and replacing records and searching for missing records. However, Murray and Topley (1974) and Elbourne *et al.* (1987) found that when the women carried their own antenatal records there was considerable saving of records clerks' time. In this study 24% of the records could not be found, but in Murray and Topley's (1974) study only one set of records was lost during 10000 pregnancies. In the randomized controlled trial carried out by Lovell *et al.* (1986) of 'record carrying' versus the standard hospital practice of giving the woman a co-operation card and retaining the records in the hospital, none of the record-carrying women ever lost her records whereas 26% of the women in the control group reported that their records had been lost or mislaid at some time during their pregnancy. Bryant (personal communication) stated that in her 13 years experience in providing health care in Pakistan not one woman failed to attend the hospital with her antenatal records. Work in developing countries has demonstrated that women are perfectly capable of looking after their child's 'Road to Health' chart. It is suggested that retention of records during pregnancy may have allowed the medical record clerks to concentrate their efforts on maintaining the stack of old records in a more satisfactory manner. Because of the difficulties in obtaining the data the comparison with the outcomes of care provided by community midwives and obstetricians was not pursued.

Validity and reliability of data have to be considered in any study. As Bulmer and Atkinson (1979) pointed out, when a secondary source is used as a data set the original reasons for collecting the data were not designed to meet the needs of a particular research question. In this case the data were collected to satisfy medico-legal requirements, not to answer the author's question. This study demonstrated that a large number of health professionals contributed to part of the antenatal records of the women (Table 6.6). It was not possible to ascertain the number of people who had been involved in contributing to the antenatal records with respect to information on weight and urinalysis because of the large number of different signatures. It was obvious that many more contributed to the labour, delivery, postnatal, and paediatric records. It was not possible in this study to assess if those contributing to the records measured and recorded in a standard way. As in the study by Cartwright, Jacoby and Martin (1987) there were many occasions in which data were missing from relevant summary sheets and had to be searched for from the rest of the record. Cartwright, Jacoby and Martin (1987) and Oakley (personal communication) have both shown that health professionals can be inaccurate in recording facts in medical records and Cartwright, Jacoby and Martin (1987) state that 'Statistics based on extractions from hospital records will therefore tend to underestimate the frequency with which complications occur and procedures are carried out'. As already indicated doubt was raised as to the validity of the findings on the gestational age at delivery and in the postnatal records, it is possible that there were further undetected inaccuracies and omissions in the records studied in this research.

Cartwright, Jacoby and Martin (1987) describe the extraction of the information from records as a 'difficult and tedious job'. In coding and transferring data from the records to the proforma the author could have affected the validity and reliability of the data. Due to time and financial constraints it was not possible to have the data collection checked by a second person. However, ten sets of records were inadvertently coded twice, and no discrepancies were found between the two sets of coding.

Style of antenatal care at the Teaching Midwives' clinic

The aim of the TMC was to give student midwives experience of observing normal antenatal care provided by midwives, albeit Midwife Teachers. The women who were originally referred to this clinic came predominantly from the lower socio-economic groups, a relatively large proportion were primiparae, up to 20% may not have been born in this country, and 19% were teenagers. It has been recognized that women in these groups have an increased incidence of perinatal mortality and the Social Services Committee (1980, 1984) recommended that such women be referred to obstetricians. Midwives are qualified to provide antenatal care to women at low obstetric risk, but it could also be argued that they should provide care to those at high obstetric risk in greater collaboration with the obstetrician than, for example, occurred in this study. In view of the proportion of women in this group at high obstetric risk the 55% referral rate back to the obstetrician is not surprising. However, what effect did this high referral rate have on the student midwives' experience of observing normal antenatal care? Perhaps the student midwives' education would have been more satisfactory if the women had been 'booked' by midwives, their subsequent antenatal care provided by midwives and the women referred to the obstetrician only if they were at high obstetric risk or if there was a problem. Then the student midwife would have seen midwives fulfilling their role as outlined in the WHO (1966) definition of a midwife.

Continuity of care

Although the Teaching Midwives thought they were able to provide greater continuity of care this was not borne out by the findings of the study. Only 26% of women saw four or less care givers during pregnancy (Table 6.6). In reporting the findings the author describing the Sighthill project did not discuss the issue of continuity of care (McKee, 1984). However Reid, Gutteridge and McIlwaine (1983) demonstrated that 47% of those attending the Glasgow Royal Maternity hospital for antenatal care saw four or less care givers whereas 99% of women attending the community clinic in Easterhouse saw up to four obstetricians. In the Know Your Midwife Scheme (Chapter 4) even in the group provided antenatal care by a team of midwives only 10% saw five or fewer care givers. It would appear that antenatal care provided in a hospital clinic means that a large number of people will be involved in providing the care, whereas community clinics appear to provide greater continuity of care.

Detection of intra-uterine growth retardation

There were high under- and over-detection rates of IUGR in this study. Although the numbers in the study were small the detection rates found here were poorer than those in Aberdeen (Hall, Chng and MacGillivray, 1980). One of the reasons for this could have been the clinical method used to assess fetal growth. There was no indication in the records that an attempt at an objective measurement of fundal height was used. It appeared that the midwives were assessing fundal height in relation to abdominal landmarks. Crosby and Engstrom (1989) have shown that there is great variation in fundal height measurements between clinicians when using calipers and tape measures. They state that 'inter-examiner reliability of fundal height measurements is low when multiple examiners are compared'. In this study only 26% of women saw up to four care givers in pregnancy. It is possible that the absence of continuity of care was also a major contribution to the over- and under-diagnosis of IUGR. Crosby and Engstrom (1989) suggest there is a need for specific protocols on the recording of fundal heights when multiple examiners are involved. It would surely be more sensible to provide continuity of carer in the first instance so that inter-examiner differences are abolished.

Evaluation of care

Since this study was begun there have been at least two published reports (Callis, 1983; Stuart and Judge, 1984) and several personal communications of the setting up of antenatal clinics in which midwives provide the care. However, none of these changes in practice have included an evaluation of the process and outcome of the care. One evaluation of midwife-provided antenatal care has been undertaken (Flint and Poulengeris, 1987, and Chapter 4) but this was part of a total package of care provided by a team of midwives throughout the childbirth continuum. Callis (1983) and Stuart and Judge (1984) suggest that midwife-provided antenatal care for the woman with a low-risk pregnancy is better than antenatal care provided by obstetricians. The Maternity Services Advisory Committee (1982) state that a failure to utilise the skills of the midwife in the provision of antenatal care will ultimately lead to a poorer service for pregnant women. There has been no evidence so far that midwife-provided antenatal care is worse than that provided by obstetricians although there is evidence that women prefer care provided by midwives. (Flint and Poulengeris, 1987, and Chapter 4). There is a continuing need for documentation and evaluation of the different types of midwife-provided antenatal care if the standard of care provided to child-bearing women is to be improved.

ACKNOWLEDGEMENTS

I wish to thank the Division of Obstetrics at the hospital in which this study was undertaken for their permission to carry out the study. Colin Ashcroft has my grateful thanks for his computational advice and assistance. I am very grateful to Sarah Robinson for her advice on earlier drafts of this chapter.

REFERENCES

Armand-Smith, N.G. (1980) Perinatal health in the Lothians. *Edinburgh Medicine*, March, pp. 10–11.

Barnett, Z.H. (1979) The changing pattern of maternity care and the future role of the midwife. *Midwives Chronicle and Nursing Notes*, **92**(1102), 381–4.

Boyd, C., Sellars, L. (1982) *The British way of birth.* Pan Books, London.

Brain, M. (1979) Observations by a midwife, in *Report of a day conference on the reduction of perinatal mortality and morbidity*, organized by the children's committee and the Department of Health and Social Security, HMSO, London.

Bulmer, M. and Atkinson, P. (1979) The use of secondary sources. *Beginning research*, Research Methods in Education and the Social Sciences, DE304, Block 2, Part 2, Open University, Milton Keynes.

Butler, N.R. and Bonham, D.G. (1963) *Perinatal mortality, the first report of the British perinatal mortality survey.* E. & S. Livingstone, Edinburgh.

Callis, P. (1983) Midwives' clinics. *Midwives Chronicle and Nursing Notes*, **96**(1150), Supplement 2–4.

Campbell, R. and Macfarlane, A. (1987) *Where to be born. The debate and the evidence.* National Perinatal Epidemiology Unit, Oxford.

Cartwright, A., Jacoby, A., Martin, C. (1987) Problems extracting data from hospital maternity records. *Community Medicine* **9**(3), 286–93.

Central Midwives Board (1917) *Report of the work of the Central Midwives Board for the year ended March 31st, 1917.* CMB, London.

Central Midwives Board for Scotland, Northern Ireland Council for Nurses and Midwives, An Bord Altranais, Central Midwives Board (1983) *The role of the midwife.* Hymns Ancient and Modern, Norwich.

Chamberlain, G. and Cave, S. (1977) Antenatal education. *Community Health* **9**(1), 11–16.

Chng, P.K., Hall, M.H., MacGillivray, I. (1980) An audit of antenatal care: the value of the first antenatal visit. *British Medical Journal*, **281**, 1184–6.

Cochrane, A.L. (1972) *Effectiveness and efficiency, random reflections on health services.* The Nuffield Provincial Hospitals Trust, London.

Cowell, B. and Wainwright, D. (1981) *Behind the blue door. The history of the Royal College of Midwives, 1881–1981.* Balliere Tindall, London.

Crosby, M.E. and Engstrom, J.L. (1989) Inter-examiner reliability in fundal height measurement. *Midwives Chronicle and Nursing Notes*, **102**(1219), 254–6.

Department of Health and Social Security (1970) *Domiciliary midwifery and maternity bed needs, Report of the sub-committee (Peel Report).* HMSO, London.

Department of Health and Social Security (1974) *Present day practice in infant feeding (Oppe Report).* HMSO, London.

Department of Health and Social Security (1989) *Report on confidential enquiries into maternal deaths in England and Wales 1982–84.* HMSO, London.

Elbourne, D., Richardson, M., Chalmers, I., Waterhouse, I., Holt, E. (1987) The Newbury Maternity Care Study: a randomized controlled trial to assess a policy of women holding their own obstetric records. *British Journal of Obstetrics and Gynaecology,* **94**, 612–19.

Evans, F. (1987) *The Newcastle community midwifery care project: an evaluation report.* Newcastle Health Authority Community Health Unit, Newcastle General Hospital, Westgate Road, Newcastle upon Tyne, NE4 6BE.

Fisher, C. (1989) Feeding. In Bennett, V.R. and Brown, L.K. (eds) *Myles textbook for midwives.* Churchill Livingstone, Edinburgh.

Fleury, P.M. (1967) *Maternity care, mother's experiences of childbirth.* George Allen & Unwin Ltd., London.

Flint, C. (1979) A continuing labour of love. *Nursing Mirror,* **149**(20), 16–18.

Flint, C. (1982a) Make it worth the wait. *Nursing Mirror,* **155**(23), 15–16.

Flint, C. (1982b) Continuity of care. *Nursing Mirror,* **155**(25), 67.

Flint, C. and Poulengeris, P. (1987) *The 'Know Your Midwife' report.* 49, Peckarmans Wood, Sydenham Hill, London, SE26 6RZ.

Garcia, G. (1982) Women's views of antenatal care. In Enkin, M. and Chalmers, I. (eds) *Effectiveness and satisfaction in antenatal care.* Spastics International Medical Publications and William Heinemann Medical Books Ltd, London.

Graham, H. and McKee, L. (1980) *The first months of motherhood: No. 3 summary report of a survey of women's experiences of pregnancy, childbirth and the first six months after birth.* Health Education Council, London.

Hall, M. (1984) Are our accepted practices based on valid assumptions? in Zander, L. and Chamberlain, G. (eds) *Pregnancy care for the 1980's.* Royal Society of Medicine and Macmillan Press, London.

Hall, M.H., Chng, N.G., MacGillivray, I. (1980) Is routine antenatal care worthwhile? *Lancet* **12**(7), 78–80.

Hall, M.H. and Chng, P.K. (1982) Antenatal care in practice. In Enkin, M. and Chalmers, I. (eds) *Effectiveness and satisfaction in antenatal care.* Spastics International Medical Publications, London.

Hall, M., Macintyre, S., Porter, M. (1985) *Antenatal care assessed.* University Press, Aberdeen.

Hally, M.R., Bond, J., Brown, E., Crawley, J., Gregson, B.A., Philips, P., Russell, I. (1981) *A study of infant feeding: factors influencing choice of method.* Health Care Research Unit, University of Newcastle upon Tyne.

Helsing, E., and Savage King, F. (1982) *Breast-feeding in practice, a manual for health workers.* Oxford University Press, Oxford.

Hogg, C. and Hague, J. (1980) *May be I didn't ask.* Kensington, Chelsea and Westminster (South) Community Health Council, London.

Kaliszer, M. and Kidd, M. (1981) Some factors affecting attendance at antenatal clinics. *Social Science & Medicine,* **15D**, 421–4.

Kings' Community Health Council (1978) *Report on maternity care in the Kings' Community Health District (Teaching)*. Kings' Community Health Council, London.

Kirke, P.N. (1980) Mothers' views of obstetric care. *British Journal of Obstetrics & Gynaecology*, **87**(11), 1029–33.

Kitzinger, S. (ed.) (1981) *Change in antenatal care. A report of a working party set up by the National Childbirth Trust*. National Childbirth Trust, London.

Lewis, J. (1980) *The politics of motherhood*. Croom Helm, London.

Lovell, A., Zander, L.I., James, C.E., Foot, S., Swan, A.V., Reynolds, A. (1986) *St Thomas' maternity case notes study – why not give mothers their own case notes?* Cecily Northcote Trust, London.

McClure Brown, J.C. and Dixon, G. (1978) *Browne's antenatal care*. Churchill Livingstone, Edinburgh.

McKee, I.H., (1984) Community antenatal care: the Sighthill community antenatal scheme. In Zander, L. and Chamberlain, G. (eds) *Pregnancy Care for the 1980s*, Royal Society of Medicine and Macmillan Press, London.

Martin, J. (1978) *Infant feeding 1975: attitudes and practice in England and Wales*. HMSO, London.

Martin, J., and Monk, J. (1982) *Infant feeding 1980*. Office of Population Censuses and Surveys, London.

Maternity Services Advisory Committee (1982) *Maternity care in action, Part 1 – Antenatal care*. HMSO, London.

Milner, R.D.G. and Richards, B. (1974) An analysis of birthweight by gestational age of infants born in England and Wales (1967–1971). *Journal of Obstetrics and Gynaecology of the British Commonwealth*, **81**, 956–67.

Ministry of Health, Department of Health for Scotland, Ministry of Labour and National Service (1949) *Report of the Working Party on Midwives* (Chairman Mrs M.D. Stocks). HMSO, London

Morrin, H.A. (1982) Are we in danger of extinction? *Midwives Chronicle*, **95**(1128), 17.

Murray, F.A. and Topley, L. (1974) Patients as record holders. *Health and Social Services Journal*, **84**(4397), 1675.

Myles, M. (1981) *Textbook for midwives*, 9th edn. Churchill Livingstone, Edinburgh.

Nie, N.H., Hull, C.H., Jenkinson, J.G., Steinbrenner, K., Bent, D.H. (1975) *Statistical Package for the Social Sciences*. McGraw-Hill, New York.

Oakley, A. (1979) *Women confined, towards a sociology of childbirth*. Martin Robertson, Oxford.

Oakley, A. (1984) *The captured womb*. Basil Blackwell, Oxford.

O'Brien, M. and Smith, C. (1981) Women's views and experiences of antenatal care. *Practitioner*, **25**, 123–5.

Office of Population, Censuses and Surveys (1970) *Registrar General's classification of occupations*, HMSO, London.

Office of Population, Censuses and Surveys (1987) *Mortality statistics, perinatal and infant: social and biological factors*. HMSO, London.

Parsons, W. and Perkins, E. (1980) *Why don't women attend for antenatal care?* Leverhulme Health Education Project Occasional paper No. 23, University of Nottingham, Nottingham.

Perfrement, S. (1982) *Women's Information on pregnancy, childbirth and baby care*.

Centre for Medical Research, University of Sussex, Sussex.

Rajan, L. and Oakley, A. (1990) Low birth weight babies: the mother's point of view. *Midwifery*, **6**(2), 73–85.

Reid, M.E., Gutteridge, S., McIlwaine, G.M. (1983) *A comparison of the delivery of antenatal care between a hospital and a peripheral clinic.* Social Paediatric and Obstetric Research Unit, University of Glasgow, Glasgow.

Richards, I.D.G., Donald, E.M., Hamilton, F.M.W. (1970) Use of maternity care in Glasgow. In McLachlan, G. and Shegog, R. (eds) *In the beginning – studies in maternity care.* Oxford University Press, Oxford.

Robinson, S. (1985) Midwives, obstetricians and general practitioners: the need for role clarification. *Midwifery*, **1**(2), 102–13.

Robinson, S. (1989) Caring for childbearing women: the interrelationship between midwifery and medical responsibilities. In Robinson, S. and Thomson, A.M. (eds) *Midwives, Research and Childbirth, vol. 1*, Chapman and Hall, London.

Robinson, S. (1990) Maintaining the independence of the midwifery profession: a continuing struggle, in Garcia, G., Kilpatrick, R., Richards, M. (eds) *Politics of maternity care.* Oxford University Press, Oxford.

Robinson, S., Golden, J., Bradley, S. (1982) The role of the midwife in the provision of antenatal care. In Enkin, M. and Chalmers, I. (eds) *Effectiveness and satisfaction in antenatal care.* Spastics International Medical Publications, London.

Robinson, S., Golden, J., Bradley, S. (1983) *A study of the role and responsibility of the midwife.* Nursing Education Research Unit, report No. 1, University of London, London.

Roland, J. (1981) *Perinatal mortality in Manchester.* Unpublished MSc. thesis, University of Manchester, Manchester.

Royal College of Midwives (1977) *Evidence to the Royal Commission on the National Health Service.* Royal College of Midwives, London.

Simpson, H. and Walker, G. (1980) When do pregnant women attend for antenatal care? *British Medical Journal*, **281**, 104–7.

Social Services Committee (1980) *Perinatal and Neonatal Mortality, second report (Short report).* HMSO, London.

Social Services Committee (1984) *Perinatal and Neonatal Mortality. follow-up.* HMSO, London.

Stuart, B. and Judge, E. (1984) The return of the midwife? *Midwives Chronicle and Nursing Notes*, **97**(1152), 8–9.

Taylor, R.W. (1984) Community-based specialist obstetric services. In Zander, L. and Chamberlain, G. (eds) *Pregnancy care for the 1980's.* Royal Society of Medicine and Macmillan Press, London.

Thomson, A.M. (1980) Planned or unplanned? Are midwives ready for the 1980's? *Midwives Chronicle and Nursing Notes*, **93**(1106), 68–72.

Thomson, A.M. (1989) Why don't women breast feed? in Robinson, S. and Thomson, A.M. (eds) *Midwives, Research and Childbirth, Vol. 1.*, Chapman and Hall, London.

Thomson, A.M., Billewicz, W.Z., Hytten, F.E. (1968) The assessment of fetal growth. *Journal of Obstetrics and Gynaecology of the British Commonwealth*, **75**, 903–16.

Towler, J. and Butler-Manuel, R. (1973) *Modern obstetrics for student midwives.* Lloyd-Luke, London.

Turnball, C. (1984) Quality antenatal care? *Australian Journal of Advanced Nursing*, **2**(1), 32–43.

Walker, J.F. (1976) Midwife or obstetric nurse? Some perceptions of midwives and obstetricians of the role of the midwife. *Journal of Advanced Nursing*, **1**(2), 129–38.

Wood, A. (1963) The development of the midwifery services in Great Britain. *International Journal of Nursing Studies*, **1**, 51–8.

World Health Organization (1966) The midwife in maternity care. *Technical Report Series*, No. 331. WHO, Geneva.

Zander, L. (1982) The challenge of antenatal care: a perspective from general practice. In Enkin, M. and Chalmers, I. (eds) *Effectiveness and satisfaction in antenatal care.* Spastics International Medical Publications and William Heinemann Medical Books Ltd, London.

Zander, L., Watson, M., Taylor, R., Morrell, D.C. (1978) Integration of general practitioner and specialist antenatal care. *Journal of the Royal College of General Practitioners*, **28**, 455–8.

CHAPTER SEVEN

Antenatal education: evaluation of a post-basic training course

Tricia Murphy-Black

INTRODUCTION

The need for evaluation, whether in health care or education, has assumed importance during the 1980s as the pace of change and demand for cost effectiveness has increased. This chapter describes an evaluation study in the post-basic education of midwives and health visitors; it is known as the Parent Craft Education Project and was funded by the Health Education Council (HEC).

Evaluation is undertaken to estimate the value or effectiveness of health care provision, implementation of a policy or an educational programme. Donabedian (1969) suggested a tri-partite approach to evaluation of health care provision, namely examination of structure, process and outcome. Evaluation of structure focuses on an examination of the system, the resources used to provide care and the manner in which they are organized. The process concentrates on the way in which professionals use resources and how care is given. Using outcome as a measure of effectiveness explores the end results; in the case of health care a measure of the health and satisfaction of the client.

When these principles are applied to education the structure consists of facilities for teaching, the process examines what goes on during training and the outcome is the way in which the course attenders are able to use the information or skills that they gained from the course. A process and outcome evaluation in education can be linked to the formative and summative methods of evaluation suggested by Stufflebeam (1971). He suggested that evaluation for decision making (for instance, should we continue to use this new course?) is formative or proactive, while evaluation for accountability (this course does teach what it is intended to teach) is summative or retroactive. In practical terms, the major difference between formative and summative evaluation is that formative evaluation has built into it the possibility of change in response to reactions of attenders during the course, whereas this does not occur in a summative evaluation as this concentrates on the end phase of the course. While the former approach is relevant for a course of some length, it is not appropriate for the short post-basic course that was the focus of this study; and a summative evaluation was adopted. Stufflebeam (1983) also suggests that evaluators should be involved in the design and conduct of the evaluation in such a way as to assist the teaching staff to plan and implement the course.

A single measure is often used to evaluate a part or the whole of an educational programme. This may take place following a lecture, a short course, or a whole education programme and often is only a test of the amount of knowledge that a group of students has retained, such as an examination for a professional qualification. As new methods of teaching and different systems of education are introduced, greater attention has been paid to the value of courses, asking if these methods or systems are more effective than the former ones or if the students are able to benefit from the new or additional material. An example in nursing is provided by the recommendation that the then Joint Board of Clinical Nursing Studies (JBCNS) courses were the subject of both formative and summative evaluation. During each course continuous evaluation took place, with both students and teachers completing a range of instruments. At the end of the course, both the planning team and the students evaluated the whole of the course. While this evaluation package was useful when either the staff or the course were new, the JBCNS teachers felt its main use was to confirm the judgements that they had already made and the main disadvantage was that it was so time consuming (Leyton Jones *et al.*, 1981).

Structure, process and outcome evaluation have been used, either in combination or singly, to evaluate courses in nursing and midwifery. Two studies using outcome measures only were employed to assess the 12-month and 18-month midwifery courses. Some 1800 student midwives in England and Wales were sent a questionnaire, shortly after they qualified, that asked for their views on various aspects of their education (Robinson, 1986); the findings of this study are the subject of Chapter 10 in this volume. A survey of the 18-month course in Scotland, that involved sending questionnaires to both newly and longer-qualified midwives, revealed a need for more clinical teaching, preparation for management and the delegation of progressive responsibility (Pope, 1986). Process and outcome measures were used to evaluate the training of nursing assistants (Narayanasamy, 1985) while Harrison, Sanders and Sims (1977) used structure and outcome to examine a change in first level nurse education. This involved looking at ward staffing levels and interviewing a small number of students. Both process and outcome measures were used in the study discussed in this chapter.

BACKGROUND TO THE STUDY

The Health Education Council (HEC) became involved in the education of health professionals participating in antenatal teaching, following the recommendations of both the Court and the Short Reports (Committee for Child Health Services, 1976; Social Services Committee, 1980). An antenatal Health Education Working Party was set up to consider the recommendations of these committees, as well as the concerns expressed by parents and those working in maternity and health education services. The points considered included a need for greater flexibility to respond to changed attitudes, expectations and life styles of parents, and recognition of the value of group work and interactive teaching methods within health education.

Two courses, one basic and one intermediate, for both midwives and health visitors involved in antenatal education, had in fact been developed by Perkins in collaboration with senior managers in two of the Nottinghamshire Health Districts as part of the Leverhulme Health Education Project (Perkins and Craig, 1981; Perkins, 1982). A teachers' manual for the basic course was produced and distributed and was based on the idea that 'good antenatal teaching involves staff being responsive to the needs of individual women and their partners' (Perkins and Craig, 1981, p. 1). It was designed to encourage the use of small groups, with staff providing a relaxed atmosphere to encourage enjoyable teaching and learning. The manual emphasized strategies that move away from syllabus examination systems, highlight student activity and provide feedback for tutors, on the grounds that these would free health visitors and midwives from the straightjacket of their own experience and increase their confidence (Perkins and Craig, 1981).

As part of their antenatal education initiative, the HEC said that they would disseminate the Perkins and Craig manual more widely, but that it should first be evaluated. The Council made funds available for such a project and the author was appointed to carry it out. At around the same time, staff of two antenatal education centres were seeking help in evaluating revisions that they had decided to make in their own courses, and approached the HEC in this respect. After some discussion it was decided that these centres should be the subject of the evaluation project, and the process of evaluating their courses is described in this chapter.

One unusual aspect of the study was that the request for evaluation came from the health service staff responsible for antenatal education. The two centres involved (referred to as A and B) had been examining a variety of aspects of their antenatal education. For instance Centre A staff, identifying the need for information, undertook a survey of women in 1981. On the basis of this they decided that joint efforts of midwives and health visitors were required to improve the service and felt that a training programme could help to achieve this aim. After reviewing their services, staff at Centre

B changed and increased their publicity, timing and location of classes, recommended changes of content and presentation as well as developing a group work skills course. Both centres, as well as identifying problems with classes for women, realized the need for further education of their own staff, and in collaboration with the HEC agreed to use the Perkins and Craig manual as a basis for their courses.

The course was started in 1982 in Centre A and was run twice a year, while Centre B put on the course four times a year from 1981. The Perkins and Craig course structure of 5 half-days was expanded to a full week. Both centres had common material on teaching and group work skills, with additional material on teaching theory, communications and local research reports. Sessions on teaching relaxation and exercises were included at Centre A only, while Centre B had undertaken, at the request of their staff, to update them in recent developments in midwifery practice. A revised version of the training manual has been published following the evaluation reported here (Murphy-Black and Faulkner, 1987).

AIMS OF THE STUDY

The aims of the evaluation study were twofold. First, we sought to determine whether the courses would meet the expectations of the midwives and health visitors who attended them. This was undertaken by means of a series of questionnaires to evaluate the process of the course. Secondly, we attempted to assess the outcome of the course in terms of an observational study of pre- and post-course teaching sessions given by course participants. This chapter focuses primarily on the questionnaire study but also includes a summary of the observation study, full details of which can be found elsewhere (Murphy-Black, 1986).

METHODS OF DATA COLLECTION AND ANALYSIS

Both quantitative and qualitative methods of data collection were employed in order to overcome some of the deficiencies in each approach and to provide more information than would have been obtained by use of either one alone. In the questionnaire study this involved both closed and open-ended questions, while in the observation study there was a quantitative record of the interaction between the antenatal teacher and women, as well as a descriptive account of the classes. There were four courses involved in the study, one run by a professional organization which was used for the pilot study, one from a series of two a year in Centre B and two in one year from Centre A. All the courses were studied in 1983. The reason for including two courses from Centre A was that the numbers were smaller than on the Centre B courses. The courses chosen for the study were those that were organized at a convenient time in the development of the study.

The questionnaire study consisted of seven self-administered question-naires for each attender:

1. A pre-course questionnaire administered at the beginning of the course;
2. Five course questionnaires;
3. A post-course questionnaire sent to the subject six weeks after the course.

During the pilot study it was possible to discuss the questionnaires given to participants prior to course attendance and those given to them during the course, as well as examine their written responses, but verbal feedback was not available for the pilot post-course questionnaire. As the design of the questionnaires was, at times, complex and they underwent considerable modification, each questionnaire is discussed separately.

Design and analysis of the pre-course questionnaire

Closed questions were used to ascertain information about the subjects' occupation, length of service, and education for and experience of, antenatal or other teaching; differences between the two occupational groups partici-pating in the study (midwives and health visitors) were assessed using the chi square test. Reasons for attending the course and expectations of what would be gained from it were sought using open-ended questions, as this allowed the subjects greater freedom in which to express themselves. These data were subject to content analysis and the broad themes that emerged were quantified.

Design and analysis of the course questionnaire

Two approaches were employed in the course questionnaires to obtain reactions of attenders of the sessions held each day:

1. A forced choice between six pairs of course descriptors;
2. An open-ended question asking for comments on each session.

A questionnaire that had been used successfully in a similar course (Rees, 1982) was used for the pilot study. This asked attenders to give each session a score and to comment about it. The reasons for changes made to this questionnaire, following experience gained in the pilot study, were as follows:

1. The questionnaire was administered on a daily basis as opposed to a sessional basis. The respondents in the pilot study made it clear that they found having to complete a questionnaire after every session a considerable burden during a week of intensive learning. This view was expressed verbally and indicated by the low level of response after the

first day (the percentage of returns dropped from 95% on the first day to 30% on the second day).

2. Modification of the scoring system. A seven-point scoring system had been used in the pilot study so that a score could be given for each session in response to such questions as 'did you learn something from this session?' When this scoring system was applied to the whole day however, the attenders found it difficult to quantify all the sessions under the one score; some spoilt their responses by giving two different scores for morning or afternoon or by specifying which session warranted a particularly high or low score. As a result this section was revised further in the third version. This listed opposing statements that included the six course descriptors that had been used in the original questions; these were:

•	most interesting;	–	least interesting;
•	most practical;	–	least practical;
•	most useful;	–	least useful;
•	learnt most;	–	learnt least;
•	most useful group work;	–	least useful group work;
•	most productive report back;	–	least productive report back.

For each of these pairs of opposing statements the attenders were asked to name the sessions which fitted under each heading, e.g. which session was the most interesting and which the least interesting. This also caused problems, as the attenders were reluctant to specify a session for the least category of each pair. The rate of response at Centre B varied for each pair of statements, but some of the least categories had a less than 50% response rate. A third of the attenders in Centre A did not complete the categories on the first day and their verbal responses indicated their unease at completing this section. For the following days they refused to complete the 'least' category. One reason that may have contributed to this was that the course tutors, some of whom were also the course attenders' service managers, were present while they were completing these questionaires, despite assurances that the questionnaires would be returned only to the evaluator and not to the managers.

3. Removal of three questions; these were:
(a) information or skills that had been learnt;
(b) information on skills that were updating those that they already had;
(c) information on skills that would be used in their classes.

The data provided by the pilot study subjects demonstrated their difficulties in distinguishing between these three questions. Some responses were incorrect, and some repeated the list of replies given in the first question again in the second question, whereas they should have been mutually exclusive. In addition, there were questions that were only partially answered. These three questions also increased the amount of work expected of the subjects and the response rate for sessions varied from 76% to 90%. Consequently, these questions were removed following the pilot study and subsequent versions just asked the subject to comment on each session. This final form of the course questionnaire was the third version, and is included in Appendix 7.1 at the end of the chapter.

Analysis of the pilot study questionnaires presented considerable problems. A Friedman two-way analysis of variance was attempted (for the scoring section), but could not be used as there were insufficient numbers of cases within each score for the 15 sessions (see Armitage (1971) for details of this test). Measures of central tendency (mean and median) were used for the main study.

Design and analysis of the post-course questionnaire

The post-course questionnaire used a mixture of closed and open-ended questions, with a seven point Likert-type scale to quantify reactions to organizational details, such as session length. A similar system was used in relation to the aims of the course to assess whether the aims were fulfilled for each individual. The sessions held in each centre were listed and the attenders asked to rank the five that were the most useful to them and to add comments about the most useful session. Those attenders who had taught since the course, were asked to give details of any changes they had made to their classes.

Of the three questionnaires, the post-course questionnaire underwent the least change. This may have been because it was piloted by post and so there was a lack of opportunity to discuss the design and content with respondents.

FINDINGS

Profile of the course attenders

The following description refers to the 62 (94%) attenders who returned the pre-course questionnaire from the 65 distributed: 27 of the respondents were midwives and 35 were health visitors. The majority were qualified nurses. There were three direct-entry midwives and this is a high proportion (11%) in comparison with the 4.3% (180) found in a national study in England and Wales (Robinson, Golden and Bradley, 1983). While just over half of the health visitors held a midwifery qualification, only one midwife held a health visiting certificate. Chi square tests, utilizing Cochran's relaxed rule when appropriate (Cochran, 1954), demonstrated no statistically significant differences between the two groups that comprised Centre A attenders and no differences between Centre A and Centre B attenders in terms of occupations, length of service and previous teaching experience.

None of the antenatal teachers taught full time; for 50% it was part of their regular duties and 26% taught occasional sessions. The remainder said that they would be starting antenatal education in the near future or were no longer directly involved in antenatal classes. Fifteen attenders (24%) had some training that was relevant to antenatal education (10 from Centre A and 5 from Centre B). Midwives were less likely than health visitors to have had a relevant training for their teaching role (although the difference was not significant).

Information about the decision to attend the course was sought by means of a closed question with the following options given to the subjects:

1. It was suggested by a senior member of staff;
2. You asked to be sent;
3. You decided yourself.

Those who answered 2 or 3 or a combination of 2 and 3 were categorized together as self-selected. Attenders at Centre B were significantly more likely to have been manager-selected as opposed to self-selected than those at Centre A (28/36 compared with 10/26, $p = 0.004$), but this difference was not apparent between midwives and health visitors.

Expectations of the attenders

The reasons for attending the course are shown in Table 7.1. The largest category was aspects of teaching and this included wishing to update teaching skills, wanting to teach or a lack of previous training and experience. Some saw teaching as part of their role while others mentioned that they would be starting to teach in the near future.

The skills and information that attenders hoped to gain from the course are shown in Table 7.2. The greatest number of responses fell into the teaching category and included teaching relaxation and/or exercises, methods of presentation, evaluation of their own teaching and planning their classes. A need to improve communication skills was specified by 22 respondents; coping with groups and updating knowledge in midwifery were both specified by 18 respondents. When asked for their reasons for giving these replies, the attenders specified lack of training in, or little experience of teaching, wanting to improve the effectiveness of their teaching, learn new skills and gain ideas from others.

When respondents were asked which aspects of their forthcoming course they thought would be most useful, then sharing experience and exchanging

Table 7.1 Reasons given for attending the course (multiple response)

Main categories of reasons	Number (n = 65)
Aspects of teaching	25
Teaching role/new job	15
Update knowledge	14
Sent on the course	14
Exchange of ideas	10
Learn to teach relaxation & exercises	8
Other comments	7
Volunteered for the course	5

Source: Compiled by the author.

Table 7.2 Skills and information that respondents hoped to gain from the course

Skills/information	Number (n = 65)
Teaching skills	52
Communication skills	22
Conducting group work	18
Updating knowledge in midwifery	18
Other	13

Source: Compiled by the author.

ideas with others were mentioned most frequently. The themes of teaching skills and communication were also repeated. A group of 15 commented that they hoped the week's course would help to stimulate and inspire their teaching role.

Reactions to the course

Each of the 65 course attenders received a questionnaire on each day of the five-day course; 309 of the possible 325 were returned, a response rate of 95%. These questionnaires comprised a mixture of forced-choice questions and open-ended questions about various aspects of the course. The problems discussed earlier meant that this data was not as useful as it could have been. The original scoring system had disadvantages but did at least give an overall score for each session. Despite this, it may be questioned how useful that score can be to those who are trying to plan the next course, as a high score does not necessarily reflect the content of the individual sessions. For instance, the session at the end of the day might have a high score because it is interesting but alternatively the high score may only reflect that the session ended early and the attenders could get home before the rush hour.

Data from forced-choice questions

The compromise system used in this study asked the participants to say which was the 'best' session of the day using six sets of opposing statements. This meant that the sessions were only compared on a daily basis and did not allow, for example, for the 'best' session of day 2 to be compared with the 'best' session of day 3. In an attempt to overcome these problems and obtain some indication of the relative value of each session as perceived by attenders, a decision was made to summarize the results from the 'most' and 'least' of the six statements. Even this compromise was not straightforward as a number of attenders had not completed the 'least' categories. Finally, the 'most' categories alone were used to rank the sessions in the following way. Each session could potentially have been placed by all course attenders in the 'most' category for each of the following statements.

- Most interesting
- Most useful
- Most productive group work
- Most practical
- Learnt most
- Most productive report back

So, if, for example, a session on teaching methods was placed in the 'most' category by all attenders at Course B (N=36), a maximum score of 216 was possible. The actual score was calculated for each session by adding up the number of times it was placed in a 'most' category, and this score was then expressed as a percentage of the maximum potential score. The results of this analysis are shown in Table 7.3.

Data from open-ended questions

Comments made by subjects about each session were very wide ranging and provided a rich source of data on ways in which sessions were or were not perceived to be useful. The attenders varied considerably in the number of points that they made about each session: some commented briefly (e.g. 'I

Table 7.3 Ranking of percentages of sessions from the 6 'most' categories, for Centres A and B

	Centre A %	Centre B %
The environment	68.8	
Awkward people		68.6*
Presentation of topics	61.5	
Relaxation and exercises 1	56.7	
Theory into practice		50.0*
Asking questions		48.2
Free discussion	48.0	
Communications dos and don'ts		41.9
Keeping up to date 1		36.5
What preparations should be made?		
Pre-course knowledge	35.5	
Group discussion	35.4	
Teaching methods		34.7
Relaxation and exercises 2 and 3	33.3	
Relaxation and exercises — labour	28.1	
The mothers' view		27.9
Relaxation and exercises	27.1	
Triggers for discussion		26.1
Aims and objectives		23.4
Keeping up to date 2		23.1
Report by previous course members		22.1
Local research	21.9	
Aims and objectives	21.1	
'I never told them that'		20.9
Teaching a skill		18.9
Choosing teaching methods	18.9	
How do groups work		16.7
Communications	16.6	
Instructional techniques	13.3	
The importance of feedback		11.3
Creating an environment		10.8
Individual and group teaching	7.7	
Planning a session		7.2
Local research		6.5
Introduction to the course and each other		5.9
Importance of feedback	4.2	

*In Centre B there were only two sessions on day 5. This meant that there were only two options instead of four, which has given them a higher percentage than they should have. These sessions (Awkward people and Theory into practice) are marked with an asterisk above to indicate their falsely high percentage scores.
Source: Compiled by the author.

liked it' or 'Rubbish'), while others made at least three separate points (e.g. 'This was a good session; I will be able to try that out when I get back to work but the group part wasn't so good as there was a most disruptive person in my group'). The attenders also varied in their response rate; most returned a questionnaire each day but some omitted to comment on an individual session.

The following method was used to analyse the content of the comments. A broad categorization was developed during the pilot study and further refined during the main study; this related to content of the session as well as views about the speaker and other general comments. Each point made in the comments about each session was then allocated to one of these categories. This provided a means of quantification and gaining an overall impression of which sessions were perceived as most useful and why, and vice versa. However, the diversity of comments resulted in very small numbers in some of the categories and, to some extent, a suppression of the detail and complexity of respondents' views. A full description of methods employed in this analysis and the findings that emerged can be found elsewhere (Murphy-Black, 1986).

One aspect of the data is presented here and relates to whether the respondent made a positive, negative or a doubtful comment about a session; for example,

Positive – 'A really good speaker, I was interested all the time'.
Negative – 'Poor speaker'.
Doubtful – 'The speaker wasn't too bad'.

The numbers of positive, negative and doubtful comments made about a sample of the course sessions are shown in Figure 7.1. to illustrate the findings that emerged. The overall picture was one of a majority of positive comments. As demonstrated in Figure 7.1, there was considerable variation in the relative proportions of positive, negative and doubtful comments, both between and within centres for different sessions. Attenders at both centres gave the greatest number of positive comments to sessions that discussed how to deal with groups. Sessions about other aspects of group work, for instance, 'asking questions' and 'free discussion' were high in the ranking of the forced-choice section of the course questionnaires. Learning how to deal with groups had not in fact been expressed directly in the reasons for attending the course. In both the pre- and post-course questionnaires the reason given most frequently for attending the course was learning how to teach. Despite this, the various sessions relating to teaching skills (such as aims and objectives, teaching a skill or choosing teaching methods) are all in the lower half of the list in Table 7.3, unlike the group work sessions.

Direct comparisons cannot be made between the scoring and the comments. In the scoring questions, the attenders were asked only about

Figure 7.1 Numbers of positive, negative and doubtful comments made about course sessions: selected examples.

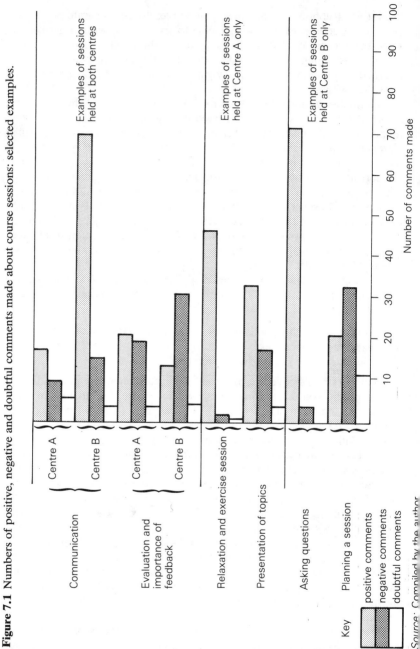

Source: Compiled by the author

sessions that occurred on one particular day, and requested comparison with the sessions held that day, whereas they were asked to comment on each session but were not asked for comparison either with that day's or other sessions. The two systems do, however, provide useful and complementary information for course planners. The scoring system provides an indication as to which sessions most need reconsidering in terms of their usefulness to participants, and the comments provide an indication as to the nature of changes that may be necessitated.

Post-course findings

The post-course questionnaire comprised a combination of closed and open-ended questions to examine the organization of the courses, how well the courses had fulfilled their specified aims, whether or not the attenders had resumed teaching and if they had made any changes, their view of midwives' and health visitors' roles in antenatal education and their overall impression of the courses. This was the only postal questionnaire and had a lower response rate (51/65, 78%) than either the pre-course or the daily question-naires. The majority of course attenders answered the questionnaire within 10 weeks of receipt, and by the time of return 73% had taught in antenatal classes.

Course organization

Although the post-course questionnaire examined the organization of the courses, the findings are not reported in full here as they are specific to the two study centres and not generalizable to other courses. Aspects that are, however, relevant to other courses include pre-course information and course length. Nearly half the respondents thought that the information was satisfactory; suggestions for improvement included more general or more specific information, while a small number found the travel directions difficult to follow. A pre-course meeting was organized by some of the health authorities within Centre B and this was appreciated; those who did not have this opportunity said that they would have liked one.

As the course had been changed from the Perkins and Craig (1981) version of five half-days at weekly intervals to a week's course, the attenders were asked how they felt about the arrangements of the course, in terms of length, timing and venue. Just under half were happy with the length. Others had opposing views; either the course was not long enough or it was too long. Some wanted more time for group work. One of those who felt it was too long expressed her limited expectations; she only wanted to learn relaxa-tion and exercises, while a health visitor complained that her case load had to be put aside for a week while she attended the course but the work would still be waiting on her return. Those who were sent on the course felt that there was too much time for individual sessions and that much was a 'waste of time', while those who had chosen to go on the course appreciated the flexibility of the timing, as it allowed discussion to continue if it was particularly interesting.

Meeting expectations

The final section of the post-course questionnaire investigated the satisfaction of attenders with the course. Each centre had specified the aims of the course and these were printed in the programme distributed prior to course commencement. These aims were incorporated in the post-course questionnaire and the midwives and health visitors asked to give a score between 1 and 7 as to how well the aims had been met in their view. This was a section of the questionnaire that worked well and responses showed differences between the two centres. One of the aims of the Centre A courses was to teach relaxation and exercises. The organizers knew that this was a need within the Health Authority; it was expressed by the attenders in the pre-course questionnaire and an indication that this need was met was reflected by both the high means (6.1) and medians (7) in the findings (see Figure 5.13 in Murphy-Black, 1986 for further details). Although the overall means for the course aims at Centre B were higher, this may have been because these aims did not include such long-term goals as the reduction of perinatal and maternal morbidity, which was one of the stated aims of the Centre A courses.

The post-course questionnaire included a list of sessions in each centre. Each attender was asked to pick the five most useful sessions and number her choice 1–5, with number 1 being the most useful. Seven of the 51 respondents did not answer this question correctly; for example, one ranked every session between 1 and 5 and another ranked five sessions as 1. Although this question had not demonstrated any problems in the pilot study of 33 subjects, this failure to complete it correctly may indicate that the directions were not stated clearly enough. In both centres the sessions that were included in response to staff needs were given high ratings (relaxation and exercises in Centre A and keeping up to date in Centre B). Relaxation and exercise sessions in Centre A were mentioned three times in the first five; the other two were 'presentation of the prepared topic' and 'choosing teaching methods'. In Centre B, the two 'keeping up to date' sessions were second and joint fifth; the other sessions chosen most frequently were visual aids, 'I never told them that', the session with the mothers ('A mother's view') and 'Teaching a skill'.

Changes to antenatal classes

Of the 73% of attenders who had taught antenatal classes since attending the course, over half had made changes, and there was no significant difference between the centres in this respect. Two people had not yet taught but commented that they were planning changes when they started their next course. Changes included shortening the content, changing the programme or topics, the timing of classes or introduction of a postnatal group. Attitudes were more flexible and informal, and more attention was paid to the needs of the 'patients'. Inclusion of team teaching involved, for example, organizing her opposite number to attend classes, or rearranging the way the two teachers took the classes. Group work changes included reducing group size or encouraging women to be more active in the classes. The small number who were unable to make changes reported that these were precluded by management, environment, staffing or peer group problems.

The course attenders were asked for their views on midwives' and health visitors' roles in antenatal education. The responses showed both co-operation and conflict between the two occupational groups. Overall, health visitors had a wider view of their role than the midwives did of theirs. In both groups, there were some who wished to limit the involvement of the other profession. For instance, some of the midwives did not think health visitors should teach about labour, while some health visitors would like to keep such a teaching session as the midwives' only contribution (for further details see Black, Booth and Faulkner, 1984).

The question on reasons for attending the course asked in the pre-course questionnaire was repeated in the post-course questionnaire. Some respondents gave as many as four reasons and as this was a greater number than the first time, it produced a wider variety of reasons and a different incidence (see Table 7.4). The most noticeable change between the two lists was that ten of the 14 who had said that they were 'sent' on the course did not give the same reason the second time.

The midwives and health visitors were asked to comment on course content in relation to their main reason for attending. An example of a reason given frequently is from a midwife who referred to exchange of ideas:

> To hear how classes are run in other areas and to gain as much information as possible to help me formulate some ideas of my own, so that I can, hopefully, take a more active part in our own classes in the near future.

(Centre B).

Comments about relaxation and exercises include this one from a health visitor:

> The relaxation sessions were interesting and useful. A little more depth could have been used in giving reason for each exercise.

(Centre A).

A health visitor who felt the need to refresh her knowledge said:

> Having been a health visitor for 15 years, I felt that I needed to be aware of current trends and methods of antenatal teaching. Although I have done this for many years, I only started group teaching 18 months ago with very little idea of what to do.

(Centre B).

A health visitor who wanted to improve her teaching commented:

> The course was structured to improve our teaching and covered many aspects of the skills needed and made us stop and think about what we are doing and what is the best way to use material.

(Centre B).

A hospital midwife starting teaching in the near future stated:

> As a midwife I was not involved in antenatal classes and I wanted to gain more experience in teaching.

(Centre B).

Less favourable comments included:
In response to a low score for relaxation and exercises:

> Not enough information given on reasons for doing exercises antenatally. I would have liked a sample programme of exercises for an 8 week session in order to avoid repetitiveness.

(Centre A).

One midwife did not feel entirely happy with the application of teaching methods:

> I thought this was well explained but would have gained more from teaching a session and then receiving advice and criticism. I felt the one session on the last day wasn't enough.

(Centre A).

One of the health visitors who felt she had been sent on the course said firmly:

> I'm sure I would have found the workshop far more interesting had I not recently attended a Health Education Certificate Course and therefore would not have requested study leave to attend this course.

(Centre B).

One health visitor gave the impression that the course was designed for the inexperienced:

> I have taught antenatal classes for nine years and wondered if updating was needed. To date I had not attended such a course and had learned

from senior colleagues. This course seemed ideal for someone setting out on antenatal teaching.
(Centre B).

The final question asked the midwives and health visitors whether they would recommend these courses to a friend or colleague. They responded enthusiastically, with 100% from Centre B and 83% from Centre A saying 'yes'.

Table 7.4 Comparison between pre- and post-course reasons for attending the course (multiple response)

Reasons	*Pre-course response (n = 62)*	*Post-course response (n = 51)*
Aspects of teaching	25	39
Teaching role/new job	15	8
Update knowledge	14	26
Learn to teach relaxation and exercises	8	22
Exchange ideas	10	25
Volunteered for course	3	0
Sent on course	14	4
Increase confidence	0	5
Improve communication	0	3
Other comments	6	9
Total number of comments made	95	141

Source: Compiled by the author.

The observation study

Although the observation study is reported in detail elsewhere (Murphy-Black, 1986) a brief summary is included here. One-third of the antenatal teachers attending the courses in both centres were observed teaching a total of 76 classes in 23 locations both pre- and post-course. They comprised a random sample stratified by study centre and by occupational group. The purpose of the observation was to record the interaction between women attending the antenatal classes and midwives or health visitors who were teaching. The objective of this part of the study was to ascertain whether there was an increase in interaction between teachers and women in the classes observed post-course compared with those observed pre-course.

The observation was undertaken by sitting just outside the teaching area and recording the nature of the teaching every three seconds on a note pad held on the knee. The method used for this recording was Flanders Inter-action Analysis Categories (Flanders, 1970). This is a series of codes designed for research into the teaching of school children, although it had been used successfully with adults and in an American study of conversa-tions between mothers and public health nurses (Kishi, 1983). The 10-point code system, which focused on initiation and response between teacher and pupil, was expanded for the antenatal classes to allow for such details as a baby crying or the teacher talking to the baby rather than the women. It was simple to use once the codes had been learnt and it was possible to record the type of questions the teacher used, the sort of responses the women gave, the type of questions the women asked and the teacher's response.

From the data it was possible to measure what went on in the class. For instance, the amount of time teachers and women spent talking was examined, as was the initiation and response between teachers and women. The content of the teaching was not examined; the focus was rather on how it occurred. When the pre-course and post-course observations were compared for the whole group, there were few differences; that is, there was very little increase in the amount of time the women talked or suggested what should be talked about. In other words, the teachers controlled what went on in the classes, yet the emphasis of the course was on encouraging the teachers to allow women to take part in the class and bring up the topics that concerned them. The group work sessions of the course were to give antenatal teachers skills to facilitate greater interaction in the class. Although the sessions on group skills were seen as useful and the teachers reported that they were trying to bring these aspects into their classes, when they were observed there was very little difference from their teaching styles before they attended the course.

There was one group whose teaching did change and this was the midwives and health visitors who had chosen to go on the course. For a variety of measures this group did not score well in the pre-course observa-tion, but after the course, had improved to a statistically significant level. For, example, one of the measures was the amount of time women spent talking in the classes. The mean percentage was 5% for the observations prior to course attendance and increased to 21% post–course; this was seen as a positive improvement in quantity of interaction in the classes.

CONCLUSION

The evaluation of a teaching and a group skills course, described in this chapter, consisted of two parts: first, questionnaires to examine the process of the course and second, observation to examine the outcome of the course in terms of changes in teaching styles. Data from questionnaires give a favourable impression. Despite criticisms of aspects of the course, both of details and organization, the attenders' responses indicated that they had learnt about teaching, leading a group and communicating with women. Some expressed enthusiasm and the inspiration to incorporate new techniques into their classes. While some were able to make the changes they desired, others found the constraints imposed by their peers, managers, the environment or shortage of staff too much to overcome.

Course tutors could examine the data from the questionnaire study and conclude that, although there were details of organization that needed changing, the course was useful for their staff. The consequence of this process evaluation could be a continuation of support for the provision of the course.

Examination of the observation data, the outcome, gives a less positive result. Differences observed in interactions between women and teachers prior to course attendance compared with those observed after course attendance were so small that the benefits of attending courses of this kind could be open to question. The self-selected group of attenders were an exception, however, in that their teaching did improve significantly post-course, indicating that greater attention should be paid to selection of staff to attend post-basic training courses. Whenever possible, staff should attend courses if they themselves perceive a need for further training. In this context it is interesting that Perkins (1981) found that those who were conscripted to the antenatal teaching courses in her study, were a 'disruptive influence'. Parnaby (1987) reported that midwives, attending statutory refresher courses, wanted to have a choice of which sessions to attend in order that their particular needs could be met. These findings have implications for the UKCC proposals to introduce refresher courses for nurses and health visitors (Nursing Times News, 1987) in that staff may be more likely to benefit from them if they themselves perceive the need for course attendance.

Difficulties in design and analysis of questionnaires, despite previous use, have been presented here to demonstrate that evaluation of short courses is not straightforward and that thorough piloting of instruments is essential. The process evaluation, even one that involves questionnaires pre-course, every day and post-course, did not offer any means of predicting the findings of the outcome of course attendance. Evaluation studies that comprise only process measures are useful to identify strengths and weaknesses of a course, and to indicate where changes are needed, but satisfaction with the course itself does not necessarily mean that there will be any change in subsequent behaviour.

ACKNOWLEDGEMENTS

This project was funded by the Health Education Council and academic supervision was by Ann Faulkner.

APPENDIX 7.1

Course questionnaire used each day in the main study

Please complete the code number with the number you were given for the pre-course questionnaire.

Section 1 Thinking about the sessions held today, please give one title under each of the following descriptions:

Most interesting	least interesting
Most practical	least practical
Most useful	least useful
Learnt most	learnt least

Section 2 Thinking about the group work you were involved with today, please give one title under each of the following:

Most useful	least useful
Most productive report back	least productive report back

Please write your answers in the space provided. Please comment about each of the sessions held today.

1st
2nd
3rd
4th
5th

Thank you for your help and co-operation.

REFERENCES

Armitage, P.O. (1971) *Statistical Methods in Medical Research.* Blackwell, Oxford.
Black, P.M., Faulkner, A. and Thomson, A.M., (1984) Antenatal classes: a selective review of the literature. *Nurse Education Today*, **3**(6), 130–3.
Black, T., Booth, K. and Faulkner, A. (1984) Co-operation or conflict? How midwives and health visitors view each other's contribution to antenatal education. *Senior Nurse*, **1**(33), 25–6.

Cochran, W.G. (1954) Some methods for strengthening the common Chi-square tests. *Biometrics*, **10**, 417–51.

Committee for Child Health Services (1976) *Fit for the future* (Chairman: Mrs J. Court). HMSO, London.

Donabedian, A. (1969) Some issues in evaluating the quality of nursing care. *American Journal of Public Health*, **59**, 1833–6.

Flanders, N.A., (1970) *Analysing teaching behaviour*. Addison Wesley Publishing Co., Massachusetts.

Harrison, J., Sanders, M.E., Sims, A. (1977) Some structural consideration in modular education for basic nursing students. *Journal of Advanced Nursing*, **2**, 383–91.

Kishi, K.I. (1983) Communication patterns of health teaching and information recall. *Nursing Research*, **32**, 230–5.

Leyton Jones, E., Bridge, W., Chatfield, K., Finn, B., and Rice, M. (1981) Course evaluation in postbasic education. *Journal of Advanced Nursing*, **6**, 179–88.

Murphy-Black, T. (1986) *The evaluation of a post basic training course for antenatal teachers*. Unpublished PhD Thesis, University of Manchester.

Murphy-Black, T. and Faulkner, A. (1987) *Antenatal group skills training – a manual of guidelines*. John Wiley and Sons, Chichester.

Murphy-Black, T. and Faulkner, A. (1990). Antenatal Education. In Faulkner, A. and Murphy-Black, T. (eds), *Midwifery, excellence in Nursing, the research route*, Volume 3. Scutari Press, London.

Narayanasamy, S.A. (1985) Evaluation of a training curriculum for nursing assistants. *Nurse Education Today*, **5**, 124–9.

Nursing Times News (1987) UKCC begin moves to make refresher schemes a must. *Nursing Times*, **83**, 35:5.

Parnaby, C.M. (1987) Surveying the opinions of midwives regarding the curriculum content of refresher courses. *Midwifery*, **3**, 133–42.

Perkins, E.R. (1979) *Parentcraft a comparative study of the teaching method.* Leverhulme Health Education Project Occasional Papers No 16. University of Nottingham.

Perkins, E.R. (1981) *Evaluating in-service training: a practical approach* Nottingham practical papers in health education, **3**. University of Nottingham, Department of Adult Education, Nottinghamshire Health Education Unit.

Perkins, E.R. (1982) Developing parentcraft teaching. Paper for limited circulation. University of Nottingham.

Perkins, E.R. and Craig, E. (1981) *Parentcraft Teaching the basic skills*. Paper for limited circulation. University of Nottingham, Department of Adult Education, Nottingham.

Perkins, E.R. and Morris, B. (1979) *Preparation for parenthood: a critique of the concept*. Leverhulme Health Education Project, Occasional Papers, No. **17**. University of Nottingham.

Pope, V. (1986) Midwifery training in Scotland: an opinion survey. *Midwives Chronicle*, **99**, 198–200.

Rees, C. (1982) '*What did we learn?*' *An assessment of an antenatal education group skills workshop*. South Glamorgan Health Authority Health Education Unit.

Robinson, S., Golden, J. and Bradley, S., (1983) *The role and responsibilities of the midwife*. NERU Report, **1**, Chelsea College, University of London.

Robinson, S. (1986) Midwifery training: the views of newly qualified midwives. *Nurse Education Today,* **6**(2), 49–59.

Social Services Committee Second Report (1980) *Perinatal and neonatal mortality.* (Chairman: Mrs R. Short) HMSO, London.

Stufflebeam, D.L. (1971) *Educational evaluation and decision-making.* Phi Delta Kappa National Study Centre on Evaluation.

Stufflebeam, D.L. (1983) The CIPP model for program evaluation. In Madaus, G.F., Scriven, M and Stufflebeam, D.L. *Evaluation models, viewpoints on educational and human services evaluation.* Kluwer-Nijhoff Publishing, Boston.

Sweet, B. (1984) Midwives in clinical practice. *Nursing Times,* **84**, 60–2.

CHAPTER EIGHT

Perineal care: a series of five randomized controlled trials

Jennifer Sleep

INTRODUCTION

One of the major contributions that midwives can make to the comfort and well-being of child-bearing women is the skilful care of the perineum during delivery and the puerperium. Such care should be based on scientifically evaluated practices. The midwife is the most senior professional person present at the majority of deliveries in the UK; she is thus responsible for managing the perineum and during normal delivery has the responsibility for deciding whether or not to perform an episiotomy. Following a change in the Central Midwives' Board's rules in 1983, midwives have increasingly taken responsibility for repair of perineal trauma. Moreover, both in hospital and at home, it is the midwife to whom women are likely to turn for advice on alleviating the distress of perineal pain. All in all, perineal management and care falls unequivocally in the midwife's sphere of responsibility and practice.

The efficacy of many of the routine procedures involved in perineal management at delivery, and subsequent care in the puerperium has not been subject to evaluation; along with other obstetric policies and practices their value has been increasingly questioned (Chalmers and Richards, 1977; Chalmers, 1978; Cochrane, 1979; Chalmers, 1989). Episiotomy has been a particular case in point. Those who advocate a liberal policy claim that this will reduce serious vaginal and perineal tears as well as longer-term problems such as stress incontinence and vaginal prolapse (Donald, 1979; Flood, 1982). On the other hand, those who advocate a more conservative approach contend that episiotomy results in unnecessary pain and in longer-term problems such as dyspareunia (House, 1981; Kitzinger and Walters, 1981; Zander, 1982).

Despite a dearth of sound scientific evidence on either the short-term or long-term effects of this procedure (Russell, 1982; Thacker and Banta,

1983), the 1970s saw a rapid increase in its incidence; from 25% in 1967 to 53% in 1978 (Macfarlane and Mugford 1984). Moreover, rates differed widely between units (House, 1983; Garcia, Garforth and Ayers 1986) and between individual midwives (Wilkerson, 1984; Logue, 1987 and Chapter 9 in this volume). Midwives expressed concern that the decision to perform an episiotomy was increasingly made by medical staff and this combined with the rising incidence meant that they were losing the skill of delivering women with an intact perineum (Wilmott, 1980; Robinson, Golden and Bradley, 1983).

Other procedures involved in perineal care, while not attracting as much public and professional concern as episiotomy, have similarly been characterized by widespread variation in practice and lack of scientific evaluation. Recent surveys have, for example, revealed considerable variation in the choice of perineal suture material and the technique used for repair (Grant, 1986) and in the therapies offered for relief of perineal pain (Sleep and Grant, 1988c). There is little available evidence to support many current practices.

The importance of minimizing morbidity post-delivery cannot be over emphasized. Pain following perineal trauma and repair and the distress and embarrassment caused by longer-term problems such as incontinence and dyspareunia can undermine women's health, their relationship with their partner, their self-confidence as well as their ability to care for their new baby, and their family. It is perhaps surprising, therefore, that there has been so little research to assess the efficacy of different policies and treatment regimes. This chapter reports a programme of clinical research into some aspects of perineal management and care. The research comprised a series of five randomized controlled trials undertaken over a three-year period at the Royal Berkshire Hospital in Reading. Each trial was undertaken as a collaborative effort between midwifery, obstetric and other staff of the hospital, and members of the National Perinatal Epidemiology Unit in Oxford. Each of the trials has been reported separately; the purpose of this chapter is to bring them together, focusing in particular on their implications for midwifery practice and education.

In the initial study, a restricted policy for performing episiotomy was compared with a liberal policy. In 1981 the Maws Midwife Scholarship was awarded for the conduct of this study, which was also supplemented by a small grant awarded through the locally organised research scheme, Oxford Region. The findings were made available at the 1983 Research and the Midwife Conference and published the following year (Sleep, 1984; Sleep, Grant, Garcia, Elbourne, Spencer and Chalmers, 1984). The women who took part in the study were followed up three years later (Sleep and Grant, 1987b). Materials used for repairing perineal trauma were evaluated in a trial comparing glycerol-impregnated chromic catgut with untreated chromic catgut (Spencer, Grant, Elbourne, Garcia and Sleep, 1986). As with the episiotomy policy study, the trial participants were followed up three years later (Grant, Sleep, Ashurst and Spencer, 1989). The subsequent series of studies was supported by a major grant awarded through the locally organized research scheme and continued for three years. This included an assessment of the effectiveness of bath additives in relieving perineal discomfort and was the subject of the next trial to be undertaken. The findings were reported at the 1987 Research and the Midwife Conference and published the following year (Sleep and Grant, 1988a, 1988b). The next trial focused on the effectiveness of pelvic floor exercise regimes in preventing postpartum urinary incontinence (Sleep and Grant 1987a) and the last one evaluated recently introduced electrical therapies for the treatment of perineal trauma (Grant, Sleep, McIntosh and Ashurst, 1989). The protocol for each of the trials was approved by the District Research and Ethics Committee.

An experimental approach was selected for each of these five studies using a randomized controlled trial design. Grant (1983) has outlined the advantages of this design in evaluating alternative policies and practices in midwifery; in particular the fact that the groups compared are free of selection bias. The various stages in conducting a trial are shown in Figure 8.1. Confidence in the findings can only be justified when trials are conducted according to certain principles:

1. Sufficient numbers of subjects are recruited to reduce the likelihood of the interpretation of findings being confused by an effect of chance;
2. Random allocation of participants after entry to the trial and no withdrawal of subjects once entered in order to minimize selection bias and to obtain comparable groups for receipt of competing treatments;
3. The allocation must not be predictable in advance;
4. Good compliance with the trial directive to minimize mergence of the treatment groups;
5. For the purpose of analysis, keeping individuals in the group to which they were allocated, irrespective of the treatment they actually received.

Readers interested in details of the design, conduct, and analysis of trials are referred to Meinart (1986).

Needless to say, trials entail a considerable degree of effort and commitment, as well as the collaboration of large numbers of personnel. As Grant (1983) explains: 'once started, the trial gathers a momentum of its own and there is no going back; it cannot be stopped and started whenever the investigator feels like it. It is prospective and observations and measurements have to be made at fixed times in the future'.

The following sections include the rationale, the design, methods of data collection, analysis, and findings, for each of the five trials. The chapter is concluded with a discussion of the implications of this programme of research for midwifery practice and education.

Figure 8.1 Randomized controlled trial—flow chart.

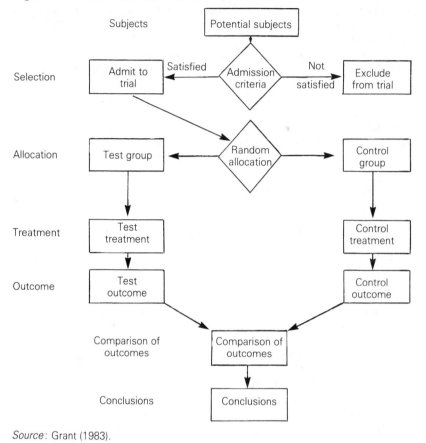

Source: Grant (1983).

TRIAL 1: LIBERAL VERSUS RESTRICTED USE OF EPISIOTOMY

In view of the contradictions concerning the short- and long-term effects of episiotomy, we mounted a randomized controlled trial to compare liberal and restricted use of episiotomy for maternal indications in women experiencing a normal vaginal delivery. In both groups the midwives were asked to minimize trauma if at all possible. The restrictive policy was defined as one in which the midwife tried to avoid an episiotomy, and to restrict its use to fetal indications only (bradycardia, tachycardia, or meconium-stained liquor). The liberal policy was defined as one in which the midwife was instructed to try and prevent a tear. The outcomes assessed were trauma at delivery, maternal morbidity at ten days and at three months post-partum terms of perineal pain, incidence of urinary incontinence, the time of resumption of sexual intercourse, and the incidence of dyspareunia. Assessment of infant morbidity was based on Apgar scores at delivery and the number of babies needing admission to the Special Care Baby Unit.

Methods

The trial size, based on the expected incidences of each of the outcomes, was preset at 1000 women (Sleep *et al.*, 1984). Power calculation indicated that a trial of this size would have a 90% chance of finding a significant difference (two tailed $\alpha = 0.05$) if, in truth, the restrictive policy doubled the incidence of an outcome expected in 5% of cases, and a 95% power of detecting an increase of 50% in an outcome expected in 20% of cases (Sleep *et al.*, 1984).

All women booked to deliver in the hospital during the five-month study period in 1982 were sent a letter towards the end of their pregnancy seeking their co-operation with research aimed at reducing pain and discomfort during delivery. On the grounds that no-one would receive a treatment known to be inferior to another, consent was implied unless stated to the contrary. Criteria for eligibility for recruitment to the trial were a live singleton fetus presenting cephalically at term, and expectation of a spontaneous vaginal delivery towards the end of the second stage of labour.

The entry criteria for the trial were met by a total of 1067 women. Sixty-seven were not recruited for various reasons: these included not having been booked for delivery at the Royal Berkshire Hospital, precipitate delivery, or sometimes the trial was forgotten. One thousand women (96% of those eligible for entry) were successfully recruited to the trial. The point of entry to the trial was when the attending midwife was confident of a spontaneous vaginal delivery, i.e. when she decided to 'scrub up'. She then noted the time and opened a sealed opaque envelope; this contained a computerized random allocation to either the restricted or the liberal episiotomy policy. In both groups the midwives were urged to conduct the delivery without any trauma if at all possible. Once the envelope was opened, the women had entered the trial, regardless of subsequent management. If the midwife failed to fulfil the directive she was asked to note the reason.

Of the thousand women entered into the trial, 498 were allocated to the restricted policy and 502 to the liberal policy. In accordance with unit policy a medio-lateral incision was used in performing episiotomies. Vaginal trauma was repaired using a continuous suture technique; interrupted stitches were used for the deeper tissues and subcuticular or interrupted sutures used to repair the perineal skin.

The degree of trauma sustained was assessed by the operator performing the repair, who was 'blind' to the trial allocation. The Apgar score of the baby at one minute was noted. Ten days after delivery women were asked to assess their residual perineal pain. The community midwife, who was 'blind' to the trial allocation recorded an assessment of perineal healing. It was also noted at this time whether the baby had been admitted to the Special Care Unit since birth. Information was returned for 88% (439) of women allocated to the restrictive episiotomy policy group and for 89% (440) of those allocated to the liberal group. Perineal discomfort, and the time of resumption of sexual intercourse were recorded by the women on a postal questionnaire sent to them at three months post-delivery. Response rates for the restrictive and liberal policy groups were 88% (438) and 91% (457) respectively. It had been decided that women who wished to know their treatment allocation should be given this information, so it was not possible to blind all trial participants during this assessment. Less than one in ten women, however, requested this information, and so the majority were in ignorance of their trial allocation when they completed their questionnaires. There was no evidence that those lost to follow-up differed between the two groups. All analyses of the specified outcomes were based on the unbiased comparisons between all women allocated to either the restrictive or liberal policy, whether or not they sustained an episiotomy or a tear. The chi-squared and Student's t-tests were used to compare discrete and continuous variables in the two groups.

Findings

Randomization generated two groups of women who were similar in a number of important respects (Table 8.1). The women were delivered by people of comparable status, the majority (94%) of whom were midwives (Table 8.2). The status of those who assessed and repaired perineal trauma in the two groups was also similar, the majority (86%) of whom were junior obstetricians.

The episiotomy rate differed considerably in the two groups; 10% of women allocated to the restrictive policy group had an episiotomy compared with 51% of those allocated to the liberal policy group ($p < 0.00001$). As shown in Table 8.3, this difference reflected the frequency of episiotomy performed for maternal reasons among both primiparae and multiparae. There was good compliance with the restrictive policy, with only 18 instances in which an episiotomy was performed for reasons other than fetal distress. These were 'thick perineum' or 'previous episiotomy' (11), large baby (3) and to prevent a tear (4).

The different episiotomy rates resulted in differing patterns of maternal trauma sustained at delivery. As anticipated, there were both more posterior tears and more intact perinea among those women allocated to the restrictive policy group (Table 8.4 $p < 0.0001$, 3 df). There were also more

Table 8.1 Episiotomy policy trial. Characteristics of the two groups of women

Characteristics	Restricted episiotomy policy (n = 498)	Liberal episiotomy policy (n = 502)
Mean maternal age (years)	26.6	26.7
Proportion who were primiparous	40% (201)	44% (219)
Proportion who were married	89% (445)	87% (435)
Mean gestational age (weeks)	39.8	39.8
Mean birth weight (grams)	3393	3367

Source: Sleep (1984).

Table 8.2 Episiotomy policy trial. Status of person undertaking delivery

Status	Restricted episiotomy policy (n = 498)		Liberal episiotomy policy (n = 502)	
	%	No.	%	No.
Midwifery sister	33	163	31	157
Staff midwife	30	150	32	161
Student midwife	30	150	31	155
Medical student	5	26	5	25
Doctor	2	9	1	4

Source: Sleep (1984).

anterior labial tears in this group (Table 8.5 $p < 0.001$, 1 df). Severe maternal trauma was less common than anticipated with only four cases in the restrictive group and one in the liberal group.

Women allocated to the liberal policy group were more likely to require suturing than those allocated to the restricted group (78% compared with 69% $p < 0.01$), and this difference was greater for primiparae (89% compared with 74%) than for multiparae (69% compared with 66%). With the exception of the four cases of severe trauma noted above, there was no evidence that trauma was more extensive in the women who actually sustained perineal injury in the restrictive policy group.

Table 8.3 Episiotomy policy trial. Incidence of episiotomy in the two groups

	Restricted episiotomy policy		Liberal episiotomy policy	
	%	No.	%	No.
All women	(n = 498)		(n = 502)	
Episiotomy rate	10	51	51	258
Maternal indications	4	18	45	228
Fetal distress	7	33	6	30
Primiparae only	(n = 201)		(n = 219)	
Episiotomy rate	18	36	67	147
Maternal indications	6	12	59	130
Fetal distress	12	24	8	17
Multiparae only	(n = 297)		(n = 283)	
Episiotomy rate	5	15	39	111
Maternal indications	2	6	35	98
Fetal distress	3	9	4	13

Source: Reproduced from Sleep *et al.* (1984). Courtesy of the British Medical Journal.

There were no significant differences in neonatal outcome. A total of 5.4% of babies born to women allocated to the restrictive policy group had Apgar scores below 7 at one minute, while the corresponding figure for the liberal policy group was 4.6%. Figures for admission to the special care baby unit in the first ten days of life were 5.7% and 7.6% for the restrictive and liberal policy groups respectively.

The incidence of perineal pain reported by the women showed little difference between the two groups at ten days after delivery and at three months postpartum (Tables 8.6 and 8.7). Overall, 90% of women had resumed intercourse within three months after delivery and, as shown in Table 8.8, the proportions were the same in the two groups. Those in the restricted group, however, were more likely to have resumed intercourse within the first month (37% compared with 27% $p < 0.01$); this difference was only partly explained by the increased proportion of women with an intact perineum in this group. Of the women who had resumed intercourse, a similar proportion in each group had experienced dyspareunia (52% and 51%). This problem persisted for 22% and 18% three months after delivery. As shown in Table 8.9, the different management policies appeared to have had no effect on the frequency of involuntary loss of urine three months after delivery, with 19% of women in both groups experiencing this problem.

Table 8.4 Episiotomy policy trial. Incidence of posterior perineal trauma

Posterior trauma	Restricted episiotomy policy (n = 498)		Liberal episiotomy policy (n = 502)	
	%	No.	%	No.
None	34	169	24	122
Episiotomy alone	9	45	45	227
Perineal tear alone	56	278	24	123
Episiotomy plus extension	1	6	6	30

Source: Sleep (1984).

Table 8.5 Episiotomy policy trial. Incidence of anterior perineal trauma

Anterior trauma	Restricted episiotomy policy (n = 498)		Liberal episiotomy policy (n = 502)	
	%	No.	%	No.
None	74	367	83	415
Labial tears	26	131	17	87

Source: Sleep (1984).

Analyses of data by status of the person who had actually conducted the delivery showed that the differential effects of the policies were little affected by the experience of the attendant. Analyses stratified by time interval between entry to the trial and delivery disclosed that, although trauma was less common in those women who delivered very soon after entry to the trial, the overall effects of the two policies were still evident in these cases.

As expected, multiparous women had fewer episiotomies, fewer anterior tears, and more intact perinea than primiparae, but they also sustained more posterior tears. They were half as likely as primiparae to have pain ten days and three months after delivery but more likely to suffer involuntary loss of urine. When the two perineal management policies were compared within parity groups, however, the pattern of the findings closely resembled that of the unstratified analysis for the total trial population; in both parity strata

Table 8.6 Episiotomy policy trial. Incidence of pain reported by women at ten days postpartum

Nature of pain experienced in last 24 hours	Restricted episiotomy policy (n = 439)		Liberal episiotomy policy (n = 446)	
	%	No.	%	No.
Mild	14	62	15	65
Moderate	8	33	8	35
Severe	1	4	0	1
Total experiencing pain	23	99	23	101

Source: Sleep (1984).

Table 8.7 Episiotomy policy trial. Incidence of pain reported by women at three months postpartum

Nature of pain experienced in last week	Restricted episiotomy policy (n = 438)		Liberal episiotomy policy (n = 457)	
	%	No.	%	No.
Mild	5	20	6	26
Moderate	2	11	2	8
Severe	1	2	0	1
Total experiencing pain	8	33	8	35

Source: Sleep (1984).

the incidences of pain and involuntary loss of urine associated with the two perineal management policies were very similar.

Discussion

The overall rate of severe maternal trauma was much lower than expected from other published studies. Nevertheless, the only justification to emerge from this study for recommending an episiotomy rate as high as 50% in

Table 8.8 Episiotomy policy trial. Incidence of resumption of sexual intercourse

Time of resumption of sexual intercourse	Restricted episiotomy policy		Liberal episiotomy policy	
	%	No.	%	No.
First month after delivery	37	162	27	123
Second month after delivery	44	193	53	242
Third month after delivery	10	44	10	46
Not yet	9	39	10	46
Total	100	438	100	457

Source: Sleep (1984).

Table 8.9 Episiotomy policy trial. Incidence of urinary incontinence at three months postpartum

Experience of loss of urine	Restricted episiotomy policy		Liberal episiotomy policy	
	%	No.	%	No.
No	81	355	81	370
Yes, but no pad necessary	13	56	13	59
Yes, and wear a pad sometimes	6	26	5	24
Yes, and wear a pad always	0	1	1	4
Total	100	438	100	457

Source: Sleep (1984).

women experiencing a normal delivery is that there were more cases of 'severe maternal trauma' among women allocated to the restrictive policy. This difference may have reflected a real effect of the restrictive policy, but despite the fact that 1000 women were entered into this trial it is still possible that the difference was due to chance. Of the five women who sustained severe trauma (four in the restrictive policy group and one in the liberal policy group) two were problem-free by three months and the other three were problem-free by 21 months.

Restricting the use of episiotomy to fetal indications resulted in neither an increase nor a major decrease in the problems experienced by women in the three months after delivery; the only difference observed was a tendency for women allocated to the restrictive episiotomy policy to resume sexual intercourse sooner. Our findings emerged from a study in which we controlled for selection bias and are in striking contrast with the findings of studies based on comparisons using observational data (Thacker and Banta, 1983; House, 1981; Kitzinger and Walters, 1981) all of which suggest that the discomfort after perineal tears is considerably less than after episiotomy.

A large proportion of women (19%) reported involuntary loss of urine three months postpartum but there is no evidence from this study that the 'liberal' use of episiotomy prevents this problem. It is still possible that it may prevent stress incontinence and vaginal prolapse in the longer term. For this reason we planned to recontact the women who participated in the trial, three years later, in order to assess the effect of both policies on subsequent recovery. Findings on recovery in the first three months after delivery suggest that the two currently opposing viewpoints are both wrong, in that tears do not appear to cause women fewer problems, and neither do episiotomies result in better healing and improved recovery. The findings also show, however, that restricting the incidence of episiotomy increases the number of women who deliver with no trauma at all.

THE FOLLOW-UP STUDY

Aims

Three years later we did, in fact, follow up the women who had participated in the original study. We considered, in particular, claims that the liberal use of episiotomy prevents urinary incontinence due to pelvic relaxation (Flood, 1982). We also investigated whether the procedure is associated with an increased prevalence of dyspareunia (Kitzinger and Walters, 1981).

Methods

The study was undertaken by means of a postal survey by questionnaire. This was the only feasible method to employ given the widespread geographical dispersion of women since the original trial. Women were asked whether they experienced urinary incontinence and if so, the degree of its severity, and whether they suffered from dyspareunia. They were also asked about their general health and whether they had had subsequent deliveries in the three years since the original study.

The procedure adopted for re-establishing the women's current whereabouts was as follows: first, approval was obtained for access to records held by the West Berkshire Family Practitioner Committee. Examination of these records indicated that just under half (481) of the original study participants had subsequently changed their address, 303 of whom were still living within the West Berkshire Health Authority. However, the new addresses of 100 of the 178 women who had moved away from the Health Authority were not known. The NHS Central Registry at Southport was able to provide the code of the family practitioner committee last known to hold the records of these women. We wrote and asked each committee for the name of the general practitioner with whom each woman was currently registered, and then wrote to the general practitioners asking them to forward a copy of the questionnaire to the women concerned. Of the 1000 women who took part in the original study, 63 proved to be untraceable, and we decided against contacting a further 15. This latter group comprised women who spoke little English, had refused to complete the three-month questionnaire or whose baby had been adopted, taken into care, or died.

A total of 674 questionnaires was returned. The response rate from women who had not changed address since the original study was much higher than for those who had moved (91% compared with 53%).

Findings

There was no evidence of a differential response rate to the follow-up study from the women in the two original trial groups; this is shown in Table 8.10. The original trial data were studied to assess the extent to which:

1. Responders differed from non-responders;
2. The two trial groups of responders matched the total trial populations.

Table 8.10 Episiotomy policy trial. Allocation to original trial groups by response to follow-up study

| Response to the three-year follow-up study | Allocation in original trial | | | |
| | Restricted episiotomy policy | | Liberal episiotomy policy | |
	%	No.	%	No.
Responded	66	329	69	345
Did not respond	34	169	31	157
Total	100	498	100	502

Source: Compiled by the author.

The findings are shown in Tables 8.11 and 8.12. The responders were slightly older on average than the non-responders, more likely to have been married at the time of the original trial and to have been delivered of a heavier baby nearer term. In terms of clinical outcome, the responders were more likely than the non-responders to have sustained trauma at delivery and to have reported perineal pain when questioned ten days postpartum.

The two trial groups of respondents were well matched; moreover, their patterns of perineal trauma sustained at delivery, subsequent pain, dyspareunia and urinary incontinence postpartum, were very similar to those reported in the total trial population in the original study. The subsequent obstetric histories of responders in the two trial groups were also similar, with 42% in the restrictive policy group and 39% in the liberal policy group having given birth since the original study. The majority of these were spontaneous vaginal deliveries. Although women in the restricted group seemed less likely to have episiotomies or require perineal suturing at subsequent deliveries, these differences were not significant.

Findings from the three-year follow-up questionnaire relating to dyspareunia and urinary incontinence are shown in Table 8.13. Similar proportions of women in the restrictive and liberal policy groups experienced dyspareunia (16% of the former and 13% of the latter). There was also no difference in the prevalence of urinary incontinence between the two groups (a total of 35% compared with a total of 37%) and the findings also show that the severity of incontinence experienced differed little. In response to a question on how they felt generally, 60% of women reported feeling very well, with a further 38% feeling quite well. The two trial groups did not differ significantly in this respect. Data for those women who had had no further children since the original study were analysed separately in order to ascertain whether their subsequent experience of dyspareunia and urinary incontinence differed from those women who had had more children. These analyses showed, however, that the experiences of these women differed little from those of the total group of respondents (details in Sleep and Grant, 1987b).

Discussion

As noted at the beginning of this chapter, a frequent claim in support of liberal use of episiotomy is that it prevents pelvic relaxation and, therefore, urinary incontinence and genital prolapse in the longer term. Although some degree of perineal stretching of the pelvic floor seems inevitable during childbirth, function of the pelvic floor muscles postnatally seems unrelated to perineal management at delivery (Gordon and Logue, 1985; Logue, Chapter 9). However, findings from the original trial indicated that restricted use of episiotomy is associated with greater incidence of anterior vaginal and labial tears (Tables 8.4 and 8.5) and this raises the possibility

Table 8.11 Episiotomy policy trial. Responders and non-responders to the follow-up study: details of the two trial groups at entry to original study

| Characteristics | Responders | | Non-responders | |
	Restricted policy (n = 329)	Liberal policy (n = 345)	Restricted policy (n = 169)	Liberal policy (n = 157)
Mean maternal age (years)	27.0	27.0	25.9	26.0
Proportion who were primiparous	41% (135)	44% (152)	39% (66)	43% (67)
Proportion who were married	91% (300)	92% (318)	86% (145)	75% (117)
Mean gestational age of baby (weeks)	39.8	40.0	39.7	39.5
Mean birth weight (grams)	3426	3407	3330	3280

Source: Reproduced from Sleep and Grant (1987b). Courtesy of the British Medical Journal.

Table 8.12 Episiotomy policy trial. Outcome measures for the two groups in total trial population and in responders to follow-up study

| | Total trial population | | | | Responders to follow-up | | | | Non-responders to follow-up | | | |
| | Restricted policy (n = 498) | | Liberal policy (n = 502) | | Restricted policy (n = 329) | | Liberal policy (n = 345) | | Restricted policy (n = 169) | | Liberal policy (n = 157) | |
	%	No.	%	No.	%	No.	%	No.	%	No.	%	No.
Posterior trauma												
None	34	169	24	122	31	102	21	73	40	67	31	49
Episiotomy alone	9	45	45	227	10	32	46	160	8	13	43	67
Perineal tear alone	56	278	24	123	58	190	27	92	52	88	20	31
Episiotomy with extension	1	6	6	30	2	5	6	20	1	1	6	10
Anterior perineal trauma (labial tears)	26	131	17	87	27	90	16	55	24	41	20	32
Perineal pain												
Pain in last 24 hours at 10 days after delivery	(n = 439)		(n = 446)		(n = 295)		(n = 315)		(n = 144)		(n = 131)	
	23	99	23	101	24	70	24	77	20	29	18	23
Pain in last week at 3 months post-partum	(n = 438)		(n = 457)		(n = 307)		(n = 338)		(n = 131)		(n = 119)	
	8	33	8	35	6	18	8	28	12	15	6	7

Table 8.12 (continued)

Dyspareunia											
at 3 months postpartum											
20	86	16	74	21	65	17	57	16	21	14	17
Urinary incontinence											
at 3 months post-partum but not requiring pad											
13	56	13	59	12	38	13	45	14	18	12	14
at 3 months post-partum requiring pad											
6	27	6	28	6	19	4	15	6	8	9	11

Source: Adapted from Sleep *et al.* (1984) and Sleep and Grant (1987b).

Table 8.13 Episiotomy policy trial. Dyspareunia and incontinence reported three years later

Symptoms of dyspareunia and incontinence	Allocation in original trial			
	Restricted episiotomy policy (n = 329)		Liberal episiotomy policy (N = 345)	
	%	No.	%	No.
Dyspareunia	(n = 324)		(n = 340)	
'ever suffering painful intercourse'	16	52	13	45
Incontinence	(n = 310)		(n = 333)	
Frequency: – less than once in past week	22	69	25	82
– once or twice in past week	12	37	10	35
– three or more time in past week	2	6	2	7
Sufficiently severe to wear a pad:				
– sometimes	8	26	7	24
– every day	2	5	1	4
Loss of urine when:				
– coughing, laughing or sneezing	33	103	32	105
– urgent desire to pass urine but no toilet nearby	13	41	12	41

Source: Adapted from Sleep and Grant (1987b).

that episiotomy may have a more specific protective effect on the bladder neck.

Our follow-up study revealed no clear differences between the two groups in respect of dyspareunia or in the prevalence of urinary incontinence. The latter finding applied even when the severity and nature of the incontinence and subsequent deliveries were taken into account. While recognizing that a more precise instrument might have shown differences in perineal outcome which our self-completed questionnaires failed to highlight, we could see no reason as to why our measurements should have been biased.

These findings related to longer-term recovery confirmed those for short-term recovery, namely that tears do not cause fewer problems, while episiotomies do not result in better healing and improved recovery. On the basis of these findings and in the absence of positive proof that the invasive procedure of episiotomy is of benefit to women, we suggest that the rationale for its use should be reappraised.

TRIAL 2: SUTURE MATERIAL FOR PERINEAL REPAIR

Perineal repair has now become part of the midwife's sphere of practice and is included in the curriculum for student midwives. While Robinson, Golden and Bradley (1983) found that in 1979 only 8% of midwives undertook this task, Garcia, Garforth and Ayers (1986 and Chapter 2 in this volume) found that by 1984 over 60% of consultant units had a policy that midwives could suture the perineum. As noted in the introduction to this chapter however, there is a dearth of evidence on which to base these newly acquired skills, and much variation in practice in choice of suture material and technique for repair (Grant, 1986).

The second trial in our series therefore focused on the important topic of suture material (Spencer *et al.*, 1986). We undertook a randomized controlled trial to compare untreated chromic catgut with a recently introduced material – glycerol-impregnated catgut (marketed as Softgut/Braun, and referred to as Softgut throughout this chapter). Outcome measures were based on both short- and longer-term maternal morbidity. The manufacturers (Davis and Geck Ltd, Gosport) claimed that 'Softgut' remained soft and supple during use and did not dry out like untreated catgut. It seemed possible, therefore, that its use might avoid longer-term problems of pain and dyspareunia known to be associated with polyglycolic acid sutures (Hansen *et al.*, 1975; Buchan and Nicholls, 1980).

Methods

The study was undertaken with the same 1000 women who participated in the episiotomy policy trial. Seven hundred and thirty seven of these women required perineal repair, and were randomly allocated to be sutured either with softgut ($n=377$) or untreated chromic catgut ($n=360$). In the hospital at this time (1982) perineal repairs were undertaken primarily by medical staff. The same material was used for all tissue layers that required repair. The vagina was repaired with a continuous suture, the deeper tissues with interrupted technique, and the perineal skin with either interrupted or subcuticular sutures according to operator preference. The operator's views on the use of the two suture materials, the time taken to carry out the repair and the amount of suture material were all recorded. The findings of the study are of considerable importance to midwives, first because perineal repair is now a midwifery responsibility and second, as the main providers of postnatal care their advice may be sought on measures to relieve discomfort that may be caused by sutures. The 10-day postpartum questionnaire used in the episiotomy trial (see section on Trial 1, page 202) included questions on perineal discomfort. It was given to each woman by the community midwife; on the same occasion she assessed healing and whether any sutures had been removed. Both the community midwife and the woman were 'blind' to the suture material allocation. The number of questionnaires returned was 89% for both the 'softgut' (335) and the catgut group (321). Data from this stage of the research enabled us to assess whether the two suture material groups differed in terms of short-term perineal discomfort, healing, and the need to remove sutures.

The three-months postpartum questionnaire assessed the incidence of perineal pain and discomfort, the time of resumption of sexual intercourse, dyspareunia, whether professional advice had been sought concerning perineal problems and whether resuturing of the perineum had been necessary. The response rate was 88% (332) for the softgut group and 90% (323) for the catgut group. These data enabled us to assess whether perineal problems experienced three months postpartum differed between the two groups.

Analyses of outcomes were based on unbiased comparisons between women allocated to either the softgut or the catgut group. Secondary analyses were also performed on the suture material actually used and the technique of perineal skin repair. Statistical comparison of discrete and continuous variables were made using chi-square and Student's t-tests respectively.

Three years later questionnaires were sent to all the women who had participated in the trial. The methods used for re-establishing contact with these women was described for the espisiotomy policy trial (see Trial 1). They were asked whether they experienced urinary incontinence and if they suffered from dyspareunia. They were also asked about their general health, and whether they had given birth again in the intervening period. A total of 516 questionnaires were returned, representing 70% of the total trial population.

Findings

Characteristics of trial groups Randomization generated two groups of women who were similar in the following respects at entry to the trial: mean maternal age; parity; marital status; gestational age, and birthweight. They were also similar with respect to type of perineal trauma sustained, status of doctor undertaking the repair, and perineal skin suture techniques (figures available in Spencer *et al.*, 1986). Over 90% of women in both groups were repaired with the suture material to which they had been allocated.

Use of suture material Questionnaires completed by 13 of the medical staff who undertook the perineal repairs showed that they found softgut easier to straighten out; it also remained softer and more supple during use. The two materials were considered equally easy to handle and to produce equally secure knots. There was no significant difference between the two materials in either the amount used or in the mean time taken to perform the repairs.

Outcomes at 10 days, 3 months and 3 years after delivery Outcomes at 10 days, 3 months and 3 years for the women who participated in the suture material trial are shown in Table 8.14. Data collected at 10 days postpartum show that women in the softgut group experienced greater prevalence of pain, and were more likely to have taken a salt bath on that day. Women in the catgut group were more likely to have had sutures removed by the 10th day usually for reasons of discomfort. The groups did not differ significantly in terms of healing by secondary intention or perineal breakdown.

By three months postpartum the prevalence of pain in the two groups was similar. As at 10 days, women in the catgut group were more likely to have had sutures removed. An equal proportion of both groups had resumed sexual intercourse by three months but those in the softgut group were more likely to have experienced both transient dyspareunia and dyspareunia persisting at three months.

Secondary analyses of the 10-day and 3-month data, based on suture material actually used, had no effect on the conclusions. Stratification by technique used to repair the perineal skin (i.e. subcuticular or interrupted sutures) indicated that differences between softgut and catgut in terms of perceived pain, dyspareunia and suture removal were more marked in women repaired with interrupted sutures although the differences were still apparent for those repaired with subcuticular sutures. Interrupted sutures were more commonly used to repair tears than to repair episiotomies and so the difference between the two suture materials was greater in the group of women who had torn spontaneously.

Table 8.14 Suture material trial. Outcomes for two groups at 10 days, 3 months and 3 years post-delivery

Outcomes	Allocated to repair with				
	softgut		catgut		
	%	No.	%	No.	
Outcomes at 10 days	(n = 335)		(n = 321)		
Degree of pain experienced within last 24 hours					
None	68	228	77	246	$p = 0.015$ (3d.f.)
Mild	21	70	14	46	
Moderate	10	32	9	29	
Severe	2	5	–	–	
Took a salt bath on 10th day	42	141	34	109	$p = 0.03$ (1d.f.)
Took oral analgesia on 10th day	4	12	2	6	NS
Healing by secondary intention	9	31	8	26	NS
Perineal breakdown	3	10	2	6	
Sutures removed	2	(8/336)	12	(37/322)	$p < 0.0001$ (1d.f.)
Outcomes at 3 months	(n = 339)		(n = 332)		
Degree of pain experienced within last 7 days					
None	91	309	93	308	NS (3d.f.)
Mild	7	22	5	17	
Moderate	2	7	2	7	
Severe	0	1	–	–	

Sutures removed	7	(23/332)	16	(53/323)	p<0.001 (1d.f.)
Resumption of sexual intercourse	88	(300/339)	88	(292/332)	NS
Occurrence of dyspareunia in women who had resumed intercourse by 3 months	(n = 300)		(n = 292)		p<0.025 (3d.f.)
None	38	114	51	148	
At first but not at 3 months	36	108	30	87	
Mild dyspareunia persisting at 3 months	23	70	18	53	
Moderate dyspareunia persisting at 3 months	3	8	1	4	
Outcomes at three years	(n = 263)		(n = 253)		
Management of first subsequent delivery	(n = 116)		(n = 97)		
Spontaneous vaginal	96	111	97	94	
Instrumental or caesarean	4	5	3	3	
Episiotomy performed in vaginal deliveries	25	(28/111)	14	(13/94)	p = 0.05 (1d.f.)
Perineum sutured in vaginal deliveries	74	(82/111)	73	(69/94)	NS
Sexual intercourse painful (all respondents)	19	51	12	29	p<0.02 (1d.f.)
Soreness		43		28	
Tightness		2		0	
Other		6		1	
Sexual intercourse painful in women with no subsequent deliveries	19	(28/146)	10	(15/155)	p<0.02 (1d.f.)
Soreness		23		14	
Tightness		1		0	
Other		4		1	

Source: Adapted from Spencer, Grant, Elbourne, Garcia and Sleep (1986) and Grant, Sleep, Ashurst & Spencer (1989).

Findings of the three-year follow-up study revealed that 44% of respondents who had been in the softgut group had had a subsequent delivery compared with 38% of those in the catgut group. Almost all the deliveries in both groups had been spontaneous and vaginal. There was a significant difference in the frequency with which episiotomy had been performed in the first delivery after the trial pregnancy, although this was not reflected in the overall frequency of perineal suturing. Women in the softgut group were significantly more likely to be experiencing dyspareunia at three years and this difference held when the analysis was limited to those who had not had a subsequent delivery. Most of the women described the dyspareunia as soreness.

Discussion

Women repaired after delivery with untreated chromic catgut were more likely to need sutures removed in the first three months after delivery than women repaired with glycerol-impregnated chromic catgut (softgut). However, the difference between the two groups in this respect is not sufficient to explain the greater prevalence in the softgut group of perineal pain at 10 days, dyspareunia at 3 months and persisting dyspareunia at 3 years. The most likely explanation is that perineal tissues reacted differently from the glycerol-impregnated catgut, possibly with increased fibrosis. The trial findings appear to reflect a true difference between the treated and untreated chromic catgut. This difference is clinically very important and indicates that softgut should not be used in perineal repair. The need to remove the untreated catgut sutures from one in six women raises further questions as to which absorbable material is most suitable for perineal repair. These issues have yet to be resolved (see Grant, 1986, 1989 for an overview of materials and suturing techniques used in perineal repair).

TRIAL 3: BATH ADDITIVES POST-DELIVERY

One in five of the women who took part in the episiotomy policy trial described above reported some degree of perineal pain at ten days postpartum (Table 8.6). In everyday midwifery care, bath additives are commonly recommended for the relief of this discomfort and a third of the women in this study were adding salt to their bath water during this initial period, thus demonstrating a widely held belief in its therapeutic properties. This in turn reflects the frequency with which perineal trauma causes discomfort.

Salt is one of the oldest remedies. It is believed to sooth discomfort and to promote healing (Watson, 1984) but a precise mode of action is unclear. Claims that it has antiseptic or antibacterial properties have not been confirmed (Ayliffe *et al.*, 1975) and there is no consensus as to the type of salt preparation, the quantity which should be used, or the length of time of immersion to produce the desired effect. Recommendations about the quantity range from a heaped tablespoon in a small bath (Marks and Ribero, 1933) to 3lb in 30 gallons of water (Houghton, 1940). Commercially prepared additives are now in increasing usage; one of the most frequently recommended is Savlon bath concentrate. It has both antiseptic and cleansing properties and is frequently used to treat inflamed or infected wounds. It has recently become available on the retail market for the first time and is packaged in 25 ml sachets, each of which contains chlorhexidine gluconate 1.5 per cent wv and cetrimide ph eur 15% wv in an aqueous solution. It is a deep orange in colour, pleasantly perfumed and foams as the bathwater is added.

As part of our programme of clinical research in perineal care, we undertook a randomized controlled trial to evaluate the usefulness or otherwise of adding salt or Savlon concentrate to the bath water in the immediate postpartum period. A control group of women was asked not to use any additive. The main hypotheses tested were that one or both additives would reduce the frequency of perineal pain and improve wound healing when assessed ten days after delivery, and would provide increased symptomatic relief during these ten days. Effects on time to resumption of sexual intercourse and dyspareunia three months after delivery were also assessed.

Methods

The trial took place over a seven-month period during 1985. Its size was preset at 1800 subjects. Power calculations indicated that in a trial of this size there would be a 90% chance of finding a statistically significant difference (2-tailed $\alpha = 0.05$) if the true effect of active treatment was a reduction by one-fifth in the frequency of perineal pain ten days postpartum, from an expected rate of 45% to 36%. The power would be 75% if the true effect is a reduction of a sixth (Sleep and Grant 1988a).

All women who had had a vaginal delivery were eligible for entry to the trial. These women were first identified from the birth register, and were then approached on the postnatal wards during the 24 hours following delivery. A verbal description of the study was given to each of the potential participants who were then invited to participate. Only when consent had been granted were the women formally given a random trial allocation, and this signalled the irrevocable entry of a woman into the trial.

The random allocation was to one of the three policies:

1. The addition of Savlon bath concentrate provided in prepacked 25 ml sachets; ten sachets were supplied for daily use over ten days;
2. The addition of crystalline table salt in measured quantities. An

adequate supply of salt to last ten days and a measure were provided. When filled to the top, each measure contained 42 g, i.e. the equivalent of two handfuls of salt;

3. No additive to be used.

During the study period, 1808 women were asked to participate. Of these, eight refused because they specifically wished to add salt during their recovery period and their wishes for their own care were respected. The remaining 1800 were randomly allocated to the three policies in equal-sized groups. At entry to the trial, descriptive data were collected from the case notes. These included variables such as maternal age, parity, mode of delivery, type of perineal trauma and method of repair, duration of gestation and baby's birth weight.

A standardized questionnaire was given to each woman by the community midwife on the tenth postnatal day. This was used to assess the following principal measures of outcome:

1. Presence and if so, degree of perineal pain (mild, moderate or severe);

2. The mother's opinion of bathing as a means of relieving perineal discomfort.

Ninety-five per cent (116) of the questionnaires were returned.

In addition the midwives recorded their observations of perineal healing, wound breakdown and infection. It was impossible to ensure that the community midwives were completely 'blind' to the trial allocation, although the women were asked not to volunteer the information. Perineal pain and its influence on the time of resumption of intercourse were assessed at three months after delivery using a standardized postal questionnaire sent to each woman.

All analyses were based on the comparisons between all women allocated to one or other of the bathing policies regardless of subsequent compliance. Indirect standardization was used to adjust for differences between the groups in a major prognostic variable. Outcome frequencies for each group were compared using the chi-square test and confidence intervals were calculated using the method recommended by Gardner and Altmann (1986).

Findings

Description of the three groups at trial entry Table 8.15 shows that the three groups generated were very similar in relation to characteristics at time of entry to the trial. Instrumental delivery was more common in the Savlon group ($p < 0.02$) and also, to a lesser extent, in the salt group ($p < 0.05$) and this was reflected in more common use of episiotomy in these

Table 8.15 Bath additives trial: Description of the three groups at entry to the trial

	Bath additive groups				
	Salt *(n = 600)*		*Savlon* *(n = 600)*		*No additive* *(n = 600)*
Mean maternal age (years)	26.5		26.5		26.9
Proportion who were primiparous	50%	299	50%	301	48% 289
Mean gestational age (weeks)	39.4		39.4		39.4
Mean birth weight (grams)	3295		3338		3332

Mode of delivery	%	No.	%	No.	%	No.
Normal	83	497	79	472	84	506
Assisted	17	103	21	128	16	94

Perineal trauma	%	No.	%	No.	%	No.
Episiotomy	40	239 [39%]	44	265 [40%]	39	233
Tear	33	199 [34%]	35	212 [38%]	37	221
No trauma requiring repair	27	161 [28%]	21	124 [22%]	24	145

Figures for salt and Savlon groups have been adjusted to take into account the differing frequencies of assisted deliveries in the three groups
Source: Sleep & Grant (1988a).

groups. For this reason, when appropriate, figures adjusted for mode of delivery have been presented in the tables, although these adjustments made little, if any, difference to the conclusions of the study.

Compliance with allocated policy Women's compliance with the bathing additive policy of the trial group to which they had been allocated was estimated on the last day of treatment (the tenth day). They were asked whether they had bathed within the 24 hours prior to completing the ten-day questionnaire and if so which additive, if any, they had used. The reason for estimating compliance on the last day of treatment was that rates were by then likely to be at their lowest. However, as the findings in Table 8.16 show, most women were following their trial instructions at this time.

Ten women (six in the salt group, three in the Savlon group and one in the no additive group) said that they had been unable to bath within the last

Table 8.16 Bath additives trial. Women's compliance with allocated policy

| | Bath additive groups | | |
	Salt (n = 569) %	Savlon (n = 566) %	No additive (n = 572) %
Bathed within 24 hours prior to completing tenth-day questionnaire	94	94	91
Bath additive of those who bathed			
— salt	89	5	7
— Savlon	2	87	1

Figures for salt and Savlon groups have been adjusted to take into account the differing frequencies of assisted deliveries in the three groups.
Source: Sleep and Grant (1988a).

24 hours. Seven of these women had no bath at home and three had received spinal taps which necessitated prolonged bed rest. The instruction to use an additive was associated with more frequent bathing on the tenth day (93.7% versus 90.7%, $p < 0.025$). Of those who bathed on the tenth day, compliance with the request to use salt or Savlon was very similar (89% and 87%); 7.9% of those who bathed in the 'no additive' group actually used an additive; this was most often salt and probably reflects the fact that salt was commonly recommended for perineal discomfort before this study was mounted (Sleep *et al.*, 1984).

Outcome at ten days after delivery The findings in relation to outcomes at ten days after delivery are shown in Table 8.17.

Oral analgesia was slightly more commonly used by women allocated to the additive policies, particularly 'salt' ($p = 0.06$). Other types of pain relief such as topical treatments, and antibiotics were equally commonly used by all three groups.

The prevalence and pattern of perineal discomfort on the tenth day of the puerperium was similar in the three groups and overall 55% of women were free of pain by this time. The adjusted frequency of the principal measure of outcome – pain on the tenth day after delivery – was very similar in the three groups. Compared with the control group, the rate was 3.8% lower in the salt group and 0.4% lower in the Savlon group. Although the relatively large sample sizes mean that these estimates are reasonably precise, it should be recognized that these are only estimates of the true effects of these policies. On the basis of this study it is possible to give a range within which the true

Table 8.17 Bath additives trial. Perineal discomfort and healing at ten days after delivery

	Bath additive groups		
	Salt (n = 576) %	Savlon (n = 566) %	No additive (n = 574) %
Use of oral analgesia on tenth day	9	7	6
Pain in last 24 hours at 10 days			
None	58	55	55
Mild	28	28	30
Moderate	12 } 42	16 } 45	13 } 45
Severe	2	1	2
Whether bathing helped over last 10 days			
A lot better	65	63	65
A little better	26	30	28
No better	6	7	8
Worse	1	1	–
Midwife's assessment of healing on tenth day			
Breaking down	2	1	1
Healing by second intention	7	9	9
Infected	3	4	3
Residual bruising	4	5	5

Figures for salt and Savlon groups have been adjusted to take into account the differing frequencies of assisted deliveries in the three groups
Source: Sleep and Grant (1988a).

effect is likely to lie. For salt this is somewhere between an increase of 2.7% and a decrease of 8.9% in perineal pain on the tenth day; and for Savlon it is somewhere between an increase of 5.4% and a decrease of 6.2% (95% confidence limits).

Overall, 93% of women reported that bathing during the first ten days after delivery had eased perineal discomfort and the rates for the three policies were very similar. Four per cent of women in the Savlon group were unhappy because Savlon tended to make the bath slippery. One per cent of women reported that salt caused skin irritation. On the other hand, 2% in each of the additive groups made especially positive comments about the additive they had used.

Wound healing as assessed by the community midwife on the tenth day, was also similar in the three groups, none of the differences observed being statistically significant.

Outcome at three months after delivery As noted 89% (1609) of women returned the questionnaire sent to them three months after delivery. The response rate in the three groups was similar and those who failed to respond at this stage did not appear to differ between the three groups. At this stage the women were asked whether they had experienced pain in the last week; they were also asked about resumption of sexual intercourse. Eleven per cent of women overall reported that they still experienced perineal pain, although for most this was described as 'mild'. As can be seen from findings in Table 8.18 there was no evidence however of an effect of the bath additives on either the incidence or the severity of this problem.

More than half of the 88% of women who had resumed sexual intercourse by three months described the experience as initially painful; for 23% intercourse was still painful at the time when they completed the questionnaire. These frequencies also appear unaffected by the bathing policy (Table 8.18).

Discussion

Overall there were no striking differences in outcome between the three bathing policies either at ten days or at three months after delivery.

If this study had been an uncontrolled descriptive study of the effects of adding salt or Savlon to bath water the interpretation of its findings might well have been different. At face value both additives appear to be popular, with 93% of women reporting that bathing with additives had made their perineal discomfort easier. The strength of this study is that it contains a 'no additive' comparison group and that the three groups were generated by random allocation. As it turned out, 93% in the 'no additive' group also felt that bathing had improved their perineal pain.

On the basis of the findings from this study there is no case for. recommending the routine use of salt or Savlon bath additives as a means of reducing maternal discomfort in the immediate postpartum period. A further question raised by this trial is the importance of regular bathing *per se* in the immediate postpartum period. Despite the fact that most women in the study (93%) felt it was beneficial, and that there is evidence that it may be beneficial for other conditions (Lindkaer Jenson, 1986) it is not possible to evaluate bathing in a bath as opposed to a shower from this study. The trial also raises questions about the use of these additives in nursing contexts. Wider generalization of the findings may not be appropriate, for

Table 8.18 Bath additives trial. Perineal pain/resumption of sexual intercourse three months after delivery

| Outcomes | Bath additive groups | | |
	Salt (n = 535) %	Savlon (n = 531) %	No additive (n = 543) %
Pain in past week, three months after delivery			
None	89	90	88
Mild	8	8	8
Moderate	3	2	3
Severe	–	0	1
Time to resumption of sexual intercourse			
In first month	32	34	31
In second month	46	45	48
In third month	9	10	9
Too painful	12	10	10
Not tried	1	1	2
Sexual intercourse painful at first	56	54	53
Sexual intercourse still painful	25	21	23

Figures for salt and Savlon groups have been adjusted to take into account the differing frequencies of assisted deliveries in the three groups
Source: Sleep and Grant (1988a).

example, to the care of grossly infected wounds. Nevertheless re-evaluation in branches of nursing now seems indicated.

TRIAL 4: URINARY INCONTINENCE AFTER DELIVERY—THE EFFECT OF PELVIC FLOOR EXERCISES

Approximately one-fifth of the women who took part in the episiotomy policy trial reported some degree of involuntary loss of urine three months after delivery (Table 8.9). When these women were followed up some three years later, 13% indicated that they were still suffering from this problem. Urinary, and also faecal incontinence represent a major source of personal and social embarrassment which can severely undermine the quality of life for a large number of women. Any measure which can help to prevent or treat the condition at an early stage will not only enhance the confidence of the individual but is also important for effective use of health service resources.

Weakness of the pelvic floor muscles caused by stretching during pregnancy and vaginal delivery has been advanced as a possible explanation for postpartum incontinence, and consequently pelvic floor exercises are often recommended as a means of prevention and treatment. Although there is some evidence that the more successfully the exercises are performed, the better the results (Shepherd, 1983), few attempts have been made to evaluate formally the role of these exercises in postnatal recovery (Mandelstam, 1978).

We decided to undertake such a study, by means of a randomized controlled trial, as part of our on-going programme of research. Our aim was to evaluate the extent to which a programme of more intensive pelvic floor exercises prevents urinary incontinence three months after delivery. As far as we know our original publication of findings from the study (Sleep and Grant 1987a) was the first report of a randomized controlled trial of the effectiveness of pelvic floor exercises in the postnatal period.

Methods

At the time the study was conducted, it was not considered acceptable to deprive women of any component of the standard postnatal exercise regime. We were not able therefore to establish a 'no treatment' control group as we had in the bath additive study. The postnatal exercises formed an implicit part of the prenatal programme offered in preparation for parenthood and in practical terms it would have been very difficult to implement such a control policy. Moreover the physiotherapists' commitment to and belief in the therapeutic effect of these exercises made them reluctant to totally omit such instruction from the pre- or postnatal programme.

We decided therefore to compare the current postnatal exercise programme in operation in the West Berkshire Health Authority with a scheme which reinforced this initial instruction during the immediate post-natal period and which also included more active participation ·by community midwives and health visitors once women returned home. Our main hypothesis was that the more intensive programme would reduce the prevalence of urinary incontinence three months after delivery. We also assessed whether the intensive programme would reduce perineal discomfort and increase the women's feelings of general well-being.

The trial size was pre-set at 1800 subjects. The anticipated rate of urinary incontinence in the control group was 20%. We felt it was important to identify a reduction by one quarter to 15% if this was the real effect of the intensive exercise programme. Such a reduction would produce a statistically significant difference (2-tailed $\alpha = 0.05$) 8 times out of 10 (a statistical power of 80% $\beta = 0.20$) in a trial with 1800 women. The severity of incontinence was also graded to further increase the statistical power (Sleep and Grant, 1987a).

The trial was conducted over a six-month period in 1985. Every morning, except Sundays, women who had had a vaginal delivery in the previous 24 hours were invited to take part in the study. A full explanation was given to each women prior to asking for her consent. All of those invited to take part in the study agreed to do so. We believe that the women recruited to the trial were representative of all those who had had a vaginal delivery in this hospital. Eighty per cent of women eligible for entry during the recruitment phase entered the trial and most of the 20% who did not, delivered on Sundays when women were not being recruited.

Prior to entry into the trial the multiparous women were asked whether or not they had experienced urinary incontinence prior to their first pregnancy; the primiparous women were asked about such episodes prior to conception. All women were questioned about urinary incontinence during their current pregnancy and whether or not they had regularly performed pelvic floor exercises within the last six months. They were then allocated at random to one of the two postnatal exercise policy groups. Once a woman had entered the study she was not withdrawn, regardless of subsequent use of exercises. All analyses are based on groups as allocated, as this is free of selection bias.

Upon entry to the trial, descriptive data were obtained from the women's case notes: these included maternal characteristics, mode of delivery and type of perineal trauma sustained. Women in both groups received initial instruction in pelvic floor exercises as currently available in the West Berkshire Health District. Practical teaching is provided as part of the antenatal education programme and after delivery this is endorsed by obstetric physiotherapists, who visit the postnatal wards once a day on Monday to Friday offering instruction to small groups of two to four women. We believe that this is in line with policy in the majority of consultant maternity units in Britain. In Reading, women are taught awareness of pelvic floor muscle contraction and advised to practise the exercise as often as they can remember, specifically in stopping the flow of urine midstream. Over 80% of the women are discharged to community midwifery care within 48 hours of delivery. If they are transferred to general practitioner units, their instruction is usually continued by a physiotherapist, whereas women transferred home rely on the community midwives' reinforcement of their initial instruction. An explanatory leaflet is usually provided. When women are discharged from midwifery care at 10–12 days postpartum, they become the responsibility of the health visitor and general practitioner.

In addition, women in the intensive exercise group were instructed individually by a midwife co-ordinator so that they received an extra exercise session daily (this included Saturdays). Prior to discharge, each woman was issued with a health diary which she was asked to complete daily over a four-week period. Such diaries have been used as a means of prospectively documenting morbidity (Verbrugge, 1980). In this study, they were intended as a memory aid to encourage compliance with the exercise programme and also to record the exercises performed by these women.

Each week the diary described a specific pelvic floor exercise. Women were asked to repeat the exercise as often as they could remember during the day. The exercises were incorporated in various daily household tasks and these were illustrated in cartoon form. It was hoped that these would provide a memory prompt so increasing motivation and compliance. In the first week postpartum when women were more likely to be resting, the exercise was gentle and suggested activities included bathing and going to the toilet. By the fourth week, they were asked to insert a finger into the vagina to feel the squeeze pressure of the muscles whilst the exercises were being performed during bathing or while taking a shower. Activities included doing the housework, standing at the sink and shopping. Each day they were asked to record whether they had complied with the regime. Community staff were able to identify women in the intensive exercise group by their possession of this diary. During the first four weeks after delivery, these women also received telephone reminders to help to motivate them in persevering with the programme. The diaries were returned at the end of this period, so there was an interval between the formal end of the intervention and the three-months postpartum assessment. The use of pelvic floor exercises was assessed at ten days and at three months after delivery.

At three months postpartum, all the women were sent a standardized postal questionnaire. This assessed the following outcome measures:

1. The prevalence and frequency of urinary incontinence;
2. The prevalence and severity of residual perineal pain;
3. The time of resumption of sexual intercourse;
4. The prevalence of dyspareunia;
5. The prevalence of faecal incontinence;
6. The woman's feelings of general well-being.

The response rate to the three month's questionnaire was slightly higher in the intensive group (91% compared with 88%) but there was no evidence that this introduced any important bias.

Findings

Characteristics of the two groups at entry to the trial Table 8.19 shows that the two groups were similar in most respects upon entry to the

Table 8.19 Pelvic floor exercises trial. Description of the two groups at entry to the trial

| Characteristics | Pelvic floor exercise groups | | | |
	Normal ($n = 900$)		Intensive ($n = 900$)	
Mean maternal age (years)	26.2		27.1	
Proportion who were primiparous	50%	(449)	49%	(440)
Mean gestational age (weeks)	39.5		39.4	
Mean birthweight (grams)	3327		3316	
During pregnancy:	%	No.	%	No.
Experienced incontinence	29	257	32	288
Undertook pelvic exercises	46	410	59	533
Mode of delivery				
Normal	84	752	80	723
Assisted	16	148	20	177
Perineal trauma				
Episiotomy	40	360	42	378
Tear	35	311	36	321
No trauma requiring repair	25	229	22	201

Source: Adapted from Sleep and Grant (1987a).

trial. Women in the intensive exercise group were more likely to report that they had urinary incontinence during the pregnancy (32% compared with 29%) and more women in this group reported using pelvic floor exercises during the pregnancy (59% compared with 46%).

Compliance with exercise policy of trial group to which allocated By the time of the community midwife's visit on the tenth postnatal day, women in the intensive exercise group were more likely to have performed their exercises than women allocated to the normal policy (78% compared with 68%). This difference was greater three months after delivery (58% compared with 42%). Judging by their entries in the diaries, women in the intensive exercise group who performed exercises persevered with the full programme.

Table 8.20 Pelvic floor exercises trial. Prevalence of urinary and faecal incontinence at three months after delivery

| Prevalence of incontinence | Pelvic floor exercise groups | | | |
| | Normal (n = 793) | | Intensive (n = 816) | |
	%	No.	%	No.
Involuntary loss of urine	22	175	22	180
Less than once a week	14	107	13	107
Once or twice a week	6	48	7	55
Three or more times a week	1	9	1	9
Not recorded	1	11	1	9
Wearing a pad for urinary incontinence				
Sometimes	4	33	4	29
Always	1	10	2	12
Occasional faecal loss	3	22	3	21

Source: Sleep and Grant (1987a).

Outcomes at three months postpartum Findings from the questionnaire sent to the two groups of women in the study at three months after delivery are shown in Tables 8.20 and 8.21. At this stage one-fifth of women overall were experiencing some degree of urinary incontinence; for some 5% of respondents this necessitated wearing a pad for some or all of the time. Occasional faecal incontinence was experienced by 3% of respondents. The incidence of both urinary and faecal incontinence did not differ appreciably between the two groups (Table 8.20). Although women who reported using pelvic floor exercises in pregnancy were somewhat more likely to have incontinence postpartum, (24% compared with 20%), statistical adjustment by indirect standardization for the imbalance between the two randomized groups in this respect had no important effect on these findings.

The majority of women had resumed intercourse at 3 months postpartum, although 12% admitted either that they had not yet attempted intercourse or that an attempt had proved too painful. Overall, 47% of women said that they experienced dyspareunia initially and for 20% this problem persisted. Again there was little difference between the two trial groups in these respects and adjustment for exercises in pregnancy made no difference.

The two groups did, however, differ in the 'pain in the last week' reported

Table 8.21 Pelvic floor exercises trial. Perineal symptoms at three months after delivery

| Symptoms | Pelvic floor exercise groups | | | |
| | Normal (n = 793) | | Intensive (n = 816) | |
	%	No.	%	No.
Pain in the past week	13	101	9	76
Mild	9	69	7	60
Moderate	4	28	2	15
Severe	1	4	0	1
Time of resumption of sexual intercourse				
In first month	33	263	31	249
In second month	44	351	47	380
In third month	8	67	10	85
Too painful	2	13	1	9
Not attempted	11	90	10	85
Not recorded	1	9	1	8
Intercourse painful at first	46	368	48	391
Intercourse still painful	19	154	20	167

Source: Sleep and Grant (1987a).

in the three months questionnaire. The chi-square test was used to compare frequencies in the two groups. The differences in severity as judged by graded categorical responses (for example, none, mild, moderate, severe pain) were assessed using the chi-square test for trend (Armitage, 1971). When the severity of the pain was taken into account, the difference was statistically significant (χ^2 for trend = 7.14; $p < 0.01$). Adjustment for exercise use in pregnancy by direct standardization, if anything, slightly increased this difference. The women's feelings of general well-being also appeared to be improved by involvement in the intensive exercise programme (Table 8.22); in particular, fewer women reported feelings of depression (χ^2 for trend = 5.30; $p < 0.05$).

Discussion

The main difficulty in the interpretation of findings from this study is

Table 8.22 Pelvic floor exercises trial. Women's feelings of well-being three months after delivery

| Women's feelings | Pelvic floor exercise groups | | | |
| | Normal (n = 793) | | Intensive (n = 816) | |
	%	No.	%	No.
How are you feeling generally?				
Very well	56	446	60	494
Quite well	40	321	38	309
Not very well	2	17	1	11
Not at all well	0	1	–	–
Not recorded	1	8	0	2
Some women feel depressed at this time.				
Do you feel:				
Very depressed	2	13	1	8
Quite depressed	9	71	8	63
Not very depressed	30	239	27	219
Not at all depressed	58	461	64	522
Not recorded	1	9	1	4

Source: Sleep and Grant (1987a).

uncertainty about the nature and extent of the difference in the use of exercises by the two groups. Although it is possible to describe the extra education and encouragement given to the women in the intensive group, it is less easy to describe the ways in which exercises were used by both groups of women. In retrospect, we should have enquired more clearly whether exercises had been performed during the previous 24 hours rather than specifically on the tenth day, as in many instances the midwife had visited early in the morning. The fact that the difference was even greater at three months suggested that the difference at ten days may be an under-estimation. Many women remarked that the discipline required to complete the daily questionnaire in their diary had helped to sustain their motivation. There was evidence to suggest that the majority found the format more helpful than the exercise sheet currently in use.

It is possible that heightened awareness of postnatal exercises within the hospital and amongst the community midwives, and contact with women in the intervention group, may have resulted in the control group performing their exercises more diligently than is usually associated with standard hospital policy. We did consider randomizing women to different postnatal wards to avoid this 'contamination', but we finally elected to allocate them within each ward because most women stay for only 24–48 hours, and because this arrangement was much simpler in practice.

The methods used to measure compliance were, anyway, not totally reliable and the responses at both ten days and three months could be biased in either direction. We did consider trying to assess whether the pelvic floor exercises were being performed properly by recording the increase in pressure transmitted through a perineometer inserted in the vagina. Other authors have reported the value of this device as a teaching aid (Kegel, 1951; Shepherd, Montgomery and Anderson, 1983). However, as the women in this study were recruited immediately following delivery, at a time when most of them will suffer varying degrees of perineal pain, it was considered aesthetically unacceptable to introduce them to such a device; furthermore, we were reluctant to assess compliance in the control group in this way because the use of a perineometer might alter the way in which exercises were subsequently performed by this group.

One of the differences observed between the two groups was in pain 'in the tail-end' three months after delivery. This was not, however, reflected in differences in dyspareunia or in the timing of resumption of sexual intercourse. The differences between the two groups in women's feelings of well-being may reflect the difference in perineal discomfort. They may also be a consequence of the greater 'social' support provided by the intensive programme. Social support interventions during pregnancy appear to have similar psychosocial benefits (Oakley, Chalmers and Elbourne, 1986).

Urinary and faecal incontinence rates in the two groups were similar in frequency and severity. This study therefore provided no support for the hypothesis that a programme of more intensive postnatal exercise education prevents these problems. There is a growing body of evidence that the risk of incontinence is not related directly to the extent of trauma to perineal tissues at delivery (Yarnell *et al.*, 1982; Sleep *et al.*, 1984; Gordon and Logue, 1985). Snooks and his colleagues (1984) have recently suggested that faecal and urinary incontinence following vaginal delivery result from damage to the innervation of pelvic floor muscles, rather than stretching of muscles. If it is true, specific exercises may be of limited value in preventing incontinence.

Although there have been no formal randomized trials, observational studies have suggested that the use of pelvic floor exercises increases perineal muscle tone (Shepherd, 1983; Gordon and Logue, 1985). This is a possible mechanism for the reduction in pain which this study suggests is caused by intensive exercises. The study does not, however, suggest that conforming to a programme of intensive pelvic floor exercises postpartum is a critical factor in preventing urinary and faecal incontinence following vaginal delivery. This in turn raises questions about the value and content of the exercise programmes currently offered to women around the time of childbirth. It is possible that the substantial resources involved could be used more effectively. At the time when this study was designed, there was considerable reluctance on the part of physiotherapists to deprive women of any component of the standard exercise programme; in the light of these findings a more flexible approach is now possible which would make such a design both acceptable and desirable.

TRIAL 5: ULTRASOUND AND PULSED ELECTROMAGNETIC ENERGY TREATMENT FOR PERINEAL TRAUMA—A RANDOMIZED PLACEBO-CONTROLLED TRIAL

Introduction

The first trial in this series revealed that during vaginal delivery 70% of women sustained perineal trauma sufficiently severe to necessitate surgical repair. The three year follow-up revealed that this trauma commonly causes pain and discomfort persisting for months. In recent years, ultrasound therapy and to a lesser extent pulsed electromagnetic therapy, have been used increasingly to treat perineal trauma. In a telephone survey of 36 randomly selected consultant maternity units that we conducted in 1987 (Sleep and Grant, 1988c), we found that ultrasound therapy was being used for this purpose in 42% (15) of these units and pulsed electromagnetic therapy in 8% (3). Both therapies have been the subject of randomized controlled trials and these have been reviewed in Grant and Sleep (1989).

For the last trial in our series undertaken at the Royal Berkshire Hospital, Reading, we undertook a randomized controlled trial comparing ultrasound and pulsed electromagnetic therapy with double-blind (placebo) treatment (Grant *et al.*, 1989b). The therapies were given to women with moderate or severe perineal trauma and begun within 24 hours after delivery.

Two main hypotheses were tested: first that either or both techniques would reduce frequency and severity of perineal pain on the 10th day post-partum; secondly, active treatment would reduce the length of time before sexual intercourse was resumed and increase the frequency of pain-free intercourse at three months. We also examined the effects of the two therapies on perineal pain at other times, use of oral analgesia, perineal oedema, bruising and haemorrhoids, and the women's feelings of well-being.

Methods

Trial entry and allocation The trial size was preset at 400, based on an expected prevalence of perineal pain 10 days after delivery in the placebo group of 50%. This size has an 80% chance of showing a statistically significant difference if active treatment reduces this prevalence by one-third.

Recruitment to the trial took place on the postnatal wards on weekdays over a 7 month period in 1986. Women were deemed to be eligible for entry to the trial if they:

1. Required operative vaginal delivery; or
2. Sustained perineal trauma involving extensive damage to the anal sphincter or damage to anal or rectal mucosa; or
3. Developed severe perineal oedema, bruising or haematoma within 24 hours of delivery.

A total of 419 women fulfilled the entry criteria and were then asked if they were willing to participate in the research; 414 agreed to do so. At entry to the trial, each woman was given a trial number and allocated a correspondingly numbered sealed opaque envelope. This contained the random treatment allocation; first either to receive ultrasound therapy or to receive pulsed electromagnetic energy therapy, and second to a number that signified random allocation to either the group to receive active treatment or to a placebo group. In keeping with the principles of randomized controlled trials, once the envelope had been opened by the physiotherapist researcher, the woman remained in her allocated group for the purpose of analysis, irrespective of subsequent management.

One hundred and thirty-five women were allocated to pulsed electromagnetic energy treatment (PEME), 140 to ultrasound treatment and a total of 139 to the two placebo groups. Therapy was usually started about 12 hours after delivery, and always within 24 hours. This was because so many women now leave hospital after two days, and also it was thought that early treatment might prevent problems in the long term. A maximum of three treatments were given during a 36-hour period. Each machine used for the trial had a specially fitted 12-number dial. Eight of the settings were active and four were placebo; the operator was blind to the setting code. The codes were changed at two-monthly intervals to minimize the risk of the operator breaking the code and thereby introducing bias. The therapists were also checked for sensitivity to the vibration of the ultrasound transmitter and it was confirmed that they could not distinguish between the active and inactive modes. All women received the treatment to which they were allocated and all but two received three treatments. The duration of each PEME therapy was 10 minutes, ultrasound was applied for more variable lengths of time depending upon the extent of trauma (mean: 8.2 minutes in the actively treated group and 7.5 minutes in the placebo group). Further details of the machines used and their mode of operation during the trial are described in Grant *et al.* (1989b).

Assessments Assessments were made before treatment, within two hours after treatment and at ten days and three months postpartum. At the pre- and post-therapy assessments the midwife co-ordinator documented the extent of oedema, bruising, haemorrhoids and any analgesia required over the course of treatment. The women were asked to rate perineal pain experienced using 10 cm linear analogue and categorical scales. After treatment they were also asked if they felt better.

Ten days after delivery a further assessment of pain and healing was made by the women and by the community midwife. Completed assessment forms were returned for 96% (129/135) of those in the pulsed electro-magnetic energy therapy group and 96% (134/140) of those in the ultra-sound therapy group and 94% (131/139) of those in the two placebo groups.

At three months after delivery, the women were sent a postal questionnaire requesting information about perineal pain, resumption of sexual intercourse and experience of dyspareunia. These questionnaires were returned by 92%, 90% and 90% of the pulsed electromagnetic energy group, the ultrasound group and the placebo groups respectively.

It was not possible to conceal from the women which type of machine was used for their treatment, but they did not know whether they were in the active treatment group or the placebo group. In most cases the research midwife and community midwives who made the assessments did not know either the type of machine to which the woman had been allocated and none of them knew whether the treatment was active or placebo.

Analysis The findings for the two placebo groups were very similar; for the purposes of analysis they were therefore amalgamated to give a single placebo group ($n = 139$) of the same size as the two actively treated groups. Differences between the groups were examined using chi-square and t-tests with one-way analysis of variance. Confidence intervals for relative risks were calculated using the method recommended by Katz *et al.* (1978).

Findings

Randomization generated three groups of women who were similar at trial entry in terms of maternal age, parity, gestational age and birthweight. Comparable proportions in each group had an instrumental or breech delivery (69% overall), extension of an episiotomy (18% overall) or third-degree perineal trauma (4% overall). Table 8.23 shows that the three groups were also comparable at trial entry in terms of the degree of perineal pain experienced and the presence of bruising, oedema and haemorrhoids.

Effects after treatment Findings from the assessments made after the women had received treatment are shown in Table 8.24. A substantial majority (over 90% in each group) felt that the treatment made them feel

Table 8.23 Perineal trauma therapy trial: pain and trauma at trial entry

Perineal trauma	Pulsed electro-magnetic energy (n = 135)		Ultrasound (n = 140)		Placebo (n = 139)	
	%	No.	%	No.	%	No.
Perineal pain						
None	4	5	6	8	6	8
Effective epidural	7	9	3	4	7	9
Mild	15	20	13	18	16	22
Moderate	52	70	56	79	51	70
Severe	23	31	22	30	21	29
Bruising	51	68	60	82	53	74
Oedema	33	45	37	52	30	42
Haemorrhoids	21	28	24	33	24	33

Source: Adapted from Grant, Sleep, McIntosh and Ashurst (1989). By courtesy of the British Journal of Obstetrics and Gynaecology.

better; and it can be seen from Table 8.24 that the proportion who said 'a little better' and the proportion who said 'a lot better' were similar for each group. The findings also showed a similar improvement for each group with regard to pain, oedema and haemorrhoids. Although the ultrasound group showed a greater improvement in the linear analogue pain scale, this was not statistically significant. The only difference to emerge at this stage after treatment was that the ultrasound group did have more bruising and showed a significantly smaller reduction in the extent of bruising over the course of treatment when compared with the placebo ultrasound group ($p < 0.05$).

Effects at 10 days and at three months At 10 days postpartum women who had received pulsed electromagnetic energy therapy were more likely to report perineal pain than women in the other two groups (Table 8.25) ($p < 0.05$, 2 d.f.). By this time the ultrasonic group had the lowest prevalence of bruising although the difference was not statistically significant. At three months postpartum (Table 8.26) there were no statistically significant differences between the three groups in the prevalence of perineal pain, urinary or faecal incontinence, dyspareunia, or in women's feelings of well-being. Overall prevalences at this stage were 15% for perineal pain, 16% for dyspareunia and urinary incontinence and 4% for faecal incontinence.

Table 8.24 Perineal trauma therapy trial. Assessment of pain and trauma within 2 hours after treatment

Pain and trauma assessments		Pulsed electro-magnetic energy (n = 135)		Ultrasound (n = 140)		Placebo (n = 139)	
		%	No.	%	No.	%	No.
Woman's assessment							
A little worse or no better		8	11	7	10	11	15
A little better		56	75	50	70	53	73
A lot better		36	49	43	60	36	50
Pain free		13	17	12	17	12	17
Improvement in linear analogue pain rating if pain at pre-treatment assessment	Mean	21.6 mm		25.3 mm		21.1 mm	
	SE	1.9 mm		1.8 mm		2.1 mm	
Bruise free		52	70	43	60	50	69
Mean reduction in bruise size (if bruised at first)	Mean	2.9 mm		0.7 mm		3.2 mm*	
	SE	0.9 mm		0.8 mm		0.8 mm	

Oedema free	81	109	79	111	78	108
Haemorrhoid free	79	107	81	114	78	108
Mean change in size (if haemorrhoid at first)						
Mean	4.1 mm		4.4 mm		4.0 mm	
SE	0.7 mm		0.8 mm		0.7 mm	

*p 0.05

Source: Reproduced from Grant, Sleep, McIntosh and Ashurst (1989). By courtesy of the British Journal of Obstetrics and Gynaecology.

Table 8.25 Perineal trauma therapy trial. Assessment of pain and trauma at 10 days after delivery

Pain and trauma assessments	Pulsed electro-magnetic energy (n = 129)		Ultrasound (n = 134)		Placebo (n = 131)	
	%	No.	%	No.	%	No.
Perineal pain in last 24 hours reported by woman						
None	26	33	40	53	37	48
Mild	44	57	37	50	34	44
Moderate	23	30	18	24	25	33
Severe	7	9	5	7	5	6
Use of pain killers in last 24 hours	24	31	22	30	19	25
Community midwife's assessment						
Perineal wound breaking down	5	6	4	6	2	3
Haemorrhoids	26	33	26	35	24	33
Bruising	17	22	10	14	14	18
Oedema	10	13	8	10	8	11

Source: Reproduced from Grant, Sleep, McIntosh and Ashurst (1989). By courtesy of the British Journal of Obstetrics and Gynaecology.

Table 8.26 Perineal trauma therapy. Assessment of pain and resumption of sexual intercourse at three months after delivery

Pain and trauma assessments	Pulsed electro-magnetic energy (n = 124)		Ultrasound (n = 126)		Placebo (n = 125)	
	%	No.	%	No.	%	No.
Perineal pain (worst in last week)						
None	82	101	90	113	83	104
Mild	11	14	5	6	16	20
Moderate	6	8	6	7	1	1
Severe	1	1	–	0	–	0
Resumed sexual intercourse	82	101	74	93	80	100
Pain-free sexual intercourse	33	41	26	33	30	37

Source: Reproduced from Grant, Sleep, McIntosh and Ashurst (1989). By courtesy of the British Journal of Obstetrics and Gynaecology.

Discussion

The women who participated in this trial were at high risk of persistent perineal pain. Compared with the women who took part in the first trial they were 3 times more likely to experience pain at 10 days after delivery (66%, compared with 23%) and twice as likely to do so 3 months postpartum (15% compared with 8%). Assessment of the effectiveness of ultrasound and pulsed electromagnetic energy treatments to reduce this pain showed little clear benefit of either treatment. Women in the pulsed electromagnetic energy group had more pain 10 days after delivery, but there were no differences in pain between the three groups at 3 months postpartum. Bruising was more extensive immediately following ultrasound therapy, but also seemed to disappear more rapidly afterwards, although this latter difference was not statistically significant.

For all other assessments made after treatment, at 10 days and at 3 months after delivery, no significant differences emerged between the two therapy groups or between the therapy groups and the placebo groups. Further discussion of possible explanations for the findings of the trial are available in Grant *et al.*, 1989b. Suffice it to say here that on the basis of our findings, we suggest that current enthusiasm for these new therapies should be tempered. We also suggest that further controlled trials are needed to replicate our design, to assess different machine settings and length of treatment and to assess the usefulness of these two therapies in other obstetric settings.

CONCLUSION

The series of randomized controlled trials described in this chapter demonstrates the importance of evaluating the effectiveness of long established practices in maternity care, as well as those that have been introduced more recently. The trials also demonstrate the need for critical evaluation of products marketed for use by providers and consumers of maternity services.

Turning first to our episiotomy policy trial, despite national rates well in excess of 50% (and 70% for primiparae), we found little justification for a rate higher than 10% of normal deliveries. We found no support for the view that tears cause fewer problems than episiotomies, while the latter do not result in better healing and improved recovery. Their use should therefore be restricted to fetal indications only. The second trial demonstrated that glycerol-impregnated chromic catgut, a material in common use for perineal repair, was associated with a higher incidence of dyspareunia at three months and long lasting adverse effects for up to three years post-delivery, when compared with untreated chromic catgut. Its use in clinical care should therefore be discontinued.

The third trial focused on the efficacy of bathing additives after delivery in relieving perineal pain, promoting healing and resumption of intercourse. We found no difference between adding salt (a long-established remedy), adding Savlon bath concentrate or bathing with no additives at all. This suggests that mothers need not be actively encouraged to buy either of these additives. Findings from the fourth trial provided no support for the hypothesis that intensive pelvic floor exercise regimes after delivery prevent incontinence. The content of current postnatal exercise programmes offered to mothers should therefore be reconsidered. Finally, the fifth trial showed no clear benefit resulting from either of two recently introduced electrical therapies (ultrasound and pulsed electromagnetic energy) aimed at reducing perineal pain and trauma after delivery. Replication studies are now needed before large financial investment is made to supply this costly equipment. All five trials have important implications not only for clinical practice but also for the use of resources both in terms of professional time spent in conducting procedures of questionable benefit to recipient women and in expenditure on unefficacious therapies.

Our programme of research investigated various aspects of perineal care and management. Much, however, remains to be done. As discussed at the end of each of the preceding sections, some of our studies, or aspects of them, need to be replicated. Moreover, many other aspects of care remain unevaluated or poorly evaluated; these include different suturing techniques, the choice of suture materials and the use of topical and oral preparations for relieving perineal pain. As Grant (1986) comments, research into these topics may seem unglamorous, but is undoubtedly relevant in improving the comfort and quality of life of literally hundreds of thousands of women worldwide.

Studies such as the ones described in this chapter have important implications for midwifery practice and education. Firstly, midwives have a responsibility to base their clinical care and advice on research-based evidence, and not on tradition, personal preference or whims of fashion; only in this way will women receive the kind of care most likely to be effective and beneficial. If research-based practice is to become a reality, however, midwifery teachers must base their teaching on research findings whenever possible and encourage students to read critically. Similarly managers must foster innovation and support the implementation of research findings in the units for which they are responsible. A multi-disciplinary team approach should be actively encouraged and facilitated. A commitment to improving practice entails keeping up-to-date by reading a range of journals, discussing with colleagues ways in which relevant research can be used as the basis for change, supporting those who undertake research and maybe undertaking research oneself. The latter may take the form of a single small-scale study conducted by one or two people, or as with the research described here may be a large-scale collaborative effort over a number of years.

Secondly there is the issue of developing and maintaining midwifery skills in perineal management and care. There is evidence that in some units, the episiotomy rate is falling. At the Royal Berkshire Hospital, for example, the rate before the first trial was undertaken was 61%, whereas by 1987 it was 20%. Similarly at Northwick Park Hospital the rate was reduced from 39% in 1981 to 12% in 1987 (see Chapter 9 in this volume). Reducing the incidence of episiotomy however, is not a simple matter of throwing away the Mayo scissors. Much concern has been expressed that midwives have either never developed or have lost, the art of managing the perineum with patience, anticipation and confidence but without intervention. These special qualities need to be actively nurtured and encouraged if midwives are to develop and maintain confidence in their delivery skills. Similarly skills in undertaking perineal repair need to be fostered and, as Grant (1986) suggests, alternative teaching strategies in this respect should be evaluated.

Thirdly these studies indicate the necessity for midwives to assess the longer term implications of their care. Rigorous documentation and enquiry into the causes of maternal death have provided the basis for action resulting in a drastic reduction in mortality rates. Perhaps what we now need is to develop a system of recording morbidity. It would not be an onerous exercise for community midwives to record details of good or poor perineal healing. This would help to assess short-term recovery. The number of women needing gynaecological admission for corrective perineal surgery (e.g. Fenton's operation) and those attending physiotherapy units for electrical therapy to scar tissue would provide information on some of the longer term problems. These figures could then be discussed at ward and unit meetings as a means of auditing care and the basis for remedial action. A multi-disciplinary approach to this task should be encouraged. The longer term problems such as dyspareunia, urinary incontinence, loss of self esteem and altered body image may not be life threatening experiences but can prove to be life sentences. We have only recently become aware of the size of the problem. All aspects of perineal management and care present midwives with a challenge. Women trust in our judgement and in our care and we must ensure that this trust is not misplaced.

ACKNOWLEDGEMENTS

The conduct of such a programme of clinical research requires the help and support of a large number of people. Principally, Adrian Grant of the National Perinatal Epidemiology Unit (NPEU) in Oxford, who was responsible for the design and supervision of each of the trials; other colleagues at the NPEU – Jo Garcia, Diana Elbourne, Hazel Ashurst and Iain Chalmers, without whose encouragement and support these studies would not have been mounted. The success of the programme was also due to the hard work of the many midwives, obstetricians and obstetric physiotherapists in the West Berkshire Health District, and the women who responded so enthusiastically to our requests for information about their experiences. Funding for the work came from several sources, principally the locally organized research scheme of the Oxford Regional Health Authority; other agencies included the Maw's scholarship, ICI Pharmaceuticals Division, IMI Medical Supplies, and Davis and Geck Ltd. The NPEU is supported by a grant from the Department of Health.

REFERENCES

Armitage, P. (1971) *Statistical Methods in Medical Research*, Blackwell Scientific Publications, Oxford, pp. 363–5.

Ayliffe, G.A.B., Babb, J.R., Collins, R.J., Davies, J., Deverill, C., Varney, J. (1975) Disinfection of baths and bathwater. *Nursing Times Supplement*, **11** September, 22–3.

Buchan, P.C., Nicholls, J.A.J. (1980) Pain after episiotomy – a comparison of two methods of repair. *J.R. Coll. Gen. Pract.* **30**, 297–300.

Central Midwives Board (1983) Final report on the work of the Board p. 18. Hymns Ancient and Modern. Suffolk.

Chalmers, I. (1978) Implications of the current debate on obstetric practice. In Kitzinger, S. and Davis, J. (eds) *The place of birth*, Oxford University Press, Oxford.

Chalmers, I. (1989) Evaluating the effects of care during childbirth. In Chalmers, I., Enkin, M. and Keirse, M. (eds) *Effective Care in Pregnancy and Childbirth. Vol. 1*, Oxford University Press, Oxford.

Chalmers, I. and Richards, M. (1977) Intervention and causal inference in obstetric practice. In Chard, T. and Richards, M. (eds) *Benefits and hazards of the new obstetrics*, The Lavenham Press, Suffolk.

Cochrane, A.L. (1972) *Effectiveness and Efficiency*. Nuffield Provincial Hospitals Trust, London.

Cochrane, A.L. (1979) 1931–1971: A critical review with particular reference to the medical profession. In *Medicines for the Year 2000* (ed. G. Teeling-Smith) Office of Health Economics, London. pp.1–11.

Donald, I. (1979) *Practical obstetric problems*, London Lloyd-Luke, p. 817.

Flood, C. (1982) The real reasons for performing episiotomies. *World Medicine*, **6** February p. 51.

Garcia, J. Garforth, S. and Ayers, S. (1986) Midwives Confined? Labour ward policies and routines. In Thomson, A. and Robinson, S. (eds) *Research and the Midwife Conference Proceedings for 1985*, Nursing Research Unit, King's College, University of London.

Gardner, M.J. and Altman, D.G. (1986) Confidence intervals rather than P values: estimation rather than hypothesis testing. *British Medical Journal*, **292**, 746–50.

Grant, A. (1983) Evaluating midwifery practice: the role of the randomised controlled trial. In Thomson, A. and Robinson, S. (eds) *Research and the Midwife Conference Proceedings for 1982*. Nursing Research Unit, King's College, London University.

Grant, A. (1986) Repair of episiotomies and perineal tears. *British Journal of Obstetrics and Gynaecology*, **93**, 417–9.

Grant, A. (1989) Repair of perineal trauma after childbirth. In Chalmers, I. Enkin, M. and Keirse, M.J.N.C. (eds). *Effective Care in Pregnancy and Childbirth vol. 2*, Oxford University Press, Oxford.

Grant, A and Sleep, J. (1989) Relief of perineal pain and discomfort after childbirth. In Chalmers, I., Enkin, M. and Keirse, M.J.N.C. (eds) *Effective Care in Pregnancy and Childbirth*. Vol. 2. Oxford University Press, Oxford. pp. 1347–58.

Grant, A., Sleep, J., Ashurst, H. and Spencer, J. (1989a) Dyspareunia associated with the use of glycerol-impregnated catgut to repair perineal trauma. Report of a 3 year follow-up study. *British Journal of Obstetrics and Gynaecology*, **96**, 741–3.

Grant, A., Sleep, J., McIntosh, J. and Ashurst, H. (1989b) Ultrasound and pulsed electromagnetic energy treatment for perineal trauma. A randomized placebo controlled trial. *British Journal of Obstetrics and Gynaecology*, **96**, 434–9.

Gordon, H. and Logue, M. (1985) Perineal muscle function after childbirth. *Lancet*, 20 July, 123–5.

Hansen, M.K., Selnes, A., Simonsen, E., Sorensen, K.M., Pedersen, G.T. (1975) Polyglycolic acid (Dexon) used as suture material for the repair of episiotomies. *Ugeskrift For Laeger*, **137**, 617–20.

Houghton, M. (1940) *Aids to practical nursing* Balliere, Tindall and Cox. Eastbourne, Sussex.

House, M.J. (1981) To do or not to do episiotomy. In Kitzinger, S. (ed.) *Episiotomy – physical and emotional aspects*, London, National Childbirth Trust.

House, M.J. (1983) Personal communication.

Katz, D., Baptista, J., Azen, S.P. and Pike, M.C. (1978) obtaining confidence intervals for the risk ratio in cohort studies. *Biometrics*, **34**, 469–74.

Kegel, A.H. (1951) Physiologic therapy for urinary stress incontinence. *Journal of the American Medical Association*, **146**, 915–17.

Kitzinger, S. and Walters, R. (1981) *Some women's experiences of episiotomy*. National Childbirth Trust, London.

Lindkaer Jenson, S. (1986) Treatment of first episodes of acute anal fissure: prospective randomised study of lignocaine ointment versus hydrocortisone ointment or warm sitz baths plus bran. *British Medical Journal*, **292**, 1167–9.

Logue, M. (1987) Management of the perineum and perineal muscle function. In Robinson, S. and Thomson, A. (eds) *Research and the Midwife Conference Proceedings for 1986*. Nursing Research Unit, King's College, London University.

Macfarlane, A. and Mugford, M. (1984) Birth Counts: Statistics of pregnancy and childbirth, HMSO, London.

Mandelstam, D. (1978) The pelvic floor. *Physiotherapy*, **64**, 236–9.

Marks, J and Ribero, D. (1983) Silicone foam dressings. *Nursing Times*, 11 May, 58–9.

Meinart, C.L. (1986) Clinical trials: Design conduct and analysis. Oxford University Press.

Oakley, A., Chalmers, I., Elbourne, D. (1986) The effects of social interventions in pregnancy. In Papiernik, E., Breart, G. and Spira, N. (eds) *Prevention of preterm birth. New goals and new practices in prenatal care.* INSERM, Paris.

Robinson, S., Golden, J. and Bradley, S. (1983) A study of the role and responsibilities of the midwife. NERU Report No 1, King's College, London University.

Russell, J.K. (1982) Episiotomy. *British Medical Journal,* **284,** 200.

Shepherd, A.M. (1983) Management of urinary incontinence – prevention or cure. *Physiotherapy,* **69,** 109–10.

Shepherd, A.M., Montgomery, E., Anderson, R.S. (1983) A pilot study of a pelvic exerciser in women with stress incontinence. *Journal of Obstetrics and Gynaecology,* **3,** 201–2.

Sleep, J. (1984) The West Berkshire episiotomy trial. In Thomson A and Robinson, S. (eds) *Research and the Midwife conference Proceedings for 1983.* Department of Nursing, Manchester University.

Sleep, J. and Grant, A. (1987a) Pelvic floor exercises in postnatal care. *Midwifery* **3,** 158–64.

Sleep, J. and Grant, A. (1987b) West Berkshire perineal management trial: three year follow-up. *British Medical Journal,* **295,** 749–51.

Sleep, J. and Grant, A. (1988a) Salt in Bathwater. A randomized controlled trial to compare routine addition of salt or Savlon bath concentrate during bathing in the immediate post-partum period. In Robinson, S. and Thomson, A. (eds) *Research and the Midwife Conference Proceedings for 1987.* Nursing Research Unit, King's College, London University.

Sleep, J. and Grant, A. (1988b) Effects of salt and Savlon bath concentrate postpartum. *Nursing Times Occasional Paper,* **84,** 55–7.

Sleep, J. and Grant, A. (1988c) Relief of perineal pain following childbirth: A survey of midwifery practice. *Midwifery,* **4** 118–22.

Sleep, J., Grant, A., Garcia, J., Elbourne, D., Spencer, J. and Chalmers, I. (1984) West Berkshire perineal management trial. *British Medical Journal,* **289**(8), 587–90.

Snooks, S.J., Setchell, M., Swash, M., and Henry, M.M. (1984) Injury to innervation of pelvic floor sphincter musculature in childbirth *Lancet,* **ii,** 546–50.

Spencer, J., Grant, A., Elbourne, D., Garcia, J., and Sleep, J. (1986) A randomized controlled comparison of glycerol-impregnated catgut with untreated chromic catgut for the repair of perineal trauma. *British Journal of Obstetrics and Gynaecology,* **93,** 426–30.

Thacker, S.E. and Banta, H.D. (1983) Benefits and risks of episiotomy: an interpretative review of the English language and literature 1860–1980. *Obstetrical and Gynaecological Survey,* **38,** 322–38.

Verbrugge, L.M. (1980) Health Diaries. *Medical Care,* **18,** 73–95.

Watson, M. (1984) Salt in the Bath. *Nursing Times,* **14,** 57–9.

Wilkerson, V.A. (1984) The use of episiotomy in normal delivery *Midwives Chronicle and Nursing Notes,* **97**(1155), 106–10.

Wilmott, J. (1980) Too many episiotomies. *Midwives Chronicle and Nursing Notes,* **93,** 46–8.

Yarnell, J.W.G., Voyle, G.J., Sweetnam, P.M., Milbank, J., Richards C.J. and Stephenson, T.P. (1982) Factors associated with urinary incontinence in women. *Journal of Epidemiology and Community Health,* **36,** 58–63.

Zander, L. (1982) Episiotomy: has familiarity bred contempt? *Journal of the Royal College of General Practitioners,* **32,** 400–1.

CHAPTER NINE

Putting research into practice: perineal management during delivery

Margaret Logue

Complaints voiced about research often include a lack of widespread dissemination of findings to practitioners and a reluctance to change practice on the basis of research, even when findings are available. The research described in this chapter, however, was undertaken in a unit where there has long been a tradition of midwives and obstetricians working together to evaluate practice and to make changes when these are indicated. The particular study described here focused on management of the perineum during delivery and its relationship to subsequent perineal muscle function. An account is also included of changes in midwifery practice that took place after the study was completed.

BACKGROUND TO THE STUDY

In a historical review Goodell (1871) demonstrated that prior to the middle of the 18th century very few techniques were recommended to conserve the perineum. Although treatments of a torn perineum were in abundance, the only methods used in an attempt to prevent a perineal laceration were delivery on an obstetric stool, or in the 'all-fours' position when the woman was obese; a warm bath; massage with oil; and manual dilatation of the vaginal introitus. Some internal medications such as oil of lilies, infusions of saffron, swallows' nests or of sage leaves were also used. Manual support to the perineum was not recommended until as late as 1759. This could have coincided with the involvement of the medical profession in childbirth when women were put to bed to deliver (Towler and Bramall, 1986). Goodell (1871) suggests that putting the woman on a delivery stool protected the perineum by keeping the child's head in the axis of the pelvic canal and goes on to state that this position did not allow of any manual assistance, or did he mean interference?

Goodell reports that from the middle of the 18th century the perineum was 'supported', 'guarded' or strengthened by a ring of the two thumbs meeting posteriorly and the forefingers anteriorly; or protected by directing pressure on the child's head to restrain or guide it. Sir Fielding Ould (1742) was the first to advocate a cut into the vulval outlet and despite categorical statements reported by Goodell (1871) that the perineum should be conserved, episiotomy became established practice in obstetrics at the end of the nineteenth and beginning of the twentieth centuries. As obstetricians became increasingly involved in normal childbirth (see for example Cowell and Wainwright, 1981; Robinson, Golden and Bradley, 1983; Towler and Bramall, 1986; Robinson, 1990) so episiotomy became an essentially routine procedure, especially for primiparae. By the late 1960s, midwives in many units were working within policies that dictated episiotomy for an increasing proportion of women (personal experience and communications). In the early 1970s Fox (1979) reports an episiotomy rate for hospital midwives of 40–55% for 1971–75. He reports that since the introduction of the Domino scheme in the unit in which he worked, which meant that the community midwives were conducting an increasing number of deliveries in hospital rather than at home; the community midwives' episiotomy rate rose from 4% in 1971 to 38% in 1975. However, as Inch (1982) maintains, it has been difficult to obtain figures from hospitals that will indicate the overall incidence of episiotomy. For example, Robinson, Golden and Bradley (1983) found that heads of midwifery service were able to provide annual figures for episiotomy in only 13 of the 60 districts in England and Wales that they surveyed in their study of the role of the midwife. The rate in these 13 districts averaged 43.2%. Estimates for earlier years in England and Wales suggest figures of 22% in 1968 and 37% in 1973 (Alberman, 1977). Incidence of episiotomy for primiparae appeared to reach almost 100% in some hospitals; for example, Oakley (1979) cites a rate of 98% in one London hospital in 1975/76. More recently, Garcia, Garforth and Ayers (1985) in their national study of policies and practices in England (see also Chapter 2 in this volume) demonstrated considerable variation in episiotomy rates in that 7% of consultant units reported that less than 20% of women had an episiotomy, 48% put the episiotomy rate at 20–39% of delivered women, 38% reported an episiotomy rate of 40–59% and 8% of units had a rate of 60–79%.

Advocates of episiotomy have stated that liberal use reduces the incidence of vaginal and perineal tears, reduces the incidence of longer term sequelae such as stress incontinence and vaginal prolapse and spares the baby's head from undue trauma (Donald, 1979; Flood, 1982). Such claims however are not supported by research. A study in Cardiff indicated the incidence of tears did not reduce with an increase in the number of episiotomies performed (Chalmers *et al.*, 1976), and a study in America indicated that delivery without episiotomy was not associated with poorer muscle tone (Brendsel, Peterson and Mehl 1981). Sleep *et al.*, (1984) undertook a randomized controlled trial of 1000 women comparing liberal with restricted use of episiotomy (see chapter 8); they found that liberal use of episiotomy did not reduce the incidence of urinary incontinence at three months postpartum, neither did reduced incidence of the operation increase postpartum morbidity.

In a randomized controlled trial of routine versus restricted use of episiotomy, Harrison *et al.* (1984) could find no difference in the degree of pain or discomfort reported four days post delivery between the women who had an episiotomy and those who sustained a second degree tear. However the women who experienced least pain were those who retained an intact perineum. House, Cario and Jones (1986) also compared the liberal and restricted use of episiotomy and found that symptoms on the third day post partum were, on average, reduced in the women in whom the use of episiotomy was restricted.

Practitioners have questioned high episiotomy rates (Wilmott, 1980) and some childbearing women have also indicated their dissent, claiming that an episiotomy was much more painful than a spontaneous tear in the postnatal period (Kitzinger, 1972).

RESEARCH INTO PERINEAL MANAGEMENT AT NORTHWICK PARK HOSPITAL

Northwick Park Hospital is a District General Hospital delivering 3000–3300 women annually. There is an established collaboration between midwives and obstetricians in questioning routine or customary procedures by undertaking research. Studies have been undertaken on pre-delivery vulval shaving (Romney, 1980), the routine use of enemas in labour (Romney and Gordon, 1981) and the use of a chair for delivery (Romney, 1983; Turner *et al.*, 1986).

There were three consultant obstetricians working in the maternity unit in the mid 1970s and each had a different policy with regard to management of the perineum at delivery. One required that all primiparae booked under his care have a routine episiotomy at delivery. The second felt that midwives were performing too many episiotomies and the third felt that an episiotomy should be performed if the midwife deemed it necessary. In 1973 13 out of every 20 women had an episiotomy associated with a normal delivery. The monitoring of perineal outcome of all women delivered vaginally commenced in 1981. In 1983/4 an unpublished prospective study on perineal discomfort was carried out on 1036 consecutive women who had had a vaginal delivery. Both multiparae and primiparae were included and they had sustained varying degrees of perineal trauma. A questionnaire was administered to each woman by one of three senior clinical midwives and the degree of pain they were experiencing was assessed by use of a visual analogue scale. At 24 hours, and again at five days post delivery, the proportion of women reporting perineal pain increased in relation to the degree of perineal trauma sustained. Women with an intact perineum reported less discomfort than those in any other group. Women with a second degree laceration reported considerably less pain than those with an episiotomy, both at 24 hours and five days post delivery, but at three months post delivery their pain scores were the same. When the women who had had an episiotomy for normal delivery were compared with those who had had an episiotomy with a forceps delivery, the normal delivery group reported considerably lower pain levels at five days post delivery but at three months post delivery the scores were the same. Primiparae reported considerably more pain at 24 hours than multiparae, except in the forceps group in which reported pain scores were equally high.

Perineal muscle tone

During the course of the study on perineal discomfort described above the midwives' management of the perineum changed gradually, so that there was an increase in the number of women achieving an intact perineum with normal delivery. This generated the following questions about perineal muscle function:

1. Could the perineal muscles be damaged seriously by overstretching during childbirth?
2. In the recovery of perineal muscle function was there any difference between a clean cut and a ragged tear?

As already stated the claimed advantages of episiotomy in relation to the pelvic floor are: prevention of major tears, reduction of muscle damage, improvement of healing, promotion of better long term muscle function and reduced risk of genital prolapse. In the light of this we examined the effect of perineal trauma on perineal muscle function by measuring the squeeze pressure of the levator muscles with a modification of the perineometer (Gordon and Logue, 1985). The perineometer used in the study was designed and constructed by the bioengineering department at Northwick Park Hospital. The apparatus consisted of a pressure gauge connected with rubber tubing to a solid, hollow end-piece that can be covered with a condom, inserted vaginally and inflated until the woman is just aware of the pressure. This gives the zero reading and subsequent pressure change exerted by a vaginal muscle squeeze is recorded on the gauge in centimeters of water. Five pressure readings were taken from each subject, and the mean calculated.

All the women studied were European. They had all had their first baby 12–14 months previously and were sent a letter asking them to return to the hospital for the purposes of this study. They were recruited from the women who had participated in our earlier study of perineal discomfort; these women had comprised four main groups:

- Those with an intact perineum associated with vaginal delivery;
- Those with a second degree vaginal laceration associated with vaginal delivery;
- Those with episiotomy associated with vaginal delivery;
- Those with episiotomy associated with forceps delivery.

Fourteen women were randomly selected from each of these four groups to form a sub-sample for this follow-up study. Women in the earlier study who had sustained a first degree tear were excluded from the follow-up study. Two comparison groups were also recruited, one of women who had had a caesarean section and another of nulliparous midwives. There were 14 women in each of these two groups, making a total of 84 subjects in the study. There were no significant differences between the first five groups in respect of maternal age, height, weight or baby gestational age, birthweight or head circumference.

Pressure measurements

The mean pressure score for all the women was 11.12 cm. water. The mean pressure score for each group is shown in Table 9.1. Several of the group of midwives had poor muscle tone, and a proportion of women delivered by caesarean section had poor muscle function, although the perineum had not been traumatized at the time of delivery. The women in the forceps group achieved the lowest level of vaginal squeeze pressure. However, statistical analysis, using one-way analysis of variance for multiple comparison of means showed that there was no difference between the groups (see Armitage, 1971, for details of this test). Therefore there was no relationship between the degree of perineal trauma and subsequent muscle function.

The study provided no support for the theory that episiotomy results in better perineal muscle function one year post delivery, and there was no evidence to suggest that an intact perineum at delivery gives rise to deficient muscle function due to overstretching. Perineal damage had little influence on perineal muscle function one year after delivery.

Benefits of exercise

Data on the pressure scores for each of the women in the four perineal management study groups and in the caesarean section comparison group ($n = 70$) were re-classified according to the amount of exercise that the women reported they had taken after delivery:

1. Those who performed only the hospital recommended postnatal exercises ($n = 24$) (these exercises involved breathing and leg exercises as

Table 9.1 Vaginal squeeze pressure readings for study groups

	Perineal management groups women who had:				Comparison groups	
	An intact perineum	A second degree tear	A normal delivery with episiotomy	A forceps delivery with episiotomy	Nulliparous midwives	Women who had a lower segment ceasarean section
Number of women in group	14	14	14	14	14	14
Range in pressure readings (centimetres of water)	5.0–18.4	2.6–19.2	6.8–20.8	2.8–18.0	6.6–20.0	2.4–23.8
Mean pressure reading for group (centimetres of water)	11.1	10.8	11.7	9.4	13.3	12.5

Source: Compiled by the author.

well as those for the pelvic floor, and all women were encouraged to continue these for six weeks post delivery);

2. Those who performed the hospital postnatal exercises and then continued with some form of regular formal exercise over the next year ($n = 18$);

3. Those who did not undertake any form of exercise ($n = 28$).

The chi square test indicated that there was no statistically significant difference in the type of exercise performed by the women in the different delivery/perineal management groups (Table 9.2). However, there was a statistically significant difference between the amount of vaginal squeeze pressure that the women were able to exert when they were grouped according to the amount of exercise they had undertaken since delivery (Table 9.3). The difference between the no exercise and postnatal exercise groups and the no exercise and the regular exercise groups was statistically significant ($p < 0.0001$). The difference between the postnatal exercise and the regular exercise group was the least significant ($p < 0.02$). In the no exercise group of 28 women the mean pressure measurement was 8.2 cm H_2O. This demonstrates poor muscle tone. In the regular exercise group of 18 women the mean pressure measurement of 16.1 cm H_2O demonstrates good muscle tone. Those who did not exercise achieved lower pressures than

Table 9.2 Perineal management study group by exercise group

| | Study groups – women who had: | | | | |
	An intact perineum	A second degree tear	A normal delivery with episiotomy	A forceps delivery with episiotomy	A lower segment caesarean section
No exercise	4	5	6	5	8
Postnatal exercises only	6	5	4	8	1
Postnatal exercises and regular exercise	4	4	4	1	5
Number in group	14	14	14	14	14

Source: Compiled by the author.

Table 9.3 Vaginal squeeze pressure readings for groups classified according to type of exercise taken after delivery

| | *Type of exercise taken after delivery:* | | |
	No exercise	*Hospital postnatal exercises only*	*Hospital postnatal exercises and regular exercise*
Number of women in group	28	24	18
Range in pressure readings (centimetres of water)	2.4–18.4	7.2–19.2	8.0–23.8
Mean pressure reading for group (centimetres of water)	8.2	10.8	16.1

Source: Compiled by the author.

those who only did postnatal exercises and those who exercised regularly achieved the highest squeeze pressures. Half of those who took regular exercise went to keep fit classes, walked, ran, jogged, swam, did yoga or danced. The woman with the highest vaginal squeeze pressure skipped, ran on the spot to a count of 600, jumped up and down to a further count of 300, and also contracted her perineal muscles 50–100 times daily depending on available energy! From the findings of this study it appears that any type of general exercise improves perineal muscle function.

Perineal exercises

Perineal exercises alone were not practised extensively by the women in this study (only three out of the 18 women in the regular exercise group exercised their pelvic floor). It seems that either women are not aware of the supposed benefit of these exercises or the exercises are too tedious. Specific exercises for the pelvic floor are rarely mentioned in books on physical fitness. It is therefore not surprising that women have little or no knowledge of exercises involving this area.

In certain cultures, however, the ability to contract the vaginal muscles is encouraged and regarded as a highly prized asset. For example, among some African tribes young girls are not permitted to marry until they can demonstrate good strength in the perineal muscles. Kegel (1948) reports a personal communication from Van Skolkvik who found that it was the duty of the midwife (usually the mother or mother-in-law) to ensure that good perineal muscle function returned postpartum. Exercise by contraction of vaginal muscles on distended fingers were commenced several days after birth and continued for several weeks until the desired strength was obtained. Kegel introduced the concept of perineal muscle exercises as an important factor in the prevention of pelvic floor relaxation, but did not appear to have a control group in his studies (Kegel, 1948; 1956), so that all his claimed improvements in perineal muscle function could have been due to the physiology of the postpartum period or, as was shown in this study, was due to the individual's general exercise.

Our study demonstrated that any form of regular exercise can contribute to good perineal muscle function. It would therefore seem sensible for educational establishments to encourage and teach forms of physical exercise that can be pursued most easily after formal education has ceased. Sleep and Grant (1987) could find no decrease in the incidence of urinary incontinence at three months post delivery in a randomized controlled trial of routine pelvic floor exercises and extra pelvic floor exercises. However, a surprise finding was that the women in the group performing extra pelvic floor exercises reported fewer incidences of postnatal depression. We suggest that women should follow some form of exercise programme that they find enjoyable and invigorating. Not only may this improve their general health, both physical and mental, but it will also improve the tone of their pelvic floor musculature.

THE APPLICATION OF THESE RESEARCH FINDINGS TO CLINICAL PRACTICE AT NORTHWICK PARK HOSPITAL

On the basis of their research, Harrison *et al.*, (1984) and Sleep *et al.* (1984) state that episiotomy may not be needed in many cases and the Northwick Park study supports this view. Findings of the unpublished study of perineal pain and that of Gordon and Logue (1985) helped to increase the confidence of the midwives in this unit and gave them encouragement to aim for an increased incidence of intact perinea.

In order to support the staff in this endeavour a planned programme of regular feedback was instituted. As team-work is very important the obstetricians, from house officer to consultant, were made aware of the continuing monitoring of perineal outcome of all vaginal deliveries. The feed-back was provided in the form of monthly perineal trauma statistics. These figures were then included in the annual clinical report (see Wilmott and Chapple, 1986 for an example). At each delivery midwives were requested to record the indication for performing an episiotomy. A set of guidelines for delivery technique was produced, although it is recognized that there is a deficiency in research evidence to support all our guidelines.

Junior staff are supervised by senior midwives, and new staff members are supervised for their first few deliveries.

In the management of the perineum, two factors warranting further investigation emerged:

1. Position for delivery;
2. Midwife's individual management.

Position for delivery

In a recent review of the literature on the management of the second stage of labour (Thomson, 1988) concluded that there is no definitive research evidence on the efficacy of different positions for delivery. She questions current policies in the UK requiring women to deliver in the semi-recumbent dorsal position, as in this position the woman is likely to slip down the bed and therefore lose any of the theoretical advantage of gravity. Moreover if the woman is lying on her back the sacrum is fixed and it is not able to take advantage of any potential outward movement which may increase the size of the pelvis (Thomson, 1988).

At Northwick Park Hospital women are encouraged to try different positions and they can adopt any position that they find comfortable. However we find that in the second stage of labour women are reluctant to change position and most deliver in the conventional position, that is with the back supported by pillows at an angle of about 40°. Currently only 3% opt for delivery in an alternative position (chair, squatting, kneeling or 'all fours') but 20% of women deliver in a lateral position with the shoulders supported by pillows. This latter position has a long history in the UK and it possibly originated in the 'London' position advocated by Smellie (1752). One of its promoters (Porteus, 1892) advocated it on grounds of ease of access for the accoucheur and being the position that was least embarrassing for the woman. It still offers some advantages in the 1980s in that it reduces the risk of aorto-caval compression, does not fix the sacrum, gives a greater view of the perineum and leads to easier delivery of the anterior shoulder. In our experience women delivered in a lateral position have an increased incidence of delivering with an intact perineum. Table 9.4 shows that 58% of primiparae delivering in the lateral position in 1985 achieved an intact perineum, compared with 33% delivering in the dorsal position ($p < 0.0001$) and with 17% in the birthing chair ($p < 0.00001$). The corresponding figures for multiparae are significant at the same levels.

In the 1970s and 1980s there has been a resurgence of interest in and use of the delivery chair. Chairs have been manufactured that attempt to provide the advantage of gravity and support to the woman, but that also allow midwives and obstetricians ease of access. As Thomson (1988) points out, the findings of the studies undertaken to evaluate the effectiveness of a

Table 9.4 Type of delivery by perineal outcome (1985 data)

Perineal outcome	Primiparae delivered in:						Multiparae delivered in:					
	Birthing chair		Dorsal position		Lateral position		Birthing chair		Dorsal position		Lateral position	
	No.	%	No.	%	No.	%	No.	%	No.	%	No.	%
Episiotomy	46	38	254	35	24	12	12	9	143	12	6	2
Laceration	55	45	233	32	60	30	74	57	430	36	92	21
Intact	21	17	240	33	117	58	44	34	622	52	200	67
Total	122	100	727	100	201	100	130	100	1195	100	298	100

Source: Compiled by the author.

delivery chair are conflicting. One study undertaken at this hospital (Northwick Park) (Turner *et al.*, 1986) found an increased incidence of postpartum haemorrhage and perineal damage in women delivered in an E-Z chair when compared with women delivered in a dorsal recumbent position. The increased incidence of perineal trauma when delivering in the chair was again found in 1985 (Table 9.4). Therefore women who insist on delivering in a birthing chair are warned of the increased incidence of morbidity found in this hospital (Romney, 1986).

Midwives' individual management

Midwives' individual management of the second stage of labour has a major influence on perineal outcome as was demonstrated by Wilkerson (1984). She examined the perineal trauma rates for 21 individual midwives over a one year period. She found that although the overall episiotomy rate was 43%, the range of rates between the midwives was 6%–67%. The rates for achieving an intact perineum ranged from 10%, for the midwife with the highest episiotomy rate, to 59% for the midwife with the lowest episiotomy rate. The rates of perineal laceration varied between 19% and 40%.

Active management of labour as described by Turner, Webb and Gordon (1986) increased the rate of normal delivery in primiparae in this hospital by 20% a year, with a halving of the caesarean section rate. Annually, Northwick Park midwives manage between 2100 and 2500 normal deliveries (72–80% of all deliveries that take place in the unit). We undertook our own study of the episiotomy rates for each of 13 experienced delivery suite midwives delivering primiparae. As in Wilkerson's (1984) study the midwives were supervising students rather than undertaking personal deliveries. Figure 9.1 shows that midwife 13 has a remarkably high rate of 73% compared with midwife 1 who has a rate of 14% – a difference of 59%. Midwife 1 achieves an intact perineum rate of 67% while midwife 13 manages only 7%. Length of clinical experience did not seem to have any bearing on the incidence of perineal trauma as a few of the experienced midwifery sisters and nearly all experienced part-time staff midwives show a high episiotomy rate. However, some junior midwives performing an equal number of deliveries, show quite a low rate. Junior staff can be influenced by their senior colleagues. If a senior midwife has a high episiotomy rate, then those constantly under her supervision are likely to be influenced by her and also show a high rate. A sister with a high intact perineal rate may enthuse her juniors with confidence and encouragement to achieve a slow gentle delivery, when possible, with a minimum of trauma to the woman and no harmful effects to the baby. There may still be a few midwives who believe it does not matter what happens to the perineum as long as the baby is alive and well, but in our experience the welfare of both the woman and her baby can be safely met.

Figure 9.1 Episiotomy rates for individual midwives at Northwick Park Hospital delivering primigravidae in 1985.

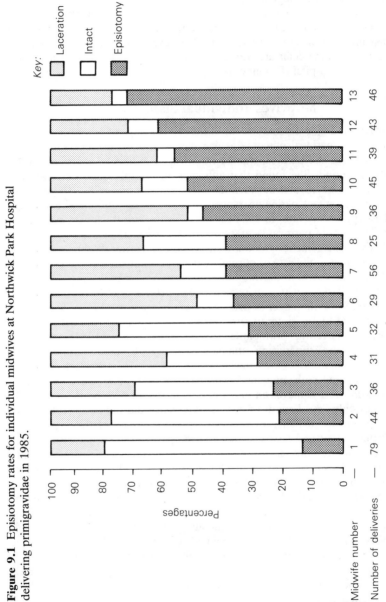

Key:
Laceration
Intact
Episiotomy

Percentages

Midwife number | 1 | 2 | 3 | 4 | 5 | 6 | 7 | 8 | 9 | 10 | 11 | 12 | 13

Number of deliveries | 79 | 44 | 36 | 31 | 32 | 29 | 56 | 25 | 36 | 45 | 39 | 43 | 46

Source: Compiled by the author.

Suggested reasons for the difference in episiotomy rates

The demonstrated differences in perineal trauma rates led the staff in the Midwifery Teaching Department to question their teaching, both in-service to qualified staff, and to student midwives (Rourke, 1986). Various reasons were suggested for the differences in episiotomy rates between individual midwives and included:

1. Lack of confidence;
2. An inexperienced midwife;
3. Reflection of training and previous practice;
4. Fear of major perineal laceration resulting in litigation, or reprimand from senior staff;
5. The midwife who is impatient and cannot wait for the natural stretching of the perineum.

It was this latter suggestion that there might be differences between individual midwives that could account for the differing perineal trauma rates that led to the hypothesis that personality could affect one's ability to conserve a perineum. In order to test this hypothesis psychological profile questionnaires were completed by midwives working in the Delivery Suite. Analysis of the data by a psychologist produced inconsistent findings. Moreover, it appeared that midwives gave the answer they thought was required rather than a true statement. We could not therefore demonstrate a personality difference between midwives who had a low perineal trauma rate and those with a high rate.

Performing an episiotomy may sometimes be an easy way out. As research to date, however, shows no benefit from episiotomy (Chalmers *et al.*, 1976; Brendsel, Peterson and Mehl, 1981, Harrison *et al.*, 1984; Sleep *et al.*, 1984; Gordon and Logue, 1985; House, Cario and Jones, 1986) it would seem unkind to subject a woman to unnecessary perineal pain in the early puerperium when she should be expending her energy on getting to know her baby. Keeping a perineum intact involves great patience and concentration, and can be really hard but satisfying work. A high episiotomy rate cannot be reduced overnight as educating staff to aim for an increased intact perineal rate takes time. In our experience a few extensive lacerations can be expected initially but when midwives have developed expertise the amount of extensive trauma becomes negligible. The annual production of the episiotomy rates for individual midwives permits staff to review their own performance. Although the graphs for all midwives are published in the unit without names, the midwives are given their individual rates in confidence. Performance monitoring then leads to practical benefits for women.

Sometimes what initially appears to be a thick and rigid perineum may stretch and allow normal delivery without trauma. The perineum is like the cervix; first it effaces or thins, then the vulval outlet dilates to allow delivery of the baby. In most cases this is a normal function of the perineum. Midwives who use scissors frequently, rarely see a perineum stretch sufficiently to accommodate the emerging head. It would seem therefore that what is a rigid perineum to some midwives is not necessarily so to others.

Prevention of major trauma

One of the supposed advantages of episiotomy is prevention of damage to the anal sphincter. However, in 1985 half of the 30 third degree and four fourth degree lacerations sustained by women delivering in the unit (see World Health Organisation (1977) for definitions of third and fourth degree tears) occurred in association with an episiotomy. The provision of a large diagram (located on the wall at the midwives' station in the delivery suite) outlining when, where and how to make the incision appears to have helped reduce the number of episiotomy extensions to a minimum.

Episiotomy rate still falling

Figure 9.2 shows the result of efforts aimed at decreasing perineal discomfort in postnatal women. The overall episiotomy rate dropped from 39% in 1981 to 17% in 1986, and in 1987 is down to 12%. Intact perinea increased by an equal proportion but the laceration rate remains relatively unchanged. However, guidelines on preservation of the perineum may also have helped reduce the amount of trauma as now half of the lacerations are only first degree. The episiotomy rate for primiparae in 1981 was a painful 63%, by 1986 this rate had dropped to 32% and in 1987 this rate is down to 22%. This fall has been achieved by the concentrated effort and caring attitude of all the midwives.

CONCLUSION

Episiotomy in the short term shortens the second stage of labour but long term may cause, for some women, weeks or even months of discomfort and does not improve the pelvic floor muscular function. An intact perineum may prolong the second stage by several contractions but long term will allow newly delivered women to be more comfortable. It has been suggested that this in turn enhances mother–baby interaction and promotes early resumption of normal family life (Kitzinger and Walters, 1981). Moreover if a woman feels comfortable she may be more likely to take some form of regular exercise and our study suggests that this can contribute to good perineal muscle function. The management of the perineum is the midwives' responsibility as they are the experts in normal midwifery practice and supervise 70–80% of all deliveries in this country (Chamberlain *et al.*, 1978; Cartwright, 1979). It is important that midwives are encouraged to monitor

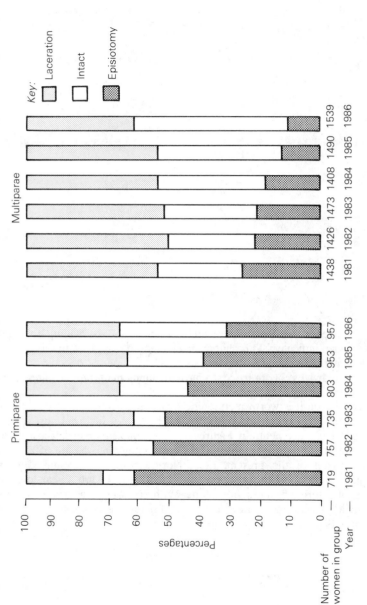

Figure 9.2 Episiotomy rates for primiparae and multiparae delivered at Northwick Park Hospital for the period 1981–1986.

Source: Compiled by the author.

Figure 9.3 Financial cost of an episiotomy (1988 prices)

Materials for the operation:
1 10 ml syringe
1 size 21 needle
10 mls lignocaine 0.5%

for the repair:
1 pair sterile gloves
200   mls cleaning lotion
1 20 ml syringe
1 size 21 needle
20 mls lignocaine 1%
2 lengths catgut
sterile pack containing — instruments
                                            drapes
                                            swabs

Itemized cost:

	£	p
Gloves		61
Sutures	2	20
Syringes		25
Needles		5
Cleansing solution		26
Lignocaine 0.5%		16
Lignocaine 1%		24
Sterile pack	2	17
	5	94

Source Compiled by the author.

their practice in the light of research findings, and be willing to make changes when indicated. This chapter has sought to demonstrate this process in one maternity unit and the way in which it depends on collaboration between midwives in practice, education and management and their obstetric colleagues.

In conclusion it is worth mentioning that the selective use of episiotomy not only benefits women and midwives but has major financial implications for hospital management. In Figure 9.3 the itemized financial cost of an episiotomy at 1988 prices is given. If the episiotomy rate was still 65% (as in 1973), instead of the present 12%, Northwick Park Hospital General Managers would need to provide an estimated extra £9306 a year to cover the cost of suturing requirements alone. With increasing financial restraints, General Managers have cause to be grateful for the cost-effectiveness of efficient midwives.

REFERENCES

Alberman, E. (1977) Facts and figures. In Chard, T. and Richards, M. (eds) *Benefits and hazards of the new obstetrics*, Lavenham Press, Lavenham, Suffolk.

Armitage, P.O. (1971) *Statistical methods in medical research*. Blackwell, Oxford.

Brendsel, C., Peterson, G., and Mehl, L. (1981) The role of episiotomy in pelvic symptomatology. In Kitzinger, S. (ed.) *Episiotomy – physical and emotional aspects*. National Childbirth Trust, London.

Cartwright, A. (1979) *The dignity of labour*, Tavistock, London.

Chalmers, I., Zlosnik, J.E., Johns, K.A., and Campbell, H. (1976) Obstetric practice and outcome of pregnancy in Cardiff residents 1965–73. *British Medical Journal*, 1, 735–8.

Chamberlain, G., Phillip, E., Howlett, B., and Master, K. (1978) British Births 1970. Vol. 2. *Obstetric Care*, William Heinemann Medical Books, London.

Cowell, B. and Wainwright, D. (1981) *Behind the blue door, the history of the Royal College of Midwives 1881–1981*, Balliere Tindall, London.

Donald, I. (1979) *Practical obstetric problems*, Lloyd-Luke, London.

Flood, C. (1982) The real reason for performing episiotomies. *World Medicine*, Feb. 6, p. 51.

Fox, J.S. (1979) Episiotomy. *Midwives Chronicle*, 92, 337–40.

Garcia, J., Garforth, S. and Ayers, S. (1985) Midwives confined? Labour ward policies and routines, In Robinson, S. and Thomson, A.M. (eds) *Research and the Midwife Conference proceedings*, Nursing Research Unit, King's College, University of London.

Goodell, W. (1871) A Critical Inquiry into the Management of the Perineum during labour. *American Journal Medical Science*, 61, 53–79.

Gordon, H. and Logue, M. (1985) Perineal Muscle Function after Childbirth. *Lancet*, ii, 123–5.

Harrison., R.F., Brennan, M., North, P.M., Reed, J.V. and Wickham, E.A. (1984) Is Routine Episiotomy Necessary? *British Medical Journal*, 288, 1971–5.

House, M.J. (1981) To do or not to do episiotomy. In Kitzinger, S. (ed.) *Episiotomy: physical and emotional aspects*, National Childbirth Trust, London.

House, M.J., Cario, G., and Jones, M.H. (1986) Episiotomy and the Perineum: A Random Controlled Trial. *Journal of Obstetrics and Gynaecology*, 7, 107–10.

Inch, S. (1982) *Birthrights, a parents' guide to modern childbirth*, Hutchinson, London.

Kegel, A.H. (1948) Progressive Resistance Exercise in the Functional Restoration of the Perineal Muscles. *American Journal of Obstetrics and Gynecology*, 56, 238–48.

Kegel, A.H. (1956), Early Genital Relaxation. New technique of Diagnosis and Non-surgical Treatment. *Obstetrics and Gynecology*, 8, 545–50.

Kitzinger, S. (1972) (ed.) *Episiotomy, physical and emotional aspects*, National Childbirth Trust, London.

Kitzinger, S. and Walters, R. (1981) *Some women's experience of episiotomy*, National Childbirth Trust, London.

Oakley, A. (1979) *Becoming a Mother*, Martin Robertson, Oxford.

Ould, F. (1742) *A Treatise of Midwifery*, J. Buckland, London.

Porteus, J.L. (1892) Posture in parturition *New York Medical Journal*, 56, 153–4.

Power, R.M.H. (1948), Embryological Development of the Levator Ani Muscle. *American Journal of Obstetrics and Gynecology*, **55**, 367–81.

Robinson, S., Golden, J. and Bradley, S. (1983) *A study of the role and responsibilities of the midwife*, Nursing Education Research Unit, University of London, London.

Robinson, S. (1990) Maintaining the independence of the midwifery profession: a continuing struggle. In Garcia, J., Richards, M. and Kilpatrick, R. (eds) *The politics of maternity care*, Oxford University Press, Oxford.

Romney, M. (1980) Pre-delivery shaving: an unjustified assault. In Robinson, S. (ed.) *Research and the Midwife Conference Proceedings*, Nursing Education Research Unit, University of London, London.

Romney, M. (1983) Chair Project. In Thomson, A.M. and Robinson, S. (eds) *Research and the Midwife Conference Proceedings*, Dept. of Nursing, University of Manchester, Manchester.

Romney, M. (1986) The birthing chair; a random controlled trial. In Robinson, S. and Thomson, A.M. (eds) *Research and the Midwife, Conference Proceedings*, Nursing Research Unit, University of London, London.

Romney, M. and Gordon, H. (1981) Is your enema really necessary? *British Medical Journal*, **282**, 1269–71.

Rourke, A. (1986) Implications of Research for the Teaching and Training of Midwives. In Robinson, S. and Thomson, A.M. (eds) *Research and the Midwife, Conference Proceedings*, Nursing Research Unit, King's College, University of London.

Sleep, J., Grant, A., Garcia, J., Elbourne, D., Spencer, J. and Chalmers, I. (1984) West Berkshire Perineal Management Trial. *British Medical Journal*, **289**, 587–90.

Sleep, J. and Grant, A. (1987) Pelvic floor exercises in postnatal care. *Midwifery*,

Smellie, W. (1752) *A Treatise on the Theory and Practice of Midwifery*, Wilson, London.

Thomson, A.M. (1988) Management of the woman in the second stage of labour: a review. *Midwifery*, **4** (2), 77–85.

Towler, J. and Bramall, J. (1986) *Midwives in history and society*. Croom Helm, London.

Turner, M.J., Romney, M.L., Webb, J.B., and Gordon, H. (1986) The Birthing Chair: an Obstetric Hazard? *Journal of Obstetrics and Gynaecology*, **6**, 232–5.

Turner, M.J., Webb, J.B., and Gordon, H. (1986) Active Management of Labour in Primigravida. *Journal of Obstetrics and Gynaecology*, **7**, 79–83.

Wilkerson, V.A. (1984) The Use of Episiotomy in Normal Delivery, *Midwives Chronicle*, **97**, 106–10.

Wilmott, J. (1980) Too many episiotomies. *Midwives Chronicle*, **93**, 46–8.

Wilmott, M. and Chapple, J. (1986) (eds) Annual Clinical Report, Northwick Park Hospital, Harrow, London.

World Health Organization (1977) *Manual of the international statistical classification of diseases, injuries, and causes of death*, WHO, Geneva.

CHAPTER TEN

Men in Midwifery: their experiences as students and as practitioners

Paul Lewis

INTRODUCTION AND BACKGROUND

The phenomenon of the modern-day male midwife in the United Kingdom is a different entity from the 'man-midwife' of old, for he enters the profession with a background in nursing and not as a doctor substitute. The discussions and controversies that have surrounded the training and practice of men as midwives are not concerned therefore with the possibility of a new breed of practitioner, but with the encroachment of men into an all-female profession and the effects that this may have on the women for whom they care.

Midwifery has traditionally been synonymous with the care of pregnant women by women, during and after childbirth (Chamberlain, 1981). However, from the 16th century, history began to record an increasing interest and involvement by men, in this previously exclusive female preserve. Donnison (1977), for example, asserts that by that time 'enough men were involved in midwifery for the term "man-midwife" to be included in the English language'. Nevertheless, women remained the principal practitioners of the art up until the 18th century (Donnison, 1977).

The subsequent rise of the 'man-midwife' in the years that followed provoked bitter inter-professional rivalry; their disparate practice was often at odds with that of female practitioners and as the social and professional status of these men rose, so that of the midwife fell (Towler and Bramall, 1986). The passing of the *Medical Acts* of 1858 and 1886 further consolidated the position of the 'man-midwife', who emerged as the forerunner of the modern day obstetric specialist. Female practitioners of midwifery were not to gain similar legal recognition until 1902, with the passing of the *First Midwives Act*. Although this prohibited the practice of midwifery by unqualified women, unqualified men, nonetheless, could continue to practise as midwives up until 1926, when the penal ban closed this loophole (Donnison, 1973).

Accordingly, a system of maternity care developed within the United Kingdom in which a predominantly male medical profession and an exclusively female midwifery profession became the main providers of care for pregnant, parturient and postpartum women. This position was further strengthened with the *Midwives Act* (1952), that prohibited men from training and practising as midwives.

However, in the late 1960s and early 1970s, a small number of male nurses voiced their dissatisfaction at the exclusion of men from midwifery and campaigned for a change in the legislation. This challenge to the exclusion of men received some support through the efforts of the Government of the day, who were attempting to introduce an Act of Parliament to prevent sex discrimination and provide equal opportunities in employment.

The question of allowing men to become midwives aroused strong feelings and fierce arguments both for and against (e.g. Clay, 1974; Banks, 1975; Blenkins, 1975; Beilby, 1977). Many of the nursing and medical organizations expressed serious reservations about such a development, whilst the Royal College of Midwives, supported by the Royal College of Obstetricians and Gynaecologists remained adamant that midwifery should remain an occupation exclusive to women. The College argued that because the midwife's role involved intimate aspects of bodily care, the majority of the public would be unwilling to accept such care from a man, unless he was chaperoned; this, they felt, would strain both manpower and financial resources. They also considered that being a woman was part of the function of the midwife and that the psychological support provided by her was objectively immeasurable; therefore no adequate assessment of the success or failure of a man in this role could be determined (Editorial, Midwives Chronicle, 1975).

In 1975, against a background of professional and mixed public opposition to men becoming midwives, the Bill to abolish sex discrimination in employment became law, and in August of that year an amendment to the Act removed the barriers to men entering the midwifery profession. However, transitional restrictions on their entry were imposed (Speak and Aitken-Swan, 1982). These restrictions confined the training and employment of men as midwives to those courses and hospitals approved by the Secretary of State. Following wide consultation, only two midwifery schools were selected to run experimental schemes; these were only monitored in order to determine the suitability of men as midwives and their acceptability to women.

In 1977 the first men entered the experimental training scheme at the Islington School of Midwifery, whilst in Scotland, owing to a lack of suitable candidates, the scheme commenced the following year at the Forth Valley Midwifery School. By 1979 when the experimental schemes were concluded, only a small number of male candidates had been accepted and had subsequently qualified as midwives. Nevertheless, the report of the experimental scheme concludes that 'male midwives were generally acceptable to mothers, husbands, midwifery and medical staff' (Speak and Aitken-Swan, 1982). The publication of the report brought no immediate Government action, although it established a reversal in the previously held position of the Royal College of Midwives, who recommended that 'the fields of midwifery should be totally opened to men' (Royal College of Midwives, 1982). Other organizations, however, criticized the Report. The Association of Nurse Administrators, for example, said 'The report, though detailed, was based on a sample size so small that it was doubtful whether it could be considered nationally representative or statistically valid' (ANA, 1982). Concern was also expressed that Government might formulate policy on its basis and some individuals and organizations called, therefore, for further studies to investigate male midwifery education and practice. Ward (1984) advocated that if there was an increased demand from men to pursue midwifery 'the profession should make every effort to retain them and to assess their progress for the benefit of the maternity services'.

On 16th March, 1983 the Secretary of State announced that the barriers contained within the Sex Discrimination Act (1975) that had restricted the training of men in midwifery were to be lifted. Thus, the amendment contained in Section 20 of the Act was removed and from 1st September, 1983 it became unlawful to discriminate in the fields of midwifery training and employment on the grounds of sex (DHSS, 1983). Men were now free to train and practise as midwives on equal terms with women.

Although the findings of the Speak and Aitken-Swan study had led to the midwifery profession opening its doors to men, the total numbers observed in the experimental schemes were extremely low, with only eight subjects in England and nine in Scotland at the completion of the study. Consequently, generalizations from the findings had to be made with caution. The authors suggested that candidates for training needed to be carefully selected and that the issue of chaperonage required further consideration. The existence of professional and individual prejudice, from midwives and doctors, was also identified as a potential difficulty in the harmonious assimilation of men into midwifery. Speak and Aitken-Swan (1982) suggested that it would be interesting to learn what motivated male nurses to apply for midwifery training and recommended that follow-up studies should be undertaken if more men entered the profession.

Although many small scale studies have looked at the male nurse within the maternity unit (Tagg, 1981; Newbold, 1984; Cooper, 1987), and the occasional article has described the experiences and perceptions of qualified male midwives (e.g. Tiller, 1980; Lewis, 1984) no in-depth evaluation of the education of male midwives or an assessment of their experiences has been undertaken. This complete absence of data about men in midwifery is surprising, in view of the controversy that had surrounded their initial introduction to the profession. Many questions remained unanswered, such as the number of men in midwifery, their continuing acceptability, the need for chaperonage, their reasons for entering or leaving the profession and their subsequent career patterns. The aim of the study described in this chapter was to provide information on these topics; it was undertaken in 1987, exactly ten years after men first entered midwifery training.

Although no previous research had been undertaken on male midwives, apart from the Speak and Aitken-Swan study, a number of studies have been undertaken of health professionals whose experience may, in some ways, be comparable. These studies were therefore drawn on in the design of questionnaires and interviews for this study of male midwives.

Robinson (1986 and Chapter 10 in this volume) and Mander (1987) have both explored the employment plans and career intentions of female midwives and found that reasons given most frequently for entering midwifery were to 'broaden experience', 'improve career prospects' and 'round off nurse training'. Robinson (1986) also found that those who had undertaken an eighteen month course were more likely to have entered midwifery with the intention of practising as a midwife than those who had taken the twelve month course. In an examination of career intentions, both the Robinson (1986) and Mander (1987) studies revealed that only a minority of those qualifying had any long term intentions of practising as midwives. A follow-up study of careers actually pursued after qualification was undertaken by both these authors (Mander, 1989, and in preparation in Volume III of this series, Robinson and Owen, 1989, providing data that can be compared with those obtained for male midwives.

A review of literature on careers of men in nursing also provided important data for comparison with men in midwifery. One of the most comprehensive studies of male nurses (Brown and Stones, 1973) found that a substantial majority (82%) of male nursing students planned to remain in nursing, most of whom in fact did so. These men also tended to have a greater expectation of promotion than their female colleagues. This expectation is born out in reality, for although men comprise only 9% of the total nursing workforce, they have attained 50% of the senior posts within the profession (Gaze, 1987). The reasons for this have been ascribed to a greater job mobility and the fact that men, unlike women, rarely take time out of the 'career ladder' (Davies and Rosser, 1986).

Several studies have examined factors that may impinge on career choices and decisions of nurses (for example Mercer and Mould, 1977; Moores, Singh and Tun 1983; Waite, 1987). One key issue that these studies have raised is the satisfaction or lack of it that nurses experience in their work and its relationship to retention. It was also concluded that moves to undertake further education, as well as family commitments, were significant contributors to wastage from the profession. Waite (1987) found that job security, levels of pay, working atmosphere, the feeling of doing a worthwhile job and the opportunity of using their abilities to the full, were all important issues that influenced nurses' decisions about whether to stay in or leave nursing.

AIMS AND METHODS

The project had three phases. The first involved sending postal question-naires to the heads of all the 171 midwifery schools in the United Kingdom. These questionnaires sought to ascertain the general level of enquiry that had been received from men interested in becoming midwives; the total number of men who had entered midwifery and those who had been accepted for a course up until September 1987. The number of students, the number who had qualified and the number in practice were also sought, together with their names and addresses in order to contact them for Phase 2 of the study.

Phase 2 also used postal questionnaires which were sent to all current male midwifery students, those men qualified and those practising. The questionnaire was in four parts; the first two applied to all subjects; the third only to those qualified, whether practising or not, and the fourth specifically to those men who were practising as midwives. This questionnaire was designed to elicit data about the types of men entering midwifery, their personal experiences of training and practice, as well as their intended and actual career patterns.

Phase 3 involved personal interviews with practising male midwives within the United Kingdom in order to explore issues in the Phase 2 questionnaire in more depth.

Phase 1: survey of midwifery schools

The aims of Phase 1 were as follows:

1. To determine the degree of interest in entering the profession shown by men who were eligible to undertake first level midwifery education;
2. To identify the total number of men who have entered, or intended to enter first level midwifery education within the United Kingdom between May 1977 and September 1987;
3. To establish the numbers of male student midwives, the number who have qualified and the number currently in practice as midwives;
4. To identify the numbers of men who have discontinued from their midwifery course and the reasons for this;
5. To obtain the names and addresses of qualified and student male midwives, in order to proceed to the second phase of the study.

A short postal questionnaire was designed to obtain information on these five topics and was sent to the head of all midwifery schools within the United Kingdom; a response rate of 100% was achieved. Both reliability and validity are hard to establish when attempting to determine the size of a previously unstudied population and the research relied heavily on the records of the midwifery schools and the memories of those involved in the selection of student midwives. The questionnaire was piloted with staff in a midwifery school that had previously taught male midwives.

In order to contact the current students and qualified male midwives the schools in the survey were asked to provide their names and addresses. This posed a dilemma over the need for confidentiality. However, 23 of the 31 schools involved in teaching male midwives complied with this request, while eight agreed to forward the questionnaires to those concerned. Information about the project published in the Nursing Times and Midwives Chronicle resulted in eight respondents contacting the author direct.

Phase 2: survey of student and qualified male midwives

The aims of the second phase of the project were as follows:

1. To obtain information on the demographic and academic background of men entering midwifery courses.
2. To ascertain reasons why men had chosen to enter midwifery.
3. To investigate problems or difficulties that they encountered during the course or while in practice, especially concerning their perceptions of the issues of acceptability to women and chaperonage.
4. To determine how the student and qualified male midwife perceived his role in relation to his female colleagues.
5. To establish the reasons given by qualified male midwives for either leaving the midwifery profession or remaining within it.
6. To establish career intentions and paths.

A questionnaire was sent to all those men identified in Phase 1 as current students or qualified male midwives. This was designed to obtain information on the topics listed above and was developed with reference to the recommendations for follow-up studies made by Speak and Aitken-Swan (1982), as well as from literature on career patterns of midwives and from the personal experience of this writer as a midwife. A combination of closed item questions and open-ended questions were included. Although the questionnaire was long and detailed, the time taken for its completion depended on the status of the respondent. Only currently practising male midwives were required to complete the whole questionnaire. The time estimated for this was 45 minutes and therefore relied heavily on the interest and commitment of respondents to ensure a satisfactory response rate.

The questionnaire was piloted three times to maximize reliability and validity; on the first occasion it was discussed with two practising male midwives, and then postal versions were sent out on two occasions to a random sample of student and qualified male midwives. Modifications were made to the questionnaire after the first and second pilot study.

In view of the small numbers of men identified in Phase 1 as having entered midwifery, the total population of current students and male

Table 10.1 Overall response rate for male midwifery questionnaires

Status	Number of men in midwifery	Number of respondents	Response rate
Student midwives	22	20	91%
Qualified non-practising midwives	31	22	71%
Practising midwives	17	16	94%
Total	70	58	83%

Source: Compiled by the author.

midwives ($n = 70$) were sent questionnaires rather than selecting a sample. As a result of the number of questionnaires sent abroad to Australia and New Zealand, six weeks were allowed before follow-up: by this time a response rate of 60% ($n = 42$) had been achieved. In order to improve this a reminder letter was sent to non-responders, increasing the response rate to 76% ($n = 53$). Finally after a further three week period, a second questionnaire and covering letter was sent to non-responders, achieving an overall response rate of 83% ($n = 58$) as shown in Table 10.1.

Five further questionnaires were returned but were unsuitable for analysis and a further three were returned, address unknown. As Table 10.1 shows, a high response rate was achieved for the two groups currently involved in midwifery, either as students or practising male midwives. Nevertheless, the lower response rate of 71% was still considered satisfactory in view of the fact that these men were no longer involved in the profession.

Phase 3: interviews with practising male midwives

In an attempt to explore in greater depth some of the issues surrounding the practice of men as midwives, face-to-face semi-structured interviews were carried out with men known to be practising as midwives within the United Kingdom and who had agreed to be interviewed. This information was elicited through the Phase 2 questionnaire and six of the eight male midwives identified as practising in the U.K. were contacted by telephone. Suitable arrangements were then made for the interviews to take place. Of the other two, one left the country before he could be interviewed and the other is the author of this chapter.

Questions in the interview schedule covered four areas of male midwifery practice.

1. The men's perceptions of their provision of care, the problems and difficulties that they had encountered and the techniques and approaches they had developed to overcome them.
2. The relationships and reactions of colleagues, women, their partners and the general public, towards men as midwives and the feelings that they might have experienced from any negative responses.
3. Their plans and hopes for the future, not only for themselves but for the future of the midwifery profession as a whole.
4. The benefits, if any, that male midwives might bring to the profession of midwifery, to women and their partners and to the profession of nursing.

Each interviewee was asked if the interview could be tape-recorded. The subjects were assured that the information divulged would be confidential and that their anonymity would be respected. Subjects were informed that if at any time during the interview they wished the tape-recorder to be turned off, this would be done immediately. They were also informed that after transcription the tape recording would be erased and the data obtained used only in the written form, without mention of the subject's name.

At the start of each interview an account of the research and its progress to date was given, as well as some personal and professional information about the researcher. In an attempt to reduce possible anxiety about answering questions and also to provide a check on the reliability of the Phase 2 questionnaires, each subject was initially asked two questions, which it was presumed would be relatively easy to answer and could be verified. The first of these checked the date of qualifying, whilst the second re-affirmed the areas in which the subjects had worked. The information received accurately reflected that given in Phase 2.

Data analysis

The questionnaires for Phase 1 and Phase 2 comprised a mixture of closed-item and open-ended questions. The latter were subject to content analysis in order to identify major themes, and were also coded to allow for quantification.

Analysis was carried out using the Statistical Package for the Social Sciences, including a multiple response analysis, and comprised frequencies, together with a cross-tabulation between data using the test of difference between proportions. Quantitative as well as qualitative data from the two surveys are presented in this chapter. The interviews were transcribed verbatim prior to content analysis.

FINDINGS FROM PHASES ONE AND TWO

Number of men in midwifery

In Phase 1 of the study, the findings revealed that 139 (81%) Schools of Midwifery had received enquiries from men interested in becoming midwives, whilst 32 (19%) had not. Of the former, only 31 (22%) had trained or were currently training men. However, nine (6%) schools did indicate that they had offered course places to male candidates who, for various reasons, either failed to accept the place offered or withdrew their applications.

In total, 90 men had entered midwifery training between May 1977 and February 1987 and Table 10.2 shows their status at that time. A further 12 men were expected to take up training by September 1987. Of the 48 qualified male midwives shown in Table 10.2 only 9 were identified as currently practising, although findings from Phase 2 indicated that the number was in fact 17 at the time that Phase 1 of the research was undertaken.

When male students had left the course without completing it, the school staff were asked for their perceptions of reasons for this event. Two principal reasons were cited: personal and family pressures, or an inability to meet the required academic standards. A discontinuation rate of nearly a quarter of the men who have entered midwifery appears somewhat excessive, and should be the subject of further study. It may reflect difficulties for men in integrating into the profession, but must also raise doubts about their selection in the first instance.

In Phase 2, a total of 64 of the 70 questionnaires sent to students and to qualified midwives was returned, of which 58 were suitable for analysis. Twelve questionnaires indicated a change in the status of some respondents

Table 10.2 The status of men in midwifery up until February 1987

Status of men	Number
Qualififed as midwives	48
Currently students	22
Failed on examination	1
Discontinued from course	19
Total	90

Source: Compiled by the author.

Table 10.3 The status of men in midwifery in July 1987

Position in midwifery	Number
Practising midwives	19
Qualified non-practising midwives	33
Current student midwives	18
Total	70

Source: Compiled by the author.

since the completion of Phase 1 of the project, four students having success-fully qualified as midwives, whilst eight previously identified in Phase One as non-practising indicated that they were currently working as midwives. Table 10.3 shows the status of men in midwifery in July 1987, as indicated by the 58 returned questionnaires and knowledge of the current status of the 12 non-respondents. Of those 19 practising male midwives shown in Table 10.3, eight were working abroad and 11 within the United Kingdom.

Demographic profile

Demographic data revealed that the majority of the 58 respondents were British, young, single, academically well qualified and had a good back-ground in nursing. Nearly half (28) were between 25 and 29 years of age on commencing midwifery training, whilst a little more than a third were younger. Ten (17%) were aged 30 years or over. In comparison, other studies (Robinson, 1986; Mander, 1987) show female midwives to be younger on average upon entering midwifery.

Only a third of the men in the study were married and just over one-fifth had children; these were primarily of pre-school age. These family commit-ments did not appear to have the same significance in terms of having to give up work as has been identified in other studies for female nurses and midwives. This has important implications for the profession of midwifery; if careers of men in its ranks are not hampered by fatherhood, then why should careers of female midwives suffer as a consequence of motherhood?

Although the majority of respondents were British, a surprising and unexpected finding revealed that over a third of the men who had entered first level midwifery education in this country held Australian or New Zealand nationality. Although the reasons for this are unclear, several respondents indicated that midwifery education in Australia, where midwives are more akin to maternity nurses, would be an inadequate preparation for the career paths that they wished to follow, such as working in the outback, with Voluntary Service Overseas or in Nurse Practitioner positions.

In the study by Speak and Aitken-Swan (1982), men entering midwifery had been described as 'academically lightweight'. This is not borne out by the findings of this study, in that half held GCE A level certificates and five had a degree.

Respondents' replies indicated extensive nursing experience. As expected, all held the SRN/RGN qualification. Just over a quarter also held a secondary basic training certificate, and one-fifth had obtained post-basic qualifications. The time spent in practice as a nurse before entering midwifery varied between respondents. Half had worked for between one and three years, a further quarter had practised for between three and ten years, and three indicated that they had worked as a nurse for longer periods. All respondents had held a staff nurse position. Eight had gone on to hold charge nurse posts and two to more senior posts.

Applying to take a midwifery course

The reasons that respondents gave for taking a midwifery course were comparable with those found for female midwives in the studies by Robinson (1986, and Chapter 10 in this volume) and Mander (1987); in that 36 (62%) said it was to broaden their experience and 29 (50%) in order to improve their career prospects. However 31 (53%) entered the course to fulfil a personal desire to become a midwife, whilst 13 (22%) did so in order to work abroad, either in a developed or a Third World country. Twelve respondents (21%), however, said that they entered midwifery as a challenge to the previous exclusion of men from the profession.

Twenty respondents (34%) claimed that when applying for a place on a midwifery course they had encountered some difficulties, although these were primarily related to information, access and entry onto available courses. However, incidences were cited which claimed that applications for a place had been ignored, replies to enquires had been hostile and interviews tended to over-emphasise the problems of a man in a female-dominated profession. When accepted for a course, respondents considered the following factors to be the most important in contributing to their acceptance: having applied to the hospital in which they had undertaken their maternity care experience; previous nursing experience, especially with women or children; determination to become a midwife; being married with a family and the willingness of the midwifery tutors to train men as midwives.

Experience of midwifery education and practice

Respondents' perceptions of various aspects of their experiences as students and as qualified midwives were sought: these included the presence or absence of other men during training; support from midwifery and medical colleagues; perceptions of differences in practice that may exist between male and female midwives; reactions of women to their care; whether they considered themselves acceptable to women; and finally, whether or not chaperonage was required. Analysis of these data takes into account the different status of the 58 respondents; data from questionnaires of four respondents who had recently qualified were included with those of the 16 current students. Of the 38 respondents who were qualified midwives, 28 had practice experience, and ten had left midwifery on qualifying. Data relating to the student experience of these qualified men were considered along with data on the experience of current students.

During training, 35 respondents (60%) had had the company of other male students and considered it welcome companionship to have other men around, enabling them to compare experiences and lend each other support. Nevertheless, those respondents who had been the only male midwife on their course felt that the absence of men was offset by the friendliness and support of other staff and that being the only man was rarely a problem. The majority of female midwives, especially when in the same peer group, were considered either 'supportive' or 'very supportive', whilst medical colleagues, although also seen to be 'supportive', were rated less so than fellow midwives. Lack of support, when evident, appeared more likely to result from student status than gender difference, except in a small minority of cases. In these, respondents cited 'blatant female chauvinism' and 'outright antagonism' by some midwives and doctors. Overall, however, it seems that the difficulties encountered by men in a female-dominated profession are less than those anticipated. These findings show that although doubts are still expressed about men as midwives (Downe, 1987), in practice they are shown a positive consideration, as might be expected from a caring profession.

In the work of any health care professional, perhaps the most important considerations arise out of the events occurring at the interface between client and practitioner. Consequently, some of the most important questions addressed in this study examined the acceptability of men as midwives and the reactions of women to their care, as perceived and experienced by male students, and by qualified and practising male midwives.

The majority of respondents considered there to be little if any difference between their practice and that of their female colleagues. Some indicated however, that in their view, men were more sympathetic, considerate and sensitive to a woman's wishes. Other comments, each made by one or two respondents, included the views that male midwives had better communication skills, that they were more likely to take decisions, and that they were more diplomatic and conscious of the need to put a woman at her ease without transgressing the fine line of over-familiarity.

The vast majority of respondents (48/58) stated that men as midwives were either 'generally' or 'wholly' acceptable to women. These findings, however, relate to the perceptions of the respondents and do not necessarily reflect the views of the women. Although some studies (Tagg, 1981; Speak and Aitken-Swan, 1982; Newbold, 1984) afford these findings credibility, others such as Sweet (1974) and more recently Cooper (1987) provide contrary findings and suggest that men are unacceptable in maternity care. Cooper's study, however, related to the male student nurse rather than the male midwife, and Sweet's findings relate to 1974 and perceptions may well have changed since that time. Moreover, her questions were possibly biased towards producing a negative response, as they emphasised the male midwife being chaperoned, and focused primarily on intimate aspects of care.

With the exception of some women from ethnic minority groups, respondents claimed to have received positive and favourable reactions to the care that they provided. Although they often showed initial surprise, women accepted and appeared comfortable with the care that they received, some even expressing a preference for men as midwives. Refusals of care that had occurred were due primarily to cultural or religious factors. Overall

Table 10.4 The chaperonage of men in midwifery

Chaperonage required	As students		As qualified midwives	
	%	No.	%	No.
All the time	3	2	–	
Only in initial training	7	4	–	
Some of the time	26	15	11	3
Only when requested by the mother	–		–	
No deliberate chaperonage provided	34	20	46	13
Chaperonage never provided	3	2	7	2
Chaperonage not considered necessary	26	15	36	10
Total	100	58	100	28

Source: Compiled by the author.

respondents identified few difficulties in their training and practice, and the issue of chaperonage, as shown in Table 10.4 posed less of a problem than had previously been anticipated. Although the findings show that chaperonage is sometimes required, it is by no means universal, with the majority of student respondents (37/58) being unchaperoned and an even greater proportion of qualified male midwives (23/28) citing that no deliberate chaperonage was provided in their hospital, or else that it was considered unnecessary.

It seems then that concerns about the need for men to be chaperoned are unfounded. It should perhaps be remembered that the majority of men entering midwifery are likely to have a background in nursing and be relatively mature; it is hoped, therefore, that they have already developed skills for making appropriate judgements about social, professional and personal interactions. Consequently, the profession should allow male midwifery students and more especially, qualified male midwives, the freedom to exercise their clinical skills and judge for themselves the necessity for chaperonage.

Career intentions and career paths

Until this time, no information has been available concerning the career intentions or patterns of employment of male midwives. Figure 10.1 shows career paths of respondents who took part in this study. Of the 38 men who had qualified as midwives ten had left without practising, and of the other 28, 12 had subsequently left, leaving 16 currently in practice. Four of the students had recently qualified, two of whom were in practice.

Half of the students indicated that they intended to practise as midwives on qualifying, if only for a short time, whilst a further quarter said that they intended to make careers in midwifery. These figures compare favourably with those found in Robinson's study (1986) and are substantially better than those for female midwifery students in the study by Mander (1987).

Data obtained from the 38 men who had qualified as midwives revealed a close association between intended and actual careers. As shown in Table 10.5, a total of 34 (89%) stated their intentions to practise as midwives if even for a short time, 28 (82%) of whom fulfilled their intentions.

Although the number of men in this study is small, these figures compare very favourably with those for female midwives identified in other studies (Robinson and Owen, 1989; Mander, 1987). The findings suggest that investment in training men is well rewarded as they are more likely to practise as a midwife, if even for a short time, than their female counterparts.

Figure 10.1 Career paths of respondents.

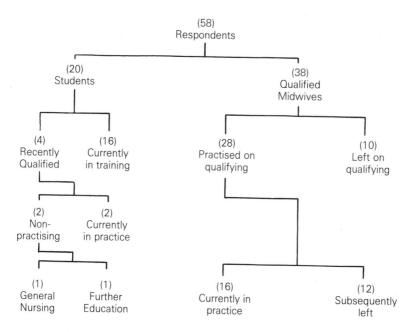

Source: Compiled by the author.

Men in midwifery practice

Of the 16 men currently in practice as midwives eight worked in the UK and eight worked abroad; they were asked to indicate the posts they had held since qualifying. The majority (13) had worked in hospitals as staff midwives, whilst four had gained promotion to Charge Midwife/Charge Nurse Midwifery. None indicated that he had attained Nursing Officer Grade. Three individuals had worked as agency midwives; a further two had held the post of Community Midwife and Independent Practitioner, respectively.

Three respondents cited other posts held; all of these were in Australia where the position of midwives is that of Nurse/Midwife. One respondent was a Flight Sister/Supervisor with the Royal Flying Doctor Service, another held a Clinical Instructor's post and one held the position of Director of Nursing responsible for nurse/midwives.

When asked why they had chosen to remain in midwifery, all 16 referred

Table 10.5 Intended and actual career paths of qualified male midwives

Career intentions prior to qualification as a midwife (n = 38)	Make a career as a midwife		Practise midwifery for some time, but not make it a career		Practise midwifery for some time, but not certain about career		Not to practise midwifery		Uncertain about practising midwifery	
	No.	%	No.	%	No.	%	No.	%	No.	%
	15	40	7	18	12	32	3	8	1	3
Actual career path										
Practised midwifery continuously	7				3					
Left midwifery, returned and now in practice	3		1		2					
Practised midwifery for a short time and then left	3		5		4					
Left midwifery on qualifying	2		1		3		3		1	

Source: Compiled by the author.

to enjoyment and satisfaction with the work. Four also said that they required the experience of midwifery practice for work that they indended to pursue in the future; two in the Australian outback, one in Africa and one in Holland. Fifteen of the men said that they intended to remain in midwifery for the foreseeable future, with one uncertain of his plans at the time of the study.

Men who have left midwifery

The ten respondents who did not practise midwifery after qualifying and the twelve who had subsequently left were asked what had led to this decision. The reason given most frequently was that at the time of qualifying the law prevented practise outside of the experimental schemes. It would be interesting to see if more men will be willing to enter the profession and remain in practice now that the legal barriers have been removed. Five respondents said they had decided that work other than midwifery would provide better career prospects, three said that they had changed their mind

Table 10.6 Positions held by qualified non-practising male midwives in 1987

Position held	*Number of respondents*
Staff nurse in intensive care unit	5
General nurse tutor	3
Staff nurse in Accident and Emergency	2
Charge nurse, Orthopaedics	1
Senior nurse, Paediatrics	1
Lecturer in Nursing and Health Studies	1
Clinical nurse specialist, Casualty	1
Student Health Visitor	1
Senior charge nurse, ITU	1
Charge nurse, Night Administration	1
Community general nurse	1
Senior clinical nurse, Gynaecology/Urology	1
Clinical nurse consultant	1
General staff nurse	1
Student general nurse tutor	1
Total	22

Source: Compiled by the author.

during training and three said that there were no midwifery vacancies in the area in which they lived. The following reasons for leaving midwifery were each cited by two respondents: family circumstances; dissatisfaction with the extent to which midwives are able to fulfil their role; poor pay and career prospects. As shown in Table 10.6, all 22 of this group of respondents held a nursing post at the time of the study. Just under two-thirds (14) said that they would 'probably not' or 'definitely not' return to midwifery.

FINDINGS FROM PHASE 3: INTERVIEWS WITH PRACTISING MIDWIVES

The interviews provided a wealth of information on the experiences and views of six of the eight male midwives practising in the United Kingdom at the time of the study. The findings are considered under the following headings:

1. Aspects of practice that are enjoyed most;
2. Aspects of practice that may present difficulties;
3. Approaches and techniques for successful practice;
4. Relationships with colleagues;
5. Acceptability to women and their partners;
6. Intended careers;
7. Views on benefits of male practitioners to the midwifery profession.

While it is impossible to generalize from findings based upon such a small number of practising male midwives, it is hoped that these interviews provide some insight into the world of men in midwifery.

Aspects of practice that are enjoyed most

In an attempt to gain some insight into the ways that practising male midwives felt towards their work, subjects were asked to indicate which aspects of midwifery practice they had enjoyed the most. Those highlighted appeared to be principally determined by either the amount of contact that the men had had with women and the possibility of continuity of care, or the degree of challenge available to them in a 'high-tech' area in which they could determine, to a greater extent, their own manner of practice.

Only one subject explicitly stated a dislike for working in a particular area, finding the postnatal wards 'routine, quiet and monotonous'. Four held some preference for labour ward work, considering it a place in which a one-to-one relationship with women was more easily developed, while at the same time providing excitement and challenge.

Whilst all subjects had at some point in the interview concentrated their attention on enjoyment of a particular aspect of midwifery practice, responses such as 'I don't think I enjoy any one area more than another — I think I enjoy and find them all rewarding in their own special way', were not uncommon. This holistic approach was frequently referred to and was summed up by one of the subjects, who declared: 'At the moment it is midwifery as a whole that interests me, rather than just delivery or antenatal care; it all inter-relates and I think that at the end of the day midwifery is the total of all the combinations, from preconception, through pregnancy and labour, to the puerperium and child care'.

An emphasis on establishing a relationship and rapport with women was also seen as of major importance in determining the amount of job satisfaction that the subjects felt, with five expressing in various ways the importance of maintaining continuity with women throughout their pregnancy, labour and the puerperium. As one subject said emotively, 'Whilst I enjoy the totality of midwifery, I think that what makes me enjoy this is the relationship you can establish with mothers and the chance to participate in the couple's growing relationship with their unborn baby and, hopefully, with their child when born'.

Aspects of practice considered as potentially problematic for male midwives

Having determined that these men enjoyed most aspects of midwifery, the interviewer attempted to elicit whether they felt that any area of midwifery practice could create problems for the male midwifery practitioner. They were also asked which aspects of care they personally found difficulties with and whether these occurred because they were men or because the situations were difficult in themselves.

The two areas considered as potentially most problematic for male midwives were providing care for women from immigrant groups and providing care in the community. Three of the respondents referred to minor difficulties when encountering women from countries in which religious and cultural backgrounds limited male involvement. The men said that they had little contact with these women out of respect for their beliefs. Two respondents described at length their reservations about male midwives in the community setting.

I initially had doubts about community. I felt OK in the hospital setting and dreaded going out into the community. When I did go out though, I had a very good community sister who was very modern in her thinking and it actually went quite well. Towards the end of my experience I was visiting women on my own, as well as conducting some GP clinics. In the end, it didn't seem a big problem. Now, as a qualified midwife, I would still have some trepidation, but I think that has more to do with being on my own and responsible, than being a man.

The only problem one might have in midwifery is in the community. In postnatal care, one can break down the barriers surrounding sexuality more easily in the hospital environment. Here people more readily accept your role within an organized, authoritarian situation, regardless of sex. I think, however, when you go into someone's home and examine them on a bed on which they probably conceived, the potential for embarrassment is going to be greater. To overcome this will take more time, which we may not have. So I think community midwifery for men is an area which will cause more problems, but probably only in the postnatal period. (Why?) ... Because examining breasts, perineums and the like, which are taboo areas for men as far as most women are concerned, could create difficulties. I think though, that being aware of problems that may occur will help us overcome them and as soon as more men are involved, I think people will come to accept that they can be midwives and these types of problems will resolve themselves.

Three subjects expressed difficulties over giving certain types of advice, although this had largely been resolved since qualifying. One man confirmed that he had found it difficult 'to offer advice about the sort of womanly things which a female would probably find easy to discuss — the type or use of a particular undergarment, for instance'. Assisting women with, and giving advice about, breast feeding had created difficulties for some of the men when they were students, and one subject also declared 'I used to find it difficult to give advice about contraception. I used to find myself going red, I don't know why, probably having to suggest alternative methods or asking about what they usually did. I've done it so many times now though that I've overcome that initial embarrassment'.

Although the issues of sex and sexuality were considered to be a potentially difficult area by all the men interviewed, it was suggested that this was only likely if one failed to be aware of it. This was graphically described by one man who said,

The sexuality of the situation isn't difficult, but you have to be more aware, open to the way the woman's feeling when you first introduce yourself as a male midwife. With so few men in midwifery it is unlikely that the woman has met a male midwife before. You need to recognize this and the sexual difference that exists and gain her confidence and trust.

I think men need to try a little harder to break down the barriers women experience when arriving in hospital and feel when meeting strangers. To do this we need to know more about our own personality, how we express ourselves and how we come across. If we don't, we are likely to create more difficulties. If we went in like some female midwives we wouldn't survive a lot of situations.

None of the practising male midwives when asked said that they would exclude men from any area in midwifery, although one expressed the view that in a situation in which someone found it offensive for a man to be present, he would if possible, go and find them a female midwife. 'If a woman is going to be unhappy or uncomfortable and would prefer a female midwife, I would make sure she got one.'

All the subjects were in agreement that no exclusion zones to male midwifery care should exist in midwifery practice, and that each individual situation needed consideration regardless of whether one was male or female, black or white. 'Decisions should be based on individual care, and men should not be excluded from any particular area, not even community work.'

Although the men could identify potentially difficult areas for the male midwife, none of them had, in practice, experienced any serious problems, and the small ones that they had, had been resolved quickly. The relatively problem-free experiences described by the interviewed subjects might well be among some of the important contributing factors to their remaining in practice.

One subject expressed his views as follows: 'Problems could occur in theory, but it depends on your approach. I think it is very much an individual response between the woman and yourself. I suppose obviously when you are performing the more intimate aspects of care they are more likely to cause problems. Not that I've actually found this'.

Another subject similarly stated: 'Vaginal examinations and post-natal checks could be problematic but not in my experience and I think approach obviates this happening'.

The question of the male midwife's approach to women for whom they are to care was explored in some detail with all the interviewees and is the subject of the next section.

Approaches and techniques for successful practice

The debates prior to men being able to train as midwives had focused on the problems that they might encounter in the course of midwifery practice. The interviewees were asked therefore 'What techniques and approaches have you developed which may have, or have, enhanced your interaction with women and possibly reduced the risk of refusal of care?'

All the men gave remarkably similar responses as to what they considered enhanced their acceptability and improved their interactions with women. This involved a heightened awareness of the psychosocial dynamics that might occur between individuals and the ability to establish explicit and clear lines of communication that enhanced rapport, confidence and trust. All the subjects declared the importance of tact and diplomacy, especially in the initial introduction stage. 'You need to be much more aware of the way you stand, your actions, what you say and the way you say it – you need to be able to control and conduct your own persona.'

One of the men interviewed considered 'Individual tasks don't create the problems, it's the way you hold yourself as a human being and whether or not you approach each aspect of your work as a whole'.

This emphasis on self-awareness was continually reiterated:

> I feel that just being aware of your own personality and image will get over many of the problems which might develop. I think though that that's the same for everyone. In this, men and women are not that different. ('What do you mean?') Well, I think that a female midwife can walk into a room and just because she's a woman, whether or not she's had children, she can identify with the woman's body, the pains of menstruation and the like. However, it doesn't mean she's going to gain the confidence of the woman if she doesn't conduct herself properly. Then she's just as likely to fail as a man.

> I think on the whole it's the way you conduct yourself which reduces the risk of refusal of care. I feel that women may only refuse men because they are aware that they can refuse them. I think if they were given the choice about refusing female midwives then some would say 'look I'm not getting on with this midwife and I don't want her to deliver my baby'. I know this sometimes does happen, but then the woman is blamed for being difficult. Men in midwifery don't have that option and they will have had to think about the problems that might occur and how they are going to deal with them … They need to discipline themselves into being more aware as individuals, both professionally and socially.

The necessity of considering potential difficulties and how one would deal with them appeared to be paramount to successful acceptance as a male midwife. 'I think on entering midwifery and being a man you've mulled over, confronted and learnt how to deal with most problems you're likely to encounter, by the time you're qualified.'

All the subjects said that they used first name terms with the majority of women for whom they cared. 'I try always to be very informal. I introduce myself by my first name and say that I'm a midwife. After the initial surprise you can get on with building a relationship which is friendlier and more supportive.'

One subject stated: 'I always try and get on first name terms. I think that's important. ('It could be considered familiar?') I suppose so, but in a situation where you are going to do intimate things with a woman, plus the fact that you're going to be talking her through situations that are stressful and embarrassing, its much more supportive if you are on first name terms rather than referring to her as 'Mrs Jones' all the time. I also think it helps in dealing with the husband, being on first name terms with him as well'.

Such friendliness and understanding was said to be underpinned by confidence and frankness about situations that facilitated open lines of communication. 'I always try to appear confident, but sometimes the impression is greater than I actually feel, but it reassures the mother and they seem happier as a result.'

'I'm not more confident than my female colleagues, but I think I come across as if I am ... I think mothers feel safe with this approach.'

Similarly, most of the subjects declared they preferred to 'ask mothers rather than tell them', they started discussions informally, on a low key, before progressing to more detailed and intimate subjects and whenever possible, they took the time to explain.

I always ask mothers if they have a particular preference and I feel it's important to explain how things are done and the reason for them ... I believe in being truthful. If I'm in a situation which isn't entirely normal I believe that you should say why you are concerned and what you're going to do about it.

The men all appeared to have a strong respect for the individuality of men and women, and an enthusiastic desire to be of help and to be involved in the remarkable event of childbirth. They felt that it was these attitudes that had led to their acceptance as midwives.

Relationships with colleagues

It was recognized by Speak and Aitken-Swan (1982), that relationships with colleagues were important to safe and satisfying practice. These were examined in the Phase 2 survey in terms of the 'support' that men had received from different staff members and these relationships were explored in greater detail in the course of the interviews.

Students. With the exception of one of the men whose hospital did not train student midwives, all subjects considered their relationship with students to be generally very good. As one male midwife explained

Student midwives are in a vulnerable situation, they are learning a new job, a new profession and they are dependent upon you and to that end they look to you for advice and help ... If they see your practice is sound and sensitive, a natural respect and friendship develops.

All the men who worked in hospitals in which midwifery students were present spoke of their interest in teaching. They all spoke of the importance to them of the informality of their relationships with students. 'I use the same approach with students as I do with mothers, very informal and on first name terms. I hope they see me not only as friendly but understanding as well.'

Another commented: 'I remember when I was a student myself, some staff midwives can be a bit intimidating, even pretty nasty. I try therefore to go out of my way to help students and I enjoy teaching them'.

Staff midwives. In identifying staff midwives as amongst the most supportive group, the interviewees corroborated findings from the Phase 2 survey. This did not appear to have been automatic and each subject gave evidence of their gradual acceptance. 'There was an obvious scepticism to begin with ... a lot of silences and things unsaid. Now people consider me as one of the team.'

The gradual accceptance and support the men received appears to have been related not only to their personalities and ability 'to get on well with others', but also to an increased recognition of their skills and abilities in practising midwifery. 'Once they see that you perform as well as a female midwife and the mothers have no objections, then you begin to be accepted as part of the team.'

Sisters. Such acceptance was also voiced in relation to midwifery sisters, whose attitudes to their male colleagues was not too dissimilar from that of staff midwives. However, two subjects did feel that older midwives and senior midwifery managers whilst not openly hostile, did resent their presence. 'They don't overtly disapprove but I feel the undercurrent and one sister asked me how soon it would be before I went back to general nursing, when I said I wasn't, she said you should, you're better off out of it.'

This interaction may perhaps be more a reflection of that midwife's exasperation with her profession than any particular reticence towards men within it.

The majority of the subjects however, declared that they were well supported by senior midwifery staff. 'They have really tried to break down the barriers and for me at least they have succeeded. They treat me very much as a midwife.' Another declared 'without exception, I have a good relationship with senior midwives, I suspect it is better than with most of my female colleagues or at least less hierarchical'.

A less hierarchical approach by management to male as opposed to female midwives may exist or it may be what these men perceived. If the former, it may reflect an ambiguity between women and men who occupy non-traditional roles.

Medical staff. Junior doctors on the whole appeared to accept the men's position as midwives and turned to them for advice and support. This resulted in part from their relative inexperience in midwifery matters, as well as it was claimed 'from a difference in attitude and approach'.

The majority of subjects interviewed acknowledged that while they were recognized by more senior medical colleagues as midwives, the fact that they were also men resulted in a difference in attitude. 'They seemed more prepared to listen to me than to my female colleagues.'

The establishment of informal, friendly and supportive relationships between the male midwives and some of their medical colleagues was also evident in the interviewees' replies and in their view had led to reduced professional barriers and improved co-operation and enhanced working relationships. This was not always the case however and particular reference was made to the hostility and resentment of general practitioners. 'When I speak to a GP on the telephone, they assume that because you're a man, you're also a doctor; when I tell them I'm a midwife their attitude changes ... 50% of them are disgustingly snobbish.'

Although two subjects had minimal contact with GPs, when they did, they described their manner as patronising and condescending. It is of interest that this was not the case with female general practitioners who were spoken of in a favourable light by the majority of the men interviewed. It is difficult to draw conclusions from such a small number of experiences but it is possible that antagonism felt by some male midwives from male general practitioners results from disputes that can occur between two groups of professionals providing the same care to the same client population. While midwives are regarded as the traditional practitioners providing care to women in normal pregnancy, labour and puerperium, GPs have increasingly encroached upon their responsibilities in this respect (Robinson, Golden and Bradley, 1983; Robinson, 1985). The predominant gender differences between midwives and general practitioners may help to obscure this take-over, but when the midwife is a man, then fundamental issues as to who is responsible for care, take on a professional rather than a sexual perspective and may result in antagonism.

Reactions of women and their partners

The reaction of women to the men as midwives was said to be one of initial surprise followed by acceptance, although as one pointed out 'it is difficult to categorize the reactions of every woman you encounter'. This is highlighted in the following response. 'Some mothers are surprised initially, some are even quite shocked sometimes. Some even say "I can't believe you're a midwife" whilst others just appear to accept it and it doesn't seem to bother them.'

The partners of women also seem to display a similar response to the men as midwives. One subject highlighted this stating 'It's funny really, many people say to me "I can see how the women may not mind, but I imagine you are going to have problems with their husbands," yet it has never happened'.

Another subject had however encountered one husband's refusal but as he was neither introduced nor able to liaise with the couple, he was unable to offer an explanation for the refusal. The majority of male midwives felt that their presence had in fact helped the partners of women to adjust to the situation that they found themselves in and that having another man around gave the partners moral support and enabled them to participate more fully in the care of their wife or girlfriend. For some of the male midwives, being a father themselves helped them to establish a rapport and relationship with the partner of the woman for whom they were providing care.

The reactions of women outside of the work setting to the idea of men as midwives appears to be, as one man claimed 'a great conversation piece'. Some women it was said, seemed to enjoy the opportunity to discuss the possible scenarios of childbirth and expressed delight at the idea of having a male midwife. Others however are uncomfortable with the thought and most of the men interviewed told of women they had encountered outside of the workplace who had implied that they would refuse male midwifery care. While the rights of women to refuse male midwifery care on an individual basis was supported by all the men interviewed, the majority were opposed to blanket objections by groups not directly involved. 'I cannot see why people have such strong objections to men as midwives just because a few anatomical pieces on his body are placed differently to the person he's looking after.'

Such opposition was viewed by the men as discriminatory and whilst three of them acknowledged that feminists might have a point in excluding men from childbirth, they also felt that in the long run, such restrictions would work against women rather than for them.

Future career plans

All the men interviewed said that they intended to remain in midwifery. Four outlined their career plans as a progression towards teaching posts, although they first intended to seek out charge midwife posts and undertake the Advanced Diploma in Midwifery. One subject intended to return to caring for the sick newborn in which area he hoped to work as a clinical teacher, and another was interested in the possibilities of management. Most of the men acknowledged that they did not wish to 'rise up the ladder too quickly' and felt that it was important to consolidate their clinical skills. 'My plan is to continue in clinical practice and to gain as much experience as a midwife as possible. I feel you cannot learn midwifery from books or non-clinical work.'

The men also had firm views about how they would like to see midwifery develop. 'I'd like to see more midwifery practitioners setting up midwifery clinics without recourse to doctors. Whilst I recognize that some medical back up in hospital is necessary, I feel that we should be practising midwifery as naturally as possible.'

This view, whilst expressed differently, was supported by all of the practising male midwives. Most were also in favour of more men entering the profession and one was 'disappointed that so few men have entered midwifery or remained in practice'.

Nevertheless, not all agreed with this point and one subject stated 'I don't think men should be encouraged to become midwives, I don't think it's a great big issue though the media and some midwives do blow it up. The opportunities are there for men to become midwives if they wish'.

The men's answers suggested that they saw themselves as midwives who have a lot to offer and who expect recognition for their skills and experience, as well as hoping that the profession will develop in line to meet their expectations.

Although not unanimously expressed, of particular interest was the longing or sense of regret that some men spoke of at never being able to experience childbirth. One man said 'I hope this doesn't sound stupid, but in some ways I feel envious that I'm never going to experience the actual process of giving birth'.

Such feelings may be part of the strong empathy that male midwives claim they have with mothers and might partly explain the high level of commitment they have towards their work. It would also be of interest to see if similar feelings are expressed by other professionals such as obstetricians or even men in general.

The benefits of men as midwives

The interviewees were asked whether they thought that their presence as men had any particular benefit for the profession of midwifery, for women and their partners or for the profession of nursing. Responses were very similar in many respects and hinged on the balance and harmony that they felt should be created between the sexes.

I've long felt that it's not good for any grouping in society to be entirely one sexed. I think a balance of the sexes makes for a much more reasonable approach and a masculine viewpoint, if there is such a thing, can redress the imbalance in midwifery.

I don't think men have inherently any particular qualities that women don't possess but I feel the way we condition and socialize our men in society as well as women, means when they are brought together, they create a balance.

The men also felt that they had contributed to easing the tension within the 'labour room' and facilitated the partner's involvement with the care of his wife or girlfriend. One of them said;

Men don't feel so much out on a limb when there is another man present. I am able to inform them about the situation and really involve them. I mean actually involved in the delivery itself, supporting his wife, holding the baby's head or even cutting the umbilical cord. As a man I would like that kind of involvement so I try and provide it for the partners of the women I care for ... mind you, so do some of my female colleagues.

The majority of the male midwives considered that their presence during pregnancy and childbirth to be of benefit in terms of a 'role model' and that the wider society could learn from their experiences.

You are able to show that a man can be a loving, caring person in a relationship. A lot of men in our society feel they have to adopt an aggressive, dominating role in relationships. Perhaps seeing a man doing successfully and with enjoyment what was once considered a woman's job may cause them to reappraise their position.

I think a greater understanding of male/female relationships can be brought about by watching how male midwives provide care for women and also work with them.

Not surprisingly one subject felt that *men naturally and more instinctively care for women than women care for women.* Yet another concluded *male midwives have the opportunity to develop a greater understanding of women and if we share this with other men it may help equality between the sexes.*

Their position as 'role models' was also considered by five out of the six men to provide encouragement for male nurses to consider careers as midwives. *'The role model function is important. Male students see you working and it breaks down barriers and doubts, they then might think about doing their midwifery.'*

CONCLUSION

The research on men in midwifery described in this chapter focused on a subject that had originally caused considerable controversy, but upon which little information was subsequently available. Although the absolute numbers in the study are small, they do comprise the substantial majority of male midwifery students on UK courses, and of the male midwives that have qualified in the UK. The findings show that many of the fears surrounding the entry of men into midwifery are unfounded. The numbers who have decided to train and have subsequently qualified are relatively small; there seems no indication, that men are entering the profession in large numbers and, as in nursing, moving towards occupying many of the senior management posts. Future plans of those currently in practice in fact emphasize careers in clinical practice and in teaching. Findings related to the career intentions and career paths of men suggest that they are a good investment, and it appears that men are making a contribution to the profession, but not taking it over as was feared by some.

The issues of acceptability of male midwives to women and the need for chaperonage have not been problematic. While it is acknowledged that in this study acceptability to women was considered only from the perspective of the men themselves, evidence available from other sources appears not to counteract their perceptions. With very few exceptions the men, both as students and as qualified midwives, received a warm welcome from their female colleagues. Findings from the interviews indicated not only the high level of satisfaction and enjoyment afforded to men by a career in midwifery but also the many and varied ways in which they felt able to contribute to the care of women and to the profession. The large number of Australasian men who, while appearing to prefer a British midwifery education, subsequently return home, raises important implications in terms of cost/return benefit to the profession in this country. Nevertheless, these men have all appeared to make good use of their qualification, if not in midwifery then within nursing, and highlights the question of whether we train midwives to benefit local, national or international needs. Overall the men who had taken up midwifery did not appear academically lightweight as had been suggested from the evaluation of experimental schemes. There was a fairly high discontinuation rate during first level education however, and it is suggested that this requires further investigation. The career paths of male midwives should also be considered for further study, as it is important to assess the continuing contribution that any group makes to the profession to which it belongs.

ACKNOWLEDGEMENTS

I would like to thank Sarah Robinson who as my research supervisor has given me invaluable advice and support, together with the King Edward's Hospital Fund for London and the Iolanthe Trust, for their generous financial support. I would also like to thank all the Schools of Midwifery, and the men who participated in this study, whose help made this research possible.

REFERENCES

Association of Nurse Administrators (1982) Manpower Male Midwives. *Health & Social Services Journal,* **92**(4799), 688.

Banks, P. (1975) Intimate duties of the midwife. *Midwives' Chronicle,* **88**(1044), 15.

Beilby, B.G. (1977) A place for the male midwife. *Midwives' Chronicle,* **90**(1079), 295–7.

Blenkins, T. (1975) Opinion: Male midwives – a feasible prospect. *Midwives' Chronicle.* **88**(1049), 191.

Brookes, F., Long, A. and Rathwell, S. (1987) *Midwives' Perceptions on the Status of Midwifery.* Nuffield Centre for Health Service Studies, Leeds University.

Brown, R. and Stones, R. (1973) *Male Nurse,* Occasional Paper on Social Admin. No.52, Bell and Son, London.

Chamberlain, M. (1981) *Old Wives' Tales,* Virago, London.

Clay, T. (1974) Male Midwives – A male nurse's point of view. *Midwife and Health Visitor,* **10**, 79–80.

Cooper, M. (1987) A Suitable Job for a Man. *Nursing Times,* **83**(34), 49–50.

Davies, C. and Rosser, J. (1986) *Processes of Discrimination.* A Report on a Study of Women Working in the NHS; DHSS, London.

Department of Health and Social Security (1983) *Male midwives.* HC(83) 15 August, HMSO, London.

Donnison, J. (1973) The sex of midwives. *New Society,* November 1st, 276–7.

Donnison, J. (1977) *Midwives and Medical Men* A History of Interprofessional Rivalry and Women's Rights, Heinemann, London.

Downe, S. (1987) Male midwives – An historical perspective. Letter. *Association of Radical Midwives Bulletin.* Winter 86/87, **33**, 7, Ormskirk, Lancashire.

Editorial (1975) Male Midwives – RCOG supports College views. *Midwives' Chronicle,* **88**(1044), 3.

Gaze, H. (1987) Man Appeal. *Nursing Times,* **82**(20) 24–7.

Lewis, P. (1984) The Inside Story. *Nursing Times,* **158**(12) 17–18.

Mander, R. (1987) Change in Employment Plans. *Midwifery,* **3**(2) 62–71.

Mander, R. (1989) Who Continue? A preliminary examination of data on continuation of employment in midwifery. *Midwifery,* **5**(1) 26–35.

Mercer, G and Mould, C. (1977) An Investigation into the level and character of labour turnover amongst trained nurses. *Journal of Advanced Nursing,* **8**, 227–35.

Moores, B., Singh, B. and Tun, A. (1983) *An Analysis of the Factors which impinge on Nurses' decisions to enter, stay in, leave or re-enter the Nursing Profession.* Dept. of Sociology, Leeds University, Leeds.

Newbold, D. (1984) The Value of Male Nurses in Maternity Care. *Nursing Times,* **80**(42) 40–3.

Robinson, S. (1985) Maternity care: a duplication of resources. *Journal of the Royal College of General Practitioners,* **35**, 346–7.

Robinson, S. (1986) Career Intentions of Newly Qualified Midwives. *Midwifery,* **2**(1), 25–36.

Robinson, S., Golden, J. and Bradley, S. (1983) A study of the role and responsibilities of the midwife. NERU Report No. 1, King's College, London University, London.

Robinson, S. and Owen, H. (1989) Career intentions and career paths of midwives. In Wilson-Barnett, J. and Robinson, S. (eds.), *Directions in nursing research: Ten years of progress at London University,* Scutari Press, London.

Royal College of Midwives (1982) Open the door to men, says RCM (Letter). *Nursing Times,* **78**(25), 1040.

Speak, M. and Aitken-Swan, J. (1982) *Male Midwives* – A Report of Two Studies, DHSS, London.

Stevens, C. (1987) A New Mother's Right Hand Man. *The Independent.* Tues, 21st July, p. 13.

Sweet, B. (1974) Patients' reactions to male midwives. *Nursing Times,* **70**(42), 1619–20.

Tagg, P. (1981) Male Nurses in Midwifery. *Nursing Times,* **77**(33), 1851–3.

Tiller, A. (1980) A Man in a Woman's World. *Woman's Realm.* Sept. 6th, 10–12.

Towler, J. and Bramall, J. (1986) *Midwives in History and Society,* Croom-Helm, London.

Waite, R. (1987) Waste Not, Want Not. *Nursing Times,* **83**(27), 24–7.

Ward, E. (1984) Men in Midwifery. *Maternal and Child Health,* **9**(2), 44, 46–7.

CHAPTER ELEVEN

Preparation for practice: the educational experiences and career intentions of newly qualified midwives

Sarah Robinson

The education provided for those who wish to practise as midwives is the bedrock upon which the profession is built. It is the nature of this experience that is likely to determine the extent to which we have competent, articulate midwives, capable not only of providing high quality care for childbearing women and their families, but also of maintaining and developing their role in a health service often characterized by inter-professional rivalries and competing demands for resources. It is perhaps surprising, therefore, that much less research has focused on the education of midwives than on either their practice or their role within the maternity services.

A recent survey of midwives' views on research developments in their profession demonstrated much concern over the paucity of studies on midwifery education and many issues felt to merit investigation were identified (Robinson, Thomson and Tickner, 1989). These included the following: alternative teaching strategies, teaching and learning in clinical settings; self-directed learning; the mentor system; continuous assessment; development needs of midwifery teachers; demand for direct entry courses; benefits or otherwise of mergers between midwifery schools, and effectiveness of management training.

The study described in this chapter was one of the first to investigate the education of student midwives in England and Wales. Motivated by the decision made in the late 1970s to increase the twelve month midwifery course for registered general nurses to eighteen months, the research sought to ascertain whether those who took the longer course were more likely to feel adequately prepared to practise midwifery, and to wish to do so, than those who had taken the shorter course. The study was undertaken by staff of the Nursing Research Unit, London University, who are funded by the Department of Health. The main findings demonstrated that both the hoped for outcomes of the longer training were to some extent achieved (Robinson, 1986, a,b,c). In this chapter these findings are brought together with a particular focus on those which have implications for recruitment policies for the course and aspects of its structure and content.

In order to place the study in context, the first section outlines other research in midwifery education and the second comprises a summary of some of the main developments in the course structure since it was first introduced. Subsequent sections focus on the aims, methods and findings of the research respectively and the chapter concludes with a discussion of the relevance of the findings to current developments and proposals for midwifery education. At the time that the first phase of the research was undertaken, the terms midwifery tutor and training were used rather than midwife teacher and education. This was reflected in the wording of the questionnaires developed at that time and is retained here in the presentation and discussion of findings.

RESEARCH INTO MIDWIFERY EDUCATION

Most of the research into midwifery education that has been undertaken has focused on continuing education rather than on the first level course leading to qualification as a registered midwife. In one of the earliest pieces of midwifery research undertaken, Kilty and Potter (1975) investigated factors related to the low pass rates among those taking the Midwife Teacher's Diploma examination. The Midwife Teacher's Diploma was also the focus of Balch's work; she explored the views of those who had taken the course in the years 1975–79 focusing in particular on their sometimes traumatic experiences of teaching practice (Balch, 1981). In a survey of midwives working in Wales, Maclean (1980) found that less than a quarter of the 147 respondents had attended a continuing education course since qualifying.

Much of the more recent research has also focused on continuing education for midwives. Concern about decreasing levels of attendance at a series of study days provided specifically for staff midwives, led Sugarman (1988) to investigate reasons for this trend. Questionnaires were sent to the 59 staff midwives employed in the district. Findings for the 43 who replied indicated that they found the study days useful and enjoyable but were often precluded from attending by family responsibilities and, to a lesser extent, by short staffing on their wards. McCrea (1989) investigated the participation of midwifery sisters and staff midwives in formal continuing education opportunities such as courses and study days as well as time spent in reading journals and using libraries. Responses from 43 midwives, representing a 72% return from a sample of those in one area health board in Northern Ireland, showed that only 13 had attended courses, other than refresher courses. The majority felt that continuing education courses should be of short duration and cover only one subject. McCrea, like Sugarman (1988), found that family responsibilities and staffing levels militated against course attendance; many of her respondents also said that encouragement from managers to attend courses was not always readily forthcoming. Other studies of continuing education for midwives have focused on specific courses, rather than on opportunities overall. A post-basic course for midwives and health visitors involved in antenatal education classes was the subject of an evaluation by Murphy-Black (1985, and Chapter 6 in this volume) Parnaby (1987) investigated midwives' views on the content of refresher courses and found that changes in midwifery practice and new policies and legislation relevant to midwifery were the areas most likely to be considered as essential for the refresher course curriculum.

Fewer studies have focused on student midwife education. Mander's longitudinal study of midwives who qualified in Scotland includes the period they spent in training (Mander, 1989 and forthcoming in volume 3 of this series). A survey of views of students and practising midwives concerning aspects of the 18 month course was undertaken by Pope (1986). More recently Davies (1988), adopting a case study approach, has explored the experiences of a set of midwives in the first three months of their course, focusing in particular on their perceptions of the role that they saw midwives fulfilling. Issues of particular relevance to the education of male midwifery students have been documented by Lewis (1987, and Chapter 10 in this volume). The feasibility of increasing the number of direct entry courses was assessed by Radford and Thompson (1988, and forthcoming in volume 3 of this series) by means of a national survey of views of people at regional, district and school level.

MIDWIFERY EDUCATION: DEVELOPMENTS IN RELATION TO RECRUITMENT AND RETENTION

It was in 1977 that the Central Midwives Board decided to extend the length of midwifery training for the registered general nurse from 12 to 18 months. This decision was inextricably bound up with issues of recruitment to and retention in the profession, as indeed were many of the changes made to the course in earlier decades. The rationale for the 1977 decision was that 12 months was insufficient time to cover the syllabus and for student midwives to obtain adequate clinical experience to feel confident (Central Midwives Board, 1977). As Stewart (1981) commented, it was hoped that the extension of time would be 'used to develop clinical skills and to give opportunities for the midwife to become confident and wish to practise as a midwife'. The newly qualified midwife's confidence in her clinical competence was regarded as an essential factor in subsequent decisions as whether to practise midwifery. This was of particular importance to a profession long dominated by concern that many of those whom it trains do not practise in the year after qualifying, with further attrition occurring in each successive year.

Lack of sufficient confidence to practise has not been the only factor in attrition from midwifery in the early years after qualification. A longer standing concern is the large number of nurses who have sought the midwifery qualification as a means of enhancing their nursing career prospects and who never intended to practise as midwives, or to do so for a short time only. This situation would not necessarily be problematic, apart from the waste of training facilities entailed, if sufficient midwives remained to staff the service adequately. Since the second world war, however, the professional and statutory bodies for midwifery have maintained that there are insufficient midwives in post. (Central Midwives Board 1957, Ministry of Health, 1959, Royal College of Midwives, 1964, 1983–88).

The problem of nurses taking midwifery training but not intending to practise midwifery has been in evidence ever since the early years of this century when the examination and registration machinery for midwives was established. Although changes made in the length and structure of training since that time have been concerned primarily with developments in maternity care, they have also been aimed at deterring nurses from qualifying for a profession in which they do not intend to practise. As early as 1913, when midwifery training for both nurses and non-nurses was of three months' duration, the Central Midwives Board expressed its view as follows:

> For some time it has been apparent to the Board that the great majority of the candidates who come up for examination from some of the best known training institutions do not seek the Board's certificate as a qualification for practising as midwives, but for collateral purposes. A maternity nurse now finds the possession of the CMB certificate a valuable asset in the practice of her calling and it has become an essential qualification in many cases for the post of Matron at a hospital or infirmary under the Local Government Board, or an appointment under the War Office. (Central Midwives Board, 1913).

A report published in 1923, as part of the Ministry of Health's investigation into the high levels of maternal mortality prevailing in the inter-war years, focused in particular on the length and content of training provided for midwives (Campbell, 1923). The training had been increased in 1916 to four months for nurses and to six months for non-nurses, and the 1923 report recommended that it be further extended to six months and one year respectively. The report's author took the view that this extension was necessary if midwives were to be adequately trained for their demanding and increasing responsibilities – particularly in the field of antenatal care – and so be able to make the maximum contribution possible to the attempt to reduce maternal mortality. By this time nurses were entering midwifery training in increasing numbers, and it was hoped that extending the training period for nurses to six months would reduce the numbers who sought the midwifery qualification only as a means of improving their nursing career prospects. Figures published by the Central Midwives Board and quoted in Campbell's 1923 report showed that on March 31st 1922, only 22% of the midwives on the Roll were practising.

In 1926 the training was increased in length as recommended, but this did not have the desired effect of reducing the number of nurses qualifying for reasons other than following a career in midwifery (Campbell, 1927). The problem was therefore considered again at the end of the decade by a government Committee, as part of their investigation into the training and employment of midwives (Ministry of Health, 1929). This committee expressed concern that 'many of the highest positions in the nursing world and a large number of positions abroad require the applicant to be a certified midwife, and that in the majority of these posts there is no reason to anticipate that the holder will ever be called upon to put into action the knowledge of midwifery she has gained'. It should be remembered, however, that at the time, many hospitals contained sizeable maternity units and possession of the midwifery certificate was regarded as an essential pre-requisite for the post of matron. The 1929 committee considered the idea that training should be restricted to those definitely wishing to practise midwifery, but rejected it on the grounds that many pupil midwives were uncertain of their future career plans at the outset of training.

The problem persisted into the 1930s. Another attempt at its resolution was made in 1938 when the training was divided into two periods, the first being spent in hospital and the second mainly in the community. There was an examination after each part and it was hoped that Part 1 would be regarded as sufficient for nursing posts that required a midwifery qualification and for entry into health visitor training. The rise in institutional confinements had reduced the number of district cases available for the training needs of pupil midwives and medical students, and it was hoped that this problem would also be overcome by reducing the numbers who wished to take the Part 2 training. However, in a review of developments in midwifery education, Bent (1982) comments that not only did this division of training fail to reduce the numbers who took both parts of the training and then did not practise, but also led to dissatisfaction with the training itself. The two parts were usually taken in different schools, and so the pupil midwife often experienced a lack of co-ordination of teaching methods. Moreover, Part 1 was regarded as too theoretical and too orientated towards abnormal midwifery to be either an appropriate basis for those who went on to Part 2 or a suitable introduction to the profession for those who did not do so.

The continuing loss of newly qualified midwives was considered in depth by the 1947 Working Party on Midwives, as part of their wider investigation into the shortage of midwives that prevailed by the late 1940s (Ministry of Health *et al.*, 1949). They considered existing data on post-enrolment wastage to be incomplete, and sometimes at variance, and so undertook their own research on the subject. A questionnaire sent to all those midwives who had qualified in England, Wales and Scotland during 1946 ($n = 2758$) showed that 29% of the 84% who responded were not in practice by August 1947. Most of those not practising as midwives were working as nurses, training for health visiting, or had left to get married. When asked why they had taken midwifery training, 51% of the respondents said it was to obtain an additional qualification which might be helpful in the future, 38% said they wanted to take up midwifery as a profession and 10% said they wanted to take up some particular work (such as health visiting) for which the State Certified Midwife's qualification was regarded as a definite asset.

A second questionnaire, sent by the Working Party to all midwives in England and Wales who had notified their intention to practise in 1944, ($n = 16374$) showed that by August 1947, 40% of the 76% who responded were working as full-time midwives, 35% held posts as district nurse/midwives, part-time midwives or supervisors of midwives, 7% were working as nurses and 16% were either working in other occupations or were not employed. Thirty-four per cent of those who held nursing posts said that they had been required to have a midwifery qualification in order to secure their nursing posts. This continuing requirement for nurses to hold the midwifery qualification was considered at length by the Midwives Working Party. They endorsed the view expressed in the Lancet in 1948 that 'the demand of employing authorities that many nurses, other than midwives, should hold a midwifery qualification wastes the hospital's staff, the nurse's time and the country's money'. As a consequence, the Midwives' Working Party recommended that all hospitals 'review their senior posts very carefully and ask themselves honestly which of them actually need a midwifery qualification'. In their report, the Working Party also drew attention to the fact that the midwifery profession had itself encouraged recruitment exclusively from the ranks of nurses, as this had been perceived as a means of raising the status of the profession. Data obtained from respondents to the two surveys showed that, for hospital midwives, pressure of work caused by short staffing was the main cause of dissatisfaction with midwifery, and this was cited as 'a powerful factor in causing wastage' (Ministry of Health *et al.*, 1949).

The Working Party considered various aspects of the recruitment of pupil midwives (Ministry of Health *et al.*, 1949). An examination of official returns showed that more young women and fewer older women were training and qualifying and attrition rates were highest among the younger age groups. At the same time, the age distribution of the population suggested that fewer young women would be available to train as midwives in the future. Furthermore, an increasing number of other occupations were now open to women. In view of this, the Working Party recommended a drive to increase recruits from the 30–45 age group. However, such a policy presented problems. Direct entrant midwives had poor career prospects in comparison to those who held a nursing qualification, and it was thought that older women with ambition would be deterred from entering midwifery if they first had to take nursing training in order to increase their career prospects as midwives.

The Working Party were of the view that direct-entry training should end, partly because it was unfair to train women for a qualification that provided them with limited career prospects and partly because they thought that midwives needed some nursing skills. The full State Registered Nurse training, however, was regarded as inappropriate as a basis for midwifery. The Working Party concluded that in the long term both nurses and midwives should share a common basic training followed by specialization. Recognizing that this was a long term objective they recommended that initially, the two-part training should be combined to form a single period of one year for nurses and two years for non-nurses. In the event, another 20 years lapsed before the single period training was introduced.

The loss of midwives after training and a shortage of midwives in practice continued through the 1950s. Figures published by the Central Midwives Board for 1949–1956 showed that about half of those who qualified each year actually notified their intention to practise and that by the second year after training this proportion had fallen to a third. In their 1957 report, the CMB referred to a 'chronic state of understaffing for the past ten years, particularly in the hospitals' (Central Midwives Board, 1957) and in the course of their investigation into the maternity services, the Cranbrook Committee expressed their concern about the effects of this staffing situation on maternity care (Ministry of Health, 1959).

Moving on to the 1960s, information about wastage after qualification and reasons for taking midwifery training were obtained by Ramsden and Radwanski (1963) in a study of the work of midwives. They sent question-naires to one in four of the midwives who had qualified in the UK in 1961, requesting information about their current occupational status. Of the 1 115 questionnaires posted, only 554 usable replies were returned; this represents a response rate of only 50% and so the findings have to be regarded with caution. Information from those who did reply showed that by 1963, 47% of those who had qualified in 1961 were practising midwifery, 36% were nursing, 5% were taking further training and 12% were housewives or in other work. In response to a question as to why they had undertaken midwifery training, 46% said it was to complete nurse training, 24% to practise midwifery, 12% to nurse overseas and 12% to gain promotion. Data on staffing levels were also obtained in the course of this study; figures provided by matrons showed that 59% of maternity units were below their establishment for staff midwives. Retention problems were also highlighted by the Royal College of Midwives in 1964, when they claimed that there were insufficient midwives in many units to cope with the increasing workload that had resulted from the rising birth rate and the increasing trend towards hospital confinement (Royal College of Midwives, 1964). In an address made during this period, the president of the College described how midwives had often been criticised for not offering adequate emotional support to mothers during childbirth, and made it clear that this was often very difficult given the pressure of work and inadequate staffing levels (Cowell and Wainwright, 1981).

During the 1970s and early 1980s the rate of attrition after midwifery training remained the same as in the two previous decades. This was demonstrated by figures for the years 1974–78 published by the Central Midwives Board (1983). The figures showed that about half of the midwives who enrolled did not notify their intention to practise in the subsequent year and that further wastage occurred in succeeding years, with about a quarter of those enrolling each year still in practice some five years later. The figures for 1979 and 1980 showed an increase in the proportion notifying their intention to practise in the year following enrolment, but still a considerable wastage in successive years (Central Midwives Board, 1983).

Returning to the issue of staffing levels, it has been shown that concern emerged in the 1940s and persisted through the 1950s and 1960s. Research findings and statements from professional bodies indicate that this concern has not subsided in the 1970s and 1980s. Data obtained in the course of a national survey on the role and responsibilities of the midwife provided an indication that at the end of the 1970s staffing levels were perceived as inadequate by the majority of hospital and community midwives (Robinson, 1980; Robinson, Golden and Bradley, 1983). Moreover, staffing figures provided by heads of midwifery service demonstrated a shortfall of every grade on 31st December, 1978 and that this was particularly acute at staff midwife level, with a discrepancy of 18% between funded establishment and whole time equivalents in post (Robinson, 1980). Similar findings were obtained in 1984 by the Royal College of Midwives from their survey of staffing levels in England and Wales (Royal College of Midwives, 1985) and in subsequent years their evidence to the Pay Review Body indicates that in their opinion, staffing levels continue to be of concern (Royal College of Midwives, 1986a, 1987a, 1988).

Against this background of continuing attrition from the profession and concern about staffing levels, the extent to which student midwives felt sufficiently confident to practise was accorded considerable importance during the 1970s. In 1968 the two part training was finally replaced by the single period course. However, in subsequent years, staff at midwifery training schools maintained that 12 months was insufficient time to cover the syllabus adequately and in particular to develop confidence in clinical skills (Central Midwives Board, 1977). As noted earlier, the Board consequently decided to extend training to 18 months for State Registered Nurses and to three years for those without nursing qualifications; the new course was introduced in September 1981. We felt, however, that if any conclusions were to be drawn as to whether the extended training did have the desired effect on midwives' confidence and career intentions, then data on these issues had first to be obtained from midwives who had taken a 12 month course, in order that a comparison could subsequently be made.

AIMS AND METHODS

The research took the form of a survey by questionnaire of two large groups of midwives; one had qualified in 1979 after a 12 month course and the other in 1983 after an 18 month course. Our objectives were as follows:

1. To obtain information from the two groups on:
    age, nationality and nursing experience at entry to midwifery training;
    reasons for training as a midwife;
    career intentions before training;
    career intentions after qualifying.
    views on aspects of the course: these included:
    amount and helpfulness of clinical and classroom teaching;
    areas in which more clinical experience is needed;
    time for private study;
    adequacy of preparation for undertaking responsibilities of practising as a midwife.
2. To determine whether a relationship existed between career intentions and demographic characteristics and between career intentions and experience of training.
3. To ascertain whether any differences existed between the two groups of qualifiers in relation to 1 and 2 above.

Questionnaires were chosen as the most appropriate and feasible data collecting instrument, given (a) the nature of the information required and (b) the geographical dispersal of newly qualified midwives. A questionnaire was designed that drew on the literature and on personal experiences of midwifery tutors. It consisted almost entirely of closed questions with pre-coded answers, although respondents were invited to make additional comments if they wished. It was piloted in 1978 with small groups of newly qualified midwives first in interviews and second by post, and then sent to a larger group. The findings were subsequently published (Golden, 1980). The revised questionnaire was then sent to 932 midwives who qualified in 1979 after a 12 month course. They comprised all those who had taken the July examination and represented a quarter of those qualifying that year.

The implementation of the 18 month training was, in fact, delayed until September 1981, and so we were not able to proceed with the comparative phase (i.e. views of those who took an 18 month course) as soon as originally intended. We decided not to send the questionnaire to the first group who took the 18 month training as their responses might have been affected by 'teething' problems with the new course, and so the second and third groups to qualify were selected. This group consisted of a similar number of midwives (*n*=931) to the 1979 qualifiers. They had taken the 1983 May/June or September/October examinations and, as with the 12 month group, they represented approximately one quarter of the midwives qualifying in that year.

On both occasions the questionnaire was accompanied by an explanatory letter and a stamped addressed envelope. One reminder letter was sent to non-respondents some four to five weeks after the initial posting and response rates of 84% (782/932) for the 1979 group and 89% (828/931) for the 1983 group were achieved. Data were analysed with the SPSS-X programme; the main statistical test used was that for the difference between proportions (Armitage, 1971) and given the large size of the two groups, the lowest level of significance accepted was $p < 0.001$ unless otherwise stated. The findings are presented in three sections:

1. Reasons for taking the course and career intentions at its outset;
2. Views on various components of the course;
3. Career intentions after qualifying and their relationship with demographic characteristics and educational experiences.

REASONS FOR TRAINING AND CAREER INTENTIONS

In response to long-standing concern over nurses seeking qualification as a midwife for purposes other than wishing to practise midwifery, the research investigated reasons for training and career intentions prior to course commencement. The findings indicated the extent to which training for collateral reasons was still prevalent among 18 month course entrants, and the extent to which this proportion had declined since the longer course was introduced. Participants were asked to indicate all of the reasons shown in Table 11.1 that had contributed to their decision to train; they were given the option of selecting more than one of the reasons listed as the pilot study findings indicated that several were usually involved.

The first three reasons listed in Table 11.1 all concern a career perspective in which obtaining a midwifery qualification is regarded as part of a nursing career. The first reason, 'to broaden my experience', was the one mentioned most frequently by those qualifying in 1979 and by those qualifying in 1983 – well over half in both years. The perception that qualifying as a midwife improves nursing career prospects appears not to have diminished in the period between the two groups starting their training; with approximately half of both groups citing this as a reason for doing so. The next two reasons

Table 11.1 Reasons for taking midwifery training

Reasons	Midwives qualifying in			
	1979 after a 12 month course (n = 782)		1983 after an 18 month course (n = 828)	
	%	No.	%	No.
To broaden my experience	58	451	63	519
As an additional qualification to improve my career prospects	49	384	53	437
I thought my training was incomplete without midwifery training	35	272	23	191
I intended to work as a midwife after qualifying	26	204	39	321
To see if I liked midwifery	14	113	17	143
I needed the qualification to work overseas	20	154	17	144
I wanted a change from nursing	8	59	11	89

Source: Compiled by the author.

listed were the most likely to show differences between the two groups. The 1983 qualifiers were less likely than the 1979 qualifiers to regard their training as incomplete without midwifery (35% compared with 23% $p < 0.00001$). Also, they were much more likely to indicate that they intended to work as a midwife after qualifying (39% compared with 26% $p < 0.00001$).

If these findings are compared with those of earlier investigations it can be seen that little has changed over time. The proportion taking midwifery training because they wanted to practise midwifery has ranged between a quarter and just over a third: 37% of those who took part in the 1947 study (Ministry of Health *et al.*, 1949); 24% of those who took part in Ramsden and Radwanski's 1963 study; 26% of those in this study who qualified in 1979 and 39% of those who qualified in 1983. Similarly, at least half of the respondents in each of the four years studied (spanning a 35 year period) gave a reason connected with a nursing career; either as an additional qualification to improve career prospects or to complete nurse training.

Subsequent studies have in some respects confirmed this trend. Mander's findings indicate that 'to complete training' was the reason cited most frequently by respondents (44%), followed by 'to satisfy interest' (43%), and 'to work abroad' (30%), with just 21% of respondents saying that they trained in order to practise midwifery (Mander, 1989). Findings for male midwives (Lewis, 1987, and Chapter 10 in this volume) showed that they were as likely as their female counterparts to take midwifery training for reasons allied to nursing in that 62% cited 'to broaden their experience' and 50% said it was 'to improve their career prospects'. Men seemed to be more likely, however, than women to give 'practising midwifery' as a reason for training, as 52% said it was 'to fulfil a personal desire to become a midwife' and 21% said it was 'as a challenge to the previous exclusion of men from midwifery'.

Findings from the Nuffield Centre Study (Brooks, Long and Rathwell, 1987) reveal a different picture in some respects in that 65% of their non-practising request sample and 48% of their non-practising random sample said that they trained in order to work as a midwife. However, these figures are probably artificially high in relation to midwives as a whole. The former sample was self-selected; it may well have over-represented those who had intended to practise midwifery and having a continuing interest in the subject volunteered to take part in the study. The second sample achieved a response rate of only 46%, and it could be argued that these respondents were more likely than the non-respondents to have intended to work as a midwife, hence their continuing interest in the subject and willingness to return a questionnaire. Even in these two samples, however, with their potential for being biased towards practising midwifery, a substantial proportion of both (53% and 65% respectively) cited 'to improve career prospects' as a reason for taking midwifery training.

Intending to work as a midwife does not necessarily entail making a career in midwifery. The newly qualified midwife may intend to work as a midwife for a short time, in order to consolidate her training before moving to another area of work. A contribution to the profession is made, however, by all those who put their training into practice albeit that this may be a short term commitment only, and so we sought to discover the proportion of newly qualified midwives who came into this category.

The range of possibilities in relation to practising midwifery is shown in Table 11.2. The first three possibilities indicate an intention to practise as a midwife, even if only for a short time, and have been sub-totalled within the table to show the overall proportion of respondents who expressed an intention to practise. Similarly, the fourth and fifth possibilities have also been sub-totalled within the table to show the overall proportion of midwives who did not express an intention to practise.

Just 3% more of the 1983 group than of the 1979 group began their course intending to make a career in midwifery: 16% compared with 13%. The largest proportion of respondents in both groups were uncertain as to whether they would practise midwifery for a short time only or for a career; 38% compared with 48%. Looking at the sub-totals for those who intended

Table 11.2 Career intentions before taking midwifery training

Career intentions before taking training in relation to practising midwifery	Midwives qualifying in			
	1979 after a 12 month course		1983 after an 18 month course	
	%	No.	%	No.
To make a career in midwifery	13	105	16	134
To practise midwifery but not sure whether for a short time or for a career	38	300	48	395
To practise for some time as a midwife, but not to make midwifery a career	14	109	14	114
Total expressing an intention to practise	66	514	78	643
Not sure whether want to practise at all as a midwife	26	206	16	137
Not to practise midwifery after qualifying	8	62	3	27
Total not expressing an intention to practise	34	268	20	164
No answer	–	–	2	21
Total	100	782	100	828

Source: Compiled by the author.

to practise midwifery, the figures show that this is the case for a substantial majority of both groups, with the figure for the 1983 qualifiers representing an increase of 12% over that for the 1979 qualifiers – 78% compared with 66% ($p < 0.00001$).

The 1979 group was more likely to enter training with a view to not practising after qualifying – 34% compared with 20% ($p < 0.00001$). This difference might reflect a reluctance to embark on the longer 18 month training by those who formerly might have sought the midwifery qualification as part of their nursing career.

EDUCATIONAL EXPERIENCES

We studied four aspects of the educational experiences of student midwives: teaching in school; teaching in clinical settings; clinical experience; and personal study. Questions were asked about each of these separately, and then respondents were asked how adequately they felt that their training had prepared them for carrying out the various responsibilities of the midwife. Finally, they were asked how much they had enjoyed the course.

Classroom and clinical teaching

The education of student midwives in England and Wales has differed from that of student nurses in that the midwifery profession has maintained that only one grade of teacher is necessary to teach in both the classroom and the clinical setting. This system is said to have a number of advantages (Roch, 1984). It produces confident teachers who have credibility with their students and other trained staff and it enables teachers to maintain some of their clinical skills. Moreover, it facilitates co-operation between service and teaching staff and this in turn facilitates the education of students. In particular, it affords teachers the opportunity to integrate theoretical and ward practices and thus helps students to apply theory to practice. Some information on the extent to which these claimed advantages occur in practice was obtained in the course of this research. The participants were asked first if they had found the amount of time spent on classroom and clinical teaching by tutors to be about right, or whether too much or too little time was devoted to it. Secondly, they were asked how helpful they had found the teaching.

It is expected that student midwives will receive teaching in clinical settings from trained staff on duty as well as from midwifery tutors, and so the study participants were also asked for their views on the amount and helpfulness of teaching provided by these staff. For sisters in particular, teaching student midwives and helping them develop confidence in their skills is regarded as an important part of their role. Studies of educational opportunities for learner nurses have indentified the ward sister as a key person in creating an environment which is conducive to learning (e.g. Fretwell, 1980; Orton, 1981). Other studies have sought to identify the characteristics of effective ward teachers and have emphasised the importance of a 'participative mode of communication' (Marson, 1982) and an 'approachable nurse learner orientated style of leadership' (Ogier, 1982). As shown in the first section of this chapter, teaching by midwifery sisters and staff midwives has not been the subject of extensive research as yet; this study provided some information on how this is perceived by newly qualified midwives.

During the period in which the two groups of midwives who took part in this project were in training, the Central Midwives Board specified that a certain number of hours should be allocated to teaching by medical staff. Participants were asked therefore for their views on the helpfulness and amount of classroom and clinical teaching that they had received from obstetricians and paediatricians. The length of time for such teaching is no longer specified and there are some indications that this component of classroom teaching has been reduced (for example, Opoku and Davies, 1988). Nonetheless, findings from this project may still be relevant, in that some aspects of present and proposed midwifery education programmes are likely to entail an input from medical staff.

Classroom teaching. The proportion of both groups of qualifiers who said that the right amount of time was spent on classroom teaching and that it was helpful or very helpful is shown in Table 11.3 for each group of staff specified. The findings differed little for the two groups and show that a substantial proportion was satisfied with the content of and amount of time spent on classroom teaching. The figures ranged from over 80% for teaching by midwifery tutors to over 60% for teaching by medical staff in paediatrics. Lower figures for the latter group were due to one-fifth of both the 1979 and the 1983 qualifiers saying they did not get enough classroom teaching from paediatricians.

Two main themes emerged from comments added by those who were not

Table 11.3 Proportion of respondents who said that the amount of time spent on classroom teaching was about right and that it was helpful or very helpful

Classroom teaching by	Midwives qualifying in			
	1979 after a 12 month course (n = 782)		*1983 after an 18 month course (n = 828)*	
	%	No.	%	No.
Midwifery tutors	83	648	84	692
Obstetric medical staff	77	603	77	638
Paediatric medical staff	62	487	66	542

Source: Compiled by the author.

satisfied with classroom teaching by midwifery tutors; these were lack of discussion and too much time spent in copying notes. The two comments made most frequently by those not satisfied with classroom teaching by medical staff were that they repeated what had already been taught by tutors, or that their views differed from those of tutors or other medical staff.

Our study did not look in detail at the content of classroom teaching. Pope (1986) however, did do so in her study of the 18 month course in Scotland, and found that students felt there was too much emphasis on anatomy, the statutory bodies and community medicine and insufficient emphasis on bereavement counselling, support groups, research and management.

Clinical teaching. The majority of respondents said that the clinical teaching provided by each group of staff specified was helpful or very helpful; this is shown in Table 11.4. There was, however, considerably less satisfaction with the amount of time spent on clinical teaching and this is shown in Table 11.5.

Turning first to clinical teaching by midwifery tutors, a total of 43% of the 1979 qualifiers and 45% of the 1983 qualifiers said that these staff either spent too little time on clinical teaching or none at all. It might have been expected that this view would be expressed by a smaller proportion of the 1983 respondents as the longer course should allow tutors more time to spend in the clinical setting, but in fact the proportion has increased slightly (although not significantly at the $p < 0.001$ level). Two main themes

Table 11.4 Proportion of respondents who said that clinical teaching was helpful or very helpful

Clinical teaching by	Midwives qualifying in			
	1979 after a 12 month course (n = 782)		1983 after an 18 month course (n = 828)	
	%	No.	%	No.
Midwifery tutors	86	672	83	689
Hospital midwives	86	675	91	752
Community midwives	91	710	93	771
Obstetric medical staff	67	526	66	549
Paediatric medical staff	59	460	61	504

Source: Compiled by the author.

Table 11.5 Views on amount of time spent on clinical teaching by various groups of staff

Amount of time spent on clinical teaching	Clinical teaching by																			
	Midwifery tutors				Hospital midwives				Community midwives				Obstetric medical staff				Paediatric medical staff			
	1979		1983		1979		1983		1979		1983		1979		1983		1979		1983	
	%	No.	%	No.	%	No.	%	No.	%	No.	%	No.	%	No.	%	No.	%	No.	%	No.
Too much time	1	11	2	14	1	3	–	1	1	8	1	5	1	11	1	4	1	7	–	3
About the right amount of time	55	427	52	430	35	274	43	359	76	591	82	676	37	290	31	258	28	215	28	231
Too little time	38	293	42	349	61	476	54	448	21	161	16	129	44	345	56	465	49	382	58	476
No time	5	37	3	27	3	20	1	9	2	16	1	10	17	130	12	95	22	171	13	111
No answer	2	14	1	8	1	9	1	11	1	6	1	8	1	6	1	6	1	7	1	7
Total	100	782	100	828	100	782	100	828	100	782	100	828	100	782	100	828	100	782	100	828

Source: Compiled by the author.

emerged from comments made on this subject. First, it was maintained that there were not enough tutors in post for them to spend sufficient time teaching in the wards and clinic; second, it was said that tutors could have spent more time with students in the clinical setting but failed to do so, some respondents also adding that there was little liaison between school and service staff. Comments made by those who felt that they had received enough clinical teaching indicated how useful they had found it.

Some evidence does exist on the adequacy of tutorial staffing levels in midwifery. For example, Standon-Batt (1979) drew attention to a deficit in the number of tutors qualifying each year. She pointed out that although an estimated 80 new tutors were needed each year in England and Wales to fill vacancies caused by 'retirement, marriage, motherhood, side stepping to administration and (hopefully) an increase in establishment', figures published by the Central Midwives Board for the years 1973–77 showed an average of only 57 new tutors qualifying each year. Data on tutorial staffing levels were obtained in the course of a national survey of the midwifery profession (Robinson, 1980) and showed that in England there was a 15% shortfall between funded establishment and tutors actually in post on 31st December, 1978, and a corresponding figure of 5% for senior tutors. Figures published annually by the Royal College of Midwives in their evidence to the Pay Review Body for the years up until 1988 indicate that the shortfall has reduced for senior tutors but not for tutors. No research to date appears to have focused on factors other than staffing shortages that may deter midwifery tutors from teaching in the clinical setting.

Table 11.5 shows that a majority of both groups claimed not to have received enough clinical teaching from hospital midwives: a total of 64% of those qualifying in 1979 and a total of 55% of those qualifying in 1983. Comments made about this lack of clinical teaching revealed the same two themes which emerged in relation to midwifery tutors: a lack of staff on duty; and an unwillingness to teach, even when opportunities were available. As shown earlier in this chapter, staffing levels have been below funded establishment throughout the late 1970s and the 1980s (Robinson, 1980; Royal College of Midwives, 1985–88). Obviously, a shortage of trained staff on duty affects the time available for teaching learners and its effect on time for teaching students is likely to be the same now as it was when this research was undertaken.

The other point made in relation to clinical teaching by hospital midwives concerned a seeming reluctance to teach. Other studies suggest that this may be because staff feel inadequately prepared for a teaching role. For example, just over a quarter of the midwives surveyed by Robinson, Golden and Bradley (1983) said that they did not feel adequately prepared for teaching responsibilities. Midwives' concerns about these responsibilities have been highlighted more recently by Parnaby (1987) who found that teaching students was one of the topics most likely to be regarded by midwives as essential for inclusion in refresher courses. Attempts to increase midwives' confidence in teaching have been made in some areas by providing teaching in clinical practice courses (Sweet, 1984) and the English National Board Course 997 (Teaching in Clinical Practice) is available to midwives as well as to nurses. Feeling inadequately prepared to teach students is not, of course, unique to midwifery. Much research has indicated that nursing staff do not always feel adequately prepared for the teaching component of their role (for example, Bendall, 1976; Pearson, 1979, Farnish, 1983; and Runciman, 1980).

More than three-quarters of both groups said that they had enough teaching from community midwives (76% in 1979 and 82% in 1983). This is not surprising as there is usually a one-to-one relationship between a midwife and her student during community experience.

A substantial majority of both groups of respondents said that in their view they received either insufficient teaching from medical staff or none at all. Sixty-one per cent of those qualifying in 1979 and 68% of those qualifying in 1983 expressed this view in relation to teaching by obstetricians and the corresponding figure in relation to paediatricians was 71% for both groups. Again, the two themes of short staffed, busy units on the one hand and a reluctance to teach on the other, were cited as the main reasons for this lack of teaching.

As with classroom teaching, comments were made about the confusing effect of contradictory views put forward in teaching by different groups of staff, and particular reference was made to differences in the content of teaching in school and practice on the wards. The existence of this situation has also been documented for general nursing (e.g. Gott, 1984).

Similar findings on classroom and clinical teaching emerged from Pope's study of the 18 month course in Scotland (Pope, 1986), in that the majority of respondents were satisfied with the content and composition of study blocks, but 66% said that they did not receive enough clinical teaching. Concerns about the lack of clinical teaching provided for student midwives and poor liaison between ward and school staff are, of course, not new. The same issues were discussed in depth nearly 40 years ago by the 1947 Working Party on Midwives which, as described in the second section of this chapter, considered various aspects of midwifery training as part of its investigation into the shortage of midwives prevailing in the 1940s. On the basis of interviews held with tutors, sisters and pupil midwives, the Working Party concluded that:

> while the formal and academic teaching is usually well carried out, there is much complaint that the ward staff are either too busy to teach or unwilling to accept their responsibilities in this connection. Relations between ward staff and teaching staff are often unco-ordinated and sometimes strained....
> (Ministry of Health *et al.*, 1949)

The Working Party was concerned that what it perceived as 'casual and rather haphazard clinical teaching' could be one of the reasons why so few pupil midwives at that time completed their course with a desire to put their training into practice.

As noted earlier the same point was advanced in the 1970s as one of the reasons for extending the training from 12 to 18 months but it is perhaps not surprising that satisfaction with the amount of clinical teaching has not increased with this extension. Neither of the two factors identified by respondents as contributing to a lack of clinical teaching, namely short staffing and an unwillingness to teach, would be affected by increasing the length of training.

Clinical experience

The student midwife's knowledge, skills and confidence are developed by clinical experience as well as by teaching. Consequently, the study participants were asked if, in their view, there were any clinical areas in which they felt they should have spent more time during training to gain sufficient experience of the work. Those who took the 18 month course were significantly less likely than those who took the 12 month course to say that they

Table 11.6 Proportion of midwives who felt they needed more time to gain sufficient experience in specified clinical areas

Clinical areas	Midwives qualifying in			
	1979 after a 12 month course (n = 782)		1983 after an 18 month course (n = 828)	
	%	No.	%	No.
Obstetric theatres	61	477	50	415
Special care baby units	54	422	37	307
Labour wards	46	362	28	228
Community	21	163	20	170
Antenatal wards	16	125	15	127
Antenatal clinics	7	53	7	60
Postnatal wards	5	37	1	10
Other	2	18	3	27

Source: Compiled by the author.

had needed more time in this respect (73% (600) compared with 85% (666) – $p < 0.00001$) but the proportion still remains a substantial majority of those who have taken the extended training. Respondents were asked to specify in which of the clinical areas listed in Table 11.6 they needed more time to gain sufficient experience.

Two main points emerge from the findings in Table 11.6: first, obstetric theatres, special care units and labour wards were the areas most likely to be specified as those in which more time was needed. Secondly, the 18 month group were significantly less likely to express this view than the 12 month group (the level of significance was $p < 0.00001$ in each case). It could be argued that both obstetric theatres and special care baby units are specialized aspects of maternity care, and that one would not expect students to gain enough experience of this work during basic training to feel confident upon qualifying. The same is not true, however, of the labour ward. Although the proportion who said that the experience was too short to gain experience of work in this area decreased from 46% in 1979 to 28% in 1983, this still remains a substantial minority.

A fifth of both groups said that they needed more time in the community. Most of the comments made referred to little or no experience of home confinements. This is, of course, not necessarily due to insufficient time but rather to the substantial decrease in the number of women delivered at home. Nonetheless, these comments suggest that for some newly qualified midwives, lack of home confinements is associated with a feeling that insufficient time had been spent in the community.

Approximately half of those who felt that there was a shortage of experience in antenatal clinics added a comment to the effect that the problem was not so much lack of time, but the inappropriate use of time. They pointed out that student midwives acted as chaperones to the medical staff and undertook tasks such as urine testing and weighing. They had no opportunity, however, to perform abdominal palpations or assess the overall course of pregnancy, as this was always done by medical staff in the clinics in which they worked.

Similar findings on clinical experience emerge from other studies of midwifery training. Mander's findings indicate that at the outset of training, only a quarter of both the 12 month and the 18 month group expected that by the end of the course they would feel confident to work in a special care baby unit (Mander, 1987). Pope (1986) found that labour wards, special care units, and the community were the areas in which students would have liked more time to have been allocated.

Time for personal study

Both groups of qualifiers were asked if in their view they were allowed enough time for personal study during midwifery training (Table 11.7).

Views of those who had taken a 12 month course were fairly evenly divided, whereas those who had taken the extended course were more likely than the former to say that they had been allowed enough time for personal study: 56% compared with 48% $(0.001 < p < 0.01)$. Nonetheless, a substantial minority (42%) of this group were of the view that they had not been allowed sufficient time.

The 1983 qualifiers were invited to amplify their answer if they wished; comments were added by 160 (46%) of the 345 who said they had insufficient time for personal study and by 78 (17%) of the 464 who felt they had been allowed enough.

Issues raised by respondents in relation to insufficient time during school 'blocks' included the following: a greater part of the study days should have been allocated to time for personal study; all the study time should not have been allocated to project work, and tutors should not have used up timetabled personal study periods in order to get through the syllabus. Some respondents also commented that tutors seemed unwilling to let students work unsupervised. The comment made most frequently about personal study time during clinical experience was that the wards were always, or nearly always, too busy for this to be feasible. Some respondents added the view that hospital staff were reluctant for students to spend time studying, even when the pressure of work would allow this, preferring domestic tasks to be performed instead. Others voiced the opinion that lack of time or personal study when working on the wards highlighted the employee/student status dilemma. However, most of the comments made by those who felt that they had had sufficient time for personal study concerned the

Table 11.7 Time for personal study during midwifery training

Time for personal study during training	Midwives qualifying in			
	1979 after a 12 month course		1983 after an 18 month course	
	%	No.	%	No.
Allowed enough time for personal study	48	375	56	464
Not allowed enough time for personal study	48	379	42	345
No answer	4	28	2	19
Total	100	782	100	828

Source: Compiled by the author.

Table 11.8 Views on adequacy of training in preparation for responsibilities of midwifery practice

Responsibilities of midwifery practice		Proportion of respondents who said that they were				
		More than adequately prepared %	Adequately prepared %	Less than adequately prepared %	No answer %	Total
Hospital care						
1. Caring for mothers attending antenatal clinics	1979	26	70	4	0	782
	1983	31	63	6	0	828
2. Caring for mothers in antenatal wards	1979	19	72	8	0	782
	1983	29	64	7	0	828
3. Caring for mothers in labour wards	1979	20	70	10	0	782
	1983	32	61	6	0	828
4. Caring for babies in labour wards	1979	12	67	20	0	782
	1983	22	66	12	1	828
5. Caring for mothers in postnatal wards	1979	39	57	4	0	782
	1983	56	43	1	0	828
6. Caring for babies in postnatal wards	1979	33	62	5	0	782
	1983	48	50	2	0	828
7. Caring for babies in special care baby units	1979	6	37	57	0	782
	1983	7	52	41	1	828

Table 11.8 contd.

	Year					
Community care						
8. Caring for mothers attending antenatal clinics	1979	30	64	6	1	782
	1983	40	55	6	1	828
9. Giving antenatal care to mothers in their own homes	1979	23	60	16	1	782
	1983	32	58	10	0	828
10. Caring for mothers during home confinement	1979	6	30	61	3	782
	1983	6	31	60	3	828
11. Caring for babies during home confinement	1979	6	33	58	4	782
	1983	6	33	58	4	828
12. Caring for mothers during postnatal period at home	1979	44	54	2	0	782
	1983	61	38	1	0	828
13. Caring for babies during postnatal period at home	1979	33	61	6	1	782
	1983	51	47	2	0	828
Teaching						
14. Teaching individual mothers in antenatal or postnatal period	1979	24	68	8	0	782
	1983	38	59	4	0	828
15. Teaching groups in parentcraft classes	1979	15	52	33	1	782
	1983	19	58	23	0	828

Source: Compiled by the author.

diligence of tutors and/or hospital midwives in ensuring that this time was available.

Since this research was completed, two of the issues raised by respondents in relation to time for personal study have been the focus of much discussion in documents produced on midwifery and on nursing education. First, the importance of encouraging learners to study independently (Royal College of Midwives, 1987b) and secondly, the desirability of supernumerary status to ensure that educational needs are not sacrificed to service demands (UKCC, 1986, Royal College of Midwives, 1986b).

Adequacy of training for undertaking responsibilities of a midwife

Findings presented so far have been concerned with separate components of the course: clinical and classroom teaching, clinical experience and personal study. In looking back on their training as a whole, both groups were asked how well they thought it had prepared them for the various responsibilities involved in practising as a midwife. They were asked whether their preparation had been adequate, less than adequate or more than adequate in relation to the components of care listed in Table 11.8. Their answers indicate that the majority felt that training had prepared them adequately or more than adequately for the various aspects of care listed, with the exception of home confinements (Items 10 and 11) and special care baby units (Item 7). It can also be seen that the 18 month group were more likely than the 12 month group to say that they felt more than adequately prepared to take responsibility for items 1 to 6, 8, 9 and 12–15. (These differences were all significant at the $p < 0.001$ level or better, except for item 1 ($p < 0.05$) and item 9 ($p < 0.005$).) Analyses of data for each group of qualifiers by whether or not training took place in a teaching hospital and by whether the course was the first, second or third extended one to be run by the school revealed no significant differences.

Answers relating to item 4 (caring for babies in labour ward) are of particular interest. The 1978 pilot study showed that 23% of respondents felt less than adequately prepared for this aspect of care, and when these data were published, (Golden, 1980) this finding was viewed with some concern by midwifery tutors and by the educational supervisors at the Central Midwives Board. Consequently, when visits were made by Board supervisors to training schools, attention was drawn to the importance of providing students with experience of caring for babies on the labour ward (personal communication). The decrease in the proportion of respondents who felt inadequately prepared in this respect may be due partly to this intervention and not entirely to the extended length of training.

Findings for special care baby units showed that just over half (57%) of the 1979 qualifiers felt less than adequately prepared for this aspect of maternity care and, as shown in Table 11.6, 54% said they had insufficient experience of this work. In the 18 month course the special care unit alloca- tion was increased to 6 weeks. The findings show that the 1983 group were more likely to say that they felt adequately, or more than adequately prepared for special care work (59% compared with 43%). As the period between 1979 and 1983 saw a continuing increase in the complexity of neonatal intensive care technology, these figures represented a considerable improvement in perceived adequacy of preparation for work in this area. Nonetheless, special care is still an area for which a substantial number of midwives feel that they require additional experience and knowledge in order to feel confident to undertake the work that it entails.

Not surprisingly, the majority of both groups felt inadequately prepared to care for mothers or babies during home confinements. The continuing decline in the proportion of women delivered at home has meant that most student midwives get little, if any, experience of home confinements. Of those midwives who qualified in 1979, 59% had not undertaken any home confinements during their training and a further 26% had only undertaken one; the corresponding figures for the 1983 respondents were 64% and 24%.

A majority from both groups felt adequately prepared to teach women on a one-to-one basis in the antenatal and postnatal periods and to teach groups in parentcraft classes. Moreover, the 1983 findings show a marked improvement on those for 1979, particularly in relation to one-to-one teaching; this may well reflect the increased emphasis placed on the principles and practice of teaching in the 18 month syllabus. Nonetheless, just under a quarter of the 1983 group felt inadequately prepared to teach groups in parentcraft classes. In recent years the need for post-basic courses in antenatal education has been recognized and many have been established (Murphy-Black in Chapter 6 of this volume). As Prince and Adams (1979) commented: 'There are so many variables in culture, education and attitudes of an antenatal group that it requires a skilled teacher to respond to all needs' (p. 109).

Findings relating to postnatal care of mothers and babies in hospital and in the community deserve particular consideration. Items in Table 11.8 relating to postnatal care (5, 6, 12 and 13) show that this was the area for which newly qualified midwives were most likely to feel able to take responsibility. Yet some evidence suggests that postnatal care is more likely than other aspects of the maternity service to be understaffed and to be the subject of consumer criticism. Midwives on postnatal wards who took part in a national survey of the profession (Robinson, Golden and Bradley, 1983) were the most likely to say that there were not enough midwives on duty to cope with the work: 67% of those on day duty and 77% of those on night duty. The main effects of short staffing cited by these respondents were insufficient time to teach and help mothers and to teach students. Women's dissatisfaction with postnatal care had been documented in a number of studies undertaken in the late 1970s and early 1980s, these included Ball (1983), Laryea (1980) and Filshie *et al.* (1981). However, the newly qualified midwives who took part in this study felt quite confident about this part of their role. Postnatal care requires interpersonal skills to help develop women's confidence in their ability to feed and care for their baby. Although most student midwives are likely to have developed relevant interpersonal skills in the course of their nurse training, it is possible that, as newly qualified midwives, they have an insufficient understanding of women's needs during the puerperium to be aware of any deficiencies in their own interpersonal skills. Deficiencies in technical and manual skills are much more readily apparent than deficiencies in interpersonal skills, and this may partly explain why those aspects of care that require the former skills are the ones about which newly qualified midwives are most likely to express feelings of inadequacy.

The 18 month course did allow for more time to be devoted to various aspects of midwifery and for students to gain more clinical experience than the 12 month course, and findings from this study suggested this has led to an increase in the proportion of newly qualified midwives who feel adequately prepared for practice. A substantial majority of the 18 month group felt adequately prepared to assume most of the responsibilities of a midwife. Findings from Pope's study (1986) also indicated that the 18 month course seemed to have been an adequate preparation for the majority of those questioned. For example, 71% of the 134 respondents considered that they were able to function as full members of the midwifery team and 99% felt that they had learned how to provide an acceptable standard of care for mothers and babies (Pope, 1986).

Enjoyment of training

Finally, the newly qualified midwives were asked to indicate how much they had enjoyed their midwifery training by rating each period on a 1 to 5 scale, in which 1=Enjoyed it very much and 5=Did not enjoy it at all. The 12 month course was divided into three discrete periods: the initial 16 weeks in hospital; community experience, and a final 19 weeks in hospital. The 18 month course was organised slightly differently in that the community experience could be divided into more than one period, and so both groups of qualifiers were asked to consider the course in terms of:

1. An initial period in hospital prior to any community experience;
2. Community experience;
3. All hospital experience other than the initial period in hospital.

The ratings given to each of the three parts of the course are shown in Table 11.9. The findings show that ratings varied little between the two

Table 11.9 Enjoyment of course

	Parts of midwifery course											
Rating of enjoyment	Initial period in hospital				Community experience				All hospital experience other than initial period			
	1979		1983		1979		1983		1979		1983	
	%	No.	%	No.	%	No.	%	No.	%	No.	%	No.
1 enjoyed it very much	17		13		47		54		33		29	
2	23		25		28		26		42		46	
3	29		34		17		13		19		19	
4	19		20		5		4		5		5	
5 did not enjoy it at all	12		8		2		2		3		–	

Source: Compiled by the author.

groups. The initial period in hospital was the least popular. The final period in hospital was less likely to be enjoyed than the community experience, but more likely to be enjoyed than the initial hospital period.

The 1983 qualifiers were invited to comment on the ratings that they gave to each part of the course and 45% did so. An analysis of these comments provided some indication of positive and negative aspects of the course as perceived by this group. Most of the comments made in relation to the initial period in hospital were concerned with reasons for not enjoying this part of the course; the one that came up most frequently was lack of recognition by staff of knowledge gained during nursing training and experience. In the words of two of them:

> During my training, student midwives were often given little credit or respect for being previously trained nurses, and were treated like girls out of school by all members of staff including the nursing auxiliary!

> I disliked the initial period very much as staff treated us as though we did not know anything. I realise that being a trained nurse does not mean we have any knowledge of midwifery but, for example, I do know how to take a blood pressure.

Other respondents said that they found it difficult to adjust to being students again, having qualified and worked as nurses:

> To begin with I was very unsettled in my midwifery training, as I had been a staff nurse on a busy surgical ward with plenty of responsibility. Suddenly, I was once again a student, and given very little respect or responsibility.

Lack of knowledge and experience required to provide care for women and babies was also given as a reason for not enjoying the initial period, for example:

> I disliked midwifery very much when I started – I felt very inadequate, unable to give simple advice to the parents, especially on the postnatal period. As my experience grew, I coped more easily and began to enjoy my work.

Other comments about lack of enjoyment of the initial hospital period referred to unfriendly ward staff, working under pressure because of staff shortages, and uncertainty at this stage of the course as to whether they wanted to become a midwife.

Community experience was the period most likely to be enjoyed; reasons given for this included having time to spend with women, providing continuity of care, learning in a one-to-one relationship with a community midwife, and having the opportunity to practise with a measure of independence. For example

Community was a great time of learning on a one-to-one basis and the most enjoyable period of training. Job satisfaction is increased through rendering continuity of care to mothers and babies.

Having a level of responsibility while on Community consolidated knowledge and confidence.

Several respondents said that the initial hospital experience made more sense after they had worked in the community, and others felt that the community experience made them feel much more confident when they returned to hospital. For example:

Initially, nothing made any sense and I think when I gained confidence in the practical aspects (mostly on community experience) I enjoyed it much better.

In the initial part of training I was expected to give advice but didn't feel qualified – e.g. on breastfeeding. However, when I was in the community, I was able to ask the community midwife about what advice to give. When I went back into hospital I felt much more confident and subsequently enjoyed it much more.

A few comments were made about hospital experience, other than the initial period, and these referred either to knowledge and experience gained on the course falling into place, or to enjoyment waning as the exams drew nearer.

At the end of the questionnaire, the 1983 qualifiers were given the opportunity to make further comments on their training if they wished to do so and just over half (52%) took up this opportunity. Comments fell into two main categories: views of the course overall, and the helpfulness of tutors. The majority of the former focused on enjoyment of the course.

Since midwifery is so different from general nursing I needed a period of time of adjustment before I developed involvement in it. After the initial period, as my knowledge and interest were building up, I enjoyed it so much and got much job satisfaction from my work.

The whole 18 month training was very interesting and worthwhile – although the study was hard work, it was very enjoyable.

Aspects of the course that were subject to critical comment included too much time spent on completing clinical experience record books, too long a gap between written and oral examinations, and inappropriate methods of assessing skills and knowledge (particularly the *viva voce*).

Forty-two respondents mentioned the helpfulness of tutorial staff, some also referring to the effect that tutors can have on students' future career plans. Nearly all of those who commented were appreciative of the quality

of teaching and support provided by tutorial staff, as the following demonstrate:

> My course was as good as it was because of the super team of midwife
> tutors we had. Their excellent teaching methods, enthusiasm, en-
> couragement and caring made a difficult course an enjoyable one. I
> know I would not have succeeded first time without their help.

> Our tutor appeared totally committed to the task of turning us into
> good, questioning and forward-thinking midwives.

> I should like to comment on the outstanding part the senior tutor has
> to play on this course. Her unflagging enthusiasm is so essential when
> students find it difficult to endure the long training. My tutor not only
> gave us the benefit of her vast experience, but every possible shred of
> information she could obtain on modern midwifery practice and
> topics. This inspired me to work harder to finish the course and
> deepened my initial wavering conviction to be a midwife.

FACTORS ASSOCIATED WITH CAREER INTENTIONS AFTER QUALIFYING

Findings presented so far have been concerned with career intentions at the
outset of the course and with views on both its practical and theoretical
aspects. This last section of findings discusses career intentions at the time of
qualification and the extent to which they varied from one group of
respondents to another.

Career intentions after qualifying

It was anticipated that respondents might change their career intentions
during their course and so they were asked to specify their career intentions
after qualifying as well as those that they had held prior to starting the
course. Career intentions held at both points in time are shown in Table
11.10 in order to facilitate a comparison.

The findings show that for both groups of qualifiers there is a 7% increase
in the number who intend to practise midwifery: from 66% to 73% in 1979
and from 78% to 85% in 1983. The 1983 qualifiers were, however, more
likely to show an increase in the proportion intending to make a career in
midwifery: from 16% to 24% compared with a corresponding increase of
13% to 17% for the 1979 group. Despite the finding that those who had
taken the longer course were more likely to opt for a career in midwifery,
24% is nonetheless very much a minority of those qualifying. It seemed
important therefore to examine whether any associations existed between

demographic profile and career intentions, and between perceptions of the adequacy of training and career intentions. Such associations, if found, may well have important policy implications for student selection and for course structure and content.

Career intentions and individual background

Data on age and years in practice as a nurse prior to midwifery training were analysed by career intentions after qualifying. Findings related to age (Table 11.11) show that those who were over 30 at the time they qualified as midwives were significantly more likely than those who were 30 or under to say that they intended to make a career in midwifery; 37% compared with 16% for the 1979 group ($p < 0.00001$) and 42% compared with 22% for the 1983 group ($p < 0.0005$). Analysis of data on age group by reasons for undertaking midwifery training showed that the over 30s were significantly more likely than the under 30s to do so because they intended to work as a midwife: 45% compared with 26% for the 1979 qualifiers ($p < 0.0001$) and 58% compared with 37% ($p < 0.001$) for the 1983 qualifiers. These findings are not unexpected, as those who commit themselves to a lengthy training later on in life are probably more likely than their younger counterparts to do so with the intention of putting it to use. No significant differences emerged when data on years in practice as a nurse prior to midwifery training were analysed by career intentions after qualifying.

Career intentions and perceptions of the course

As described at the beginning of this chapter, one of the reasons for extending midwifery training was to allow greater opportunity to prepare for the various responsibilities involved in midwifery in the hope that this, in turn, would lead to an increase in numbers deciding to make a career in the profession. Findings from this study demonstrated that those who took the longer course were significantly more likely to feel adequately prepared for most of the responsibilities of the practising midwife (Table 11.5). They also showed that the 18 month group were more likely than their counterparts who had taken the shorter course, to intend practising midwifery after qualifying and more likely to intend making it a career (Table 11.10). Both of the hoped-for benefits of the longer training were thus to some extent achieved, but to what extent, if any, were they related? In order to try and answer this question, the data were analysed to determine whether difference in career intentions were associated with particular views about the course, and whether the two groups of qualifiers differed in this respect.

Prior to carrying out this analysis, the respondents were grouped according to their intentions in relation to making a career in midwifery, not just in relation to practising midwifery. This resulted in three groups:

Table 11.10 Career intentions before taking training and after qualifying as a midwife

Career intentions in relation to practising as a midwife	Midwives qualifying in							
	1979 after a 12 month course				1983 after an 18 month course			
	Intentions before		Intentions after		Intentions before		Intentions after	
	%	No.	%	No.	%	No.	%	No.
Intending to make a career in midwifery	13	105	17	136	16	134	24	199
Intending to practise midwifery but not sure whether for a short time or for a career	38	300	40	310	48	395	49	403
Intending to practise for some time as a midwife, but not to make midwifery a career	14	109	16	127	14	114	12	102
Total expressing an intention to practise	66	514	73	573	78	643	85	704
Not sure whether want to practise at all as a midwife	26	206	15	115	16	137	7	58
Not intending to practise midwifery after qualifying	8	62	12	91	3	27	6	46
Total not expressing an intention to practise	34	268	26	206	20	164	13	104

No answer	–	–	0.4	2	3	2	21	2	20
Total	100	782	100	100	782	100	828	100	828

Source: Compiled by the author.

Table 11.11 Age at time of qualification as a midwife by career intentions at time of qualification as a midwife

Career intentions after qualifying as a midwife	Midwives qualifying in							
	1979 after a 12 month course Age at time of qualification				1983 after an 18 month course Age at time of qualification			
	30 years or under		31 years or over		30 years or under		31 years or over	
	%	No.	%	No.	%	No.	%	No.
Make a career in midwifery	16	110	37	26	22	166	42	30
Practise midwifery, but not sure whether for a short time or for a career	40	281	37	26	50	370	40	29
Practise midwifery for some time, but not to make it a career	17	122	7	5	13	97	6	4
Not sure whether want to practise midwifery at all	16	111	14	10	7	53	7	5
Not to practise midwifery	11	80	6	4	6	42	6	4
No answer	0	2	–	–	2	18	–	–
Total	100	706	100	71	100	746	100	72

Source: Compiled by the author.

1. Those who intended to make a career in midwifery (n=136 in 1979 and 199 in 1983);
2. Those who were uncertain whether they would make a career in midwifery or practise for a short time only (n=310 in 1979 and 403 in 1983);
3. Those who did not intend to make a career in midwifery: this group included those who said they intended to practise midwifery but not make it a career, those who were not sure whether they would practise at all and those who said that they would not practise were grouped together as 'not intending to make a career in midwifery' (a total of n=333 in 1979 and 206 in 1983).

Analyses were then performed to ascertain whether these three groups differed significantly in their views on clinical and classroom teaching, amount of clinical experience, time for personal study, adequacy of preparation to undertake responsibilities of a midwife and enjoyment of training. Those for the separate aspects of the course did not in fact demonstrate any consistent trends. However, such trends did emerge in relation to views on adequacy of the course and enjoyment of its three periods. Those who intended to make a career in midwifery were more likely to feel adequately prepared for each of the midwifery responsibilities listed in Table 11.8 and more likely to have enjoyed the three periods of the course than either those who were uncertain about a career in midwifery or those who had decided against one. Differences between the group who intended to make a career in midwifery and the other two groups were much more likely to reach a level of statistical significance for the 1983 qualifiers than for their 1979 counterparts (details are available in Robinson *et al.* 1988).

The interrelationship between career intentions and perceptions of the course is complex, and likely to vary from one individual to another. It may be that a 'good' course instils students with confidence and this encourages them to opt for a career in midwifery; if so then the 18 month course seems to have had a greater effect in this respect than the 12 month course. It could, however, be equally well argued that students who begin training with the intention of staying – and this was the case for more of the 1983 than of the 1979 respondents – get more out of the course than those not intending to do so. In order to pursue this issue further the extent to which career intentions had changed during the course and the extent to which this was associated with perceptions about its adequacy were investigated.

Table 11.12. shows the extent to which intentions in relation to a career in midwifery changed during training. Findings show that similar proportions of both groups of qualifiers began and ended their course intending to make a career in midwifery (11% in 1979 and 12% in 1983). The 18 month group were more likely than the 12 month group to begin and end their course uncertain about a career in midwifery ($p < 0.01$) but less likely

Table 11.12 Career intentions: static and changing

Career intentions before and after qualifying	Midwives qualifying in			
	1979 after a 12 month course		1983 after an 18 month course	
	%	No.	%	No.
Career intentions remained same				
1. Intended to make a career in midwifery before training and after qualification	10	82	12	96
2. Unsure of whether to make a career in midwifery before training and still unsure after qualifying	24	185	31	255
3. Before training and after qualifying did not intend to make a career in midwifery	30	237	14	118
Career intentions changed in a direction towards a career in midwifery				
4. Before training unsure of whether to make a career in midwifery but decided to do so after qualifying	4	31	8	64
5. Before training did not intend to make a career in midwifery, but decided to do so after qualifying	3	23	4	37
6. Before training did not intend to make a career in midwifery but unsure about this after qualifying	15	114	14	113
Career intentions changed in a direction away from a career in midwifery				
7. Before training unsure of whether to make a career in midwifery, but decided against after qualifying	11	84	9	72
8. Before training intended to make a career in midwifery, but unsure after qualifying	1	11	2	21
9. Before training intended to make a career in midwifery but decided against after qualifying	2	12	1	11
No answer	0	3	5	41
Total	100	782	100	828

Source: Compiled by the author.

to begin and end it having ruled out this option (14%: 30% $p < 0.00001$). Similar proportions of both groups demonstrated a move towards a career in midwifery practice (totals of 22% and 26%) and the same was true for a move away from a career in midwifery (totals of 14% and 13%). The data were then analysed to determine the proportion of each of the nine groups shown in Table 11.12 who felt more than adequately prepared for the various responsibilities of the practising midwife. Two main trends emerged. First, for nearly all aspects of care specified the proportion who felt more than adequately prepared was greater among those who began and ended training intending to make midwifery a career (Group 1 in Table 11.12) than those who began and ended training uncertain about (Group 2 in Table 11.12) or who had decided against (Group 3 in Table 11.12) this option. This emerged for those who had taken the 18 month course and for those who had taken the 12 month course. The second trend emerged from a comparison of those whose intentions changed from uncertainty or opposition to a career in midwifery to a decision to pursue this option (Groups 4 and 5 in Table 11.12) with those whose intentions moved in the opposite direction (Groups 7 and 9 in Table 11.12). The former two groups were much more likely than the latter two to feel more than adequately prepared for most of the midwifery responsibilities specified.

The same trends emerged when data on changing career intentions were analysed by enjoyment of training. Those who began and ended their course intending to make a career in midwifery (Group 1 in Table 11.12) were consistently more likely to have enjoyed it than those who began and ended the course uncertain about (Group 2 in Table 11.12) or decided against such a career (Group 3 in Table 11.12). Moreover, those whose intentions changed in favour of a midwifery career (Groups 4 and 5 in Table 11.12) were more likely to have enjoyed the course than whose intentions moved away from this option (Groups 7 and 9 in Table 11.12). The findings also showed that the relationships between changing career intentions and views on adequacy of the course, and between changing career intentions and enjoyment of the course were stronger among the 1983 qualifiers than among the 1979 (details are available in Robinson *et al.*, 1988).

It seems that findings from this research offer some support for both suggestions about the relationship between career intentions and perceptions of the course. First those who begin and end the course with the intention of staying in the profession are more likely to give high ratings for adequacy and enjoyment than those who begin and end it uncertain about, or decided against, a midwifery career; i.e. those who have made up their minds to become midwives are likely to get more out of the course than those who have not made this decision. Secondly, those whose intentions change in favour of midwifery are much more likely than those whose intentions change away from midwifery to have felt well-prepared and to have enjoyed the course, i.e. the quality of the course may affect career intentions. In both cases the association was stronger among respondents who had taken an 18 month course than among those who had taken the shorter course.

These findings have to be interpreted with caution. They are based on respondents' recollections of their intentions and how they felt about the course, and they are indicative, rather than conclusive, about possible relationships between career intentions and course content. They do seem to suggest, however, that there are processes at work which merit further investigation. To do so would require research of a different kind from that described here. An appropriate design would be a case study of a cohort of student midwives which explored their intentions and perceptions by means of in-depth interviews held at regular intervals from the beginning until the end of the course.

DISCUSSION

Many of the changes made this century to the structure of midwifery education were partly, as described earlier in this chapter, an attempt to reduce the number of nurses who wished to qualify as midwives for collateral purposes only. The 1981 extension to 18 months was no exception in this respect. However, our findings showed that only a minority of the 18 month group embarked on the course intending to make a career in the profession (Table 11.2), and that reasons for taking the course cited most frequently were those concerned with enhancing a nursing career (Table 11.1). Little impression appears to have been made on this long-standing pattern.

In the years since we undertook this research, there has been much discussion about the direction that midwifery education should take in the future. A recent review of these discussions (Radford and Thompson, 1988) showed that they have centred mainly around the development of direct entry training and the amalgamation of midwifery schools. The resurgence of interest in direct entry training has had two main foci. First, there has been a growing concern to emphasize that midwifery is not a branch of nursing, but a separate profession, and that consequently midwives should not necessarily be required to qualify first as nurses. Secondly, the decrease in the number of 18-year-olds from whom nursing can recruit is likely to result in a concomitant decrease in the number coming into midwifery via the post RGN route. Moreover, as successive studies have shown, including the one described in this chapter, the majority are not intending to make a career in the profession. One of the responses to this situation has been to turn attention to increasing the proportion of mature entrants. As described earlier, the same response was made by the 1949 Working Party on Midwives. Now, as then, this has been coupled with a recognition that this group is more likely to be attracted to a three year midwifery training than to a three year nursing training followed by 18 months' midwifery. At the time of writing, plans exist to establish experimental direct entry schemes. It is anticipated, however, that the post RGN route will also continue for the forseeable future.

The extent to which midwifery education in the future provides a sound foundation for practice will depend, as now, upon a successful combination of appropriate clinical and educational experiences. Findings from the 18 month group who took part in this study have drawn attention to factors that may still militate against this, and that require attention in the design and implementation of educational programmes in the future.

Lack of clinical teaching was the most striking finding, with 45% of the 18 month group saying that they had had insufficient teaching from midwifery tutors, 55% from hospital midwives, and 68% and 71% from obstetric and paediatric medical staff respectively (Table 11.5). Respondents' comments suggested that this lack was due mainly to a reluctance to teach students and to staff shortages. The former problem can be approached by providing continuing education courses on the subject of teaching students and by improving liaison between education and service staff. The second problem, however, is part of the wider issue of recruitment and retention of staff.

Some respondents commented that contradictory views about practice were espoused by different members of the teaching and service staff, and that they encountered a disparity between teaching in school and actual practice on the wards. It is unrealistic to expect that those involved in the education of student midwives will all concur in their views about details of practice. The respondents' experiences do indicate, however, the importance of basing teaching and practice on research findings whenever possible; this will not only reduce the amount of contradictory information expressed by teachers and the degree of disparity between theory and practice, but will also ensure that practice is research-based.

Forty-two per cent of the 18 month group said that they had not had sufficient time for personal study. Much discussion about professional development in recent years has focused on staff taking responsibility for keeping up to date through personal study (Royal College of Midwives, 1987). If this is to become a reality, however, it is important that opportunities for students to develop private study skills are incorporated into basic educational programmes.

Findings from the research suggested that extending the course from 12 to 18 months increased the proportion of respondents who felt that they had sufficient clinical experience (Table 11.6) and the proportion who felt adequately prepared for each of the various responsibilities involved in midwifery practice. Although many still felt insufficiently experienced in relation to obstetric theatres and special care baby units, these are specialized areas of care for which post-basic experience and education are necessary. Of those areas for which students might well hope to feel confident at the end of training, the labour ward still appeared to be the most problematic, in that 28% felt that they had insufficient experience and 12% felt less than adequately prepared to care for the baby after delivery.

Findings on the relationship between career intentions and adequacy of training indicated that a 'good' course may change intentions in favour of a career in midwifery. Moreover, respondents' comments showed how important staff attitudes may be to students' enjoyment of the course. For example, just under a third of respondents did not enjoy their initial period in hospital and this was attributed primarily to a lack of recognition of previous experience by ward staff. On the other hand, the efforts of teaching and service staff who strove to give of their best to students were recognized and appreciated.

The research demonstrated not only the extent to which extending midwifery training from 12 to 18 months for the registered general nurse achieved its hoped-for outcomes, but also drew attention to factors relevant to course design and content in the future. It did, however, relate only to views and intentions expressed at the time of qualification, and provides no indication of how good a foundation for practice the 18 month course proved to be, the extent to which career intentions were translated into reality and which respondents stayed in the profession. In order to provide this information, we are therefore following the careers of the two groups of midwives from the time that they qualified, up until 1991 (Robinson *et al.*, 1988; Robinson and Owen, 1989; Owen and Robinson, 1990, Owen and Robinson forthcoming in Volume 3 of this series).

It is hoped that the follow up study will provide information on rates of and reasons for attrition after qualification. This in turn may lead to the development of strategies to ensure that not only is there sufficient staff in post to provide care for childbearing women and their families, but also to educate and train the practitioners of the future.

ACKNOWLEDGEMENTS

I should like to thank the following: Josephine Golden who was responsible for much of the work involved in the first stage of this project, Keith Jacka for statistical and computing assistance; Jack Hayward for commenting on drafts; Sylvia Berkowitz for secretarial assistance; the Department of Health who fund the Nursing Research Unit at King's College, London University, and the midwives who completed our questionnaires.

REFERENCES

Armitage, P.O. (1971) *Statistical methods in medical research.* Blackwell, Oxford.

Balch, B. (1981) Teacher training for midwives: an investigation of the Midwife Teacher's Diploma Course 1975–79 at the Royal College of Midwives, London, with special reference to teaching practice. In *Proceedings of the 1981 Research and the Midwife Conference,* University of Manchester, Manchester.

Ball, J. (1983) Moving forward in postnatal care – some aspects of a research project. *Midwives' Chronicle and Nursing Notes,* **96,** 2, 149. Supplement pp. 14–16.

Bendall, E. (1976) Learning for reality. *Journal of Advanced Nursing,* **1,** 3–9.

Bent, E.A. (1982) The growth and development of midwifery. In Allan, P. and Jolly, M. (eds). *Nursing Midwifery and Health Visiting since 1900.* Faber and Faber, London.

Brooks, F., Long, A. and Rathwell, T. (1987) *Midwives' perceptions of the state of midwifery.* Nuffield Centre for Health Services Studies, The University of Leeds, Leeds.

Campbell, J.M. (1923) The training of midwives. *Ministry of Health reports on public health and medical subjects.* No. 21. HMSO, London.

Campbell, J.M. (1927) The protection of motherhood. *Ministry of Health reports on public health and medical subjects.* No. 48. HMSO, London.

Central Midwives Board (1913). Annual report for the year ended 31st March, 1913.

Central Midwives Board (1957) Annual report of the Board for the year ending 31.3.57. Published by Hymns Ancient & Modern Ltd, Suffolk.

Central Midwives Board (1977) Letter from Board to midwifery training schools, regional and area nursing officers, regarding the decision to extend the 12 month training to 18 months. June 1977.

Central Midwives Board (1983) Final report on the work of the Board. Published by Hymns Ancient & Modern Ltd, Suffolk

Cowell, B. and Wainwright, D. (1981) *Behind the Blue Door. The history of the Royal College of Midwives, 1881–1981.* Ballière Tindall, London.

Davies, R. (1988) *The Happy End of Nursing: An ethnographic study of initial encounters in a midwifery school.* MSc (Econ.) thesis, University of Wales.

Farnish, S. (1983) Ward sister preparation: A survey in three districts. NERU Report No. 2, Chelsea College, London University, London.

Filshie S., Williams, J., Edith, O., Osbourn, M., Symonds, E. and Backett, E. (1981) Postnatal care in hospital. *Journal of the Royal Society of Health,* **101,** 70–3.

Fretwell, J.E. (1980) An inquiry into the ward learning environment. *Nursing Times,* **76,** Occasional Papers No. 16, 69–75.

Golden, J. (1980) Midwifery training: the views of newly qualified midwives. *Midwives' Chronicle and Nursing Notes.,* **93**(1109), 190–4.

Gott, M. (1984) *Learning Nursing.* Royal College of Nursing, London.

Kilty, J.M. and Potter, F.W. (1975) *Research project on the Midwife Teacher's Diploma.* University of Surrey, Guildford.

Laryea, M.G.G. (1980). *The midwives' role in the postnatal care of primiparae and their infants in the first 28 days following childbirth.* Unpublished M. Phil. thesis. Newcastle Polytechnic, Newcastle.

Lewis, P. (1987) *Ten Years On: A study to investigate the uptake of male midwifery training within the United Kingdom and the career patterns of male midwives.*

Unpublished BSc dissertation, Dept. of Nursing Studies, King's College, London University, London.

Lewis, P. (1989) Male Midwives: Reasons for training and subsequent career paths. In Wilson-Barnett J. and Robinson S. (eds) *Directions in Nursing Research.* Scutari Press, London.

Maclean, G. (1980) *A study of the educational needs of midwives in Wales and how they could be met.* Report on study undertaken for fellowship award from National Staff Committee for Nurses and Midwives. West Glamorgan Area Health Authority.

McCrea, H. (1989) Motivation for continuing education in midwifery. *Midwifery,* 5 (3), 134–45.

Mander, R. (1989) Carers' Careers – Contingencies and crises. *Midwives Chronicle,* 102 (1212), 3–8.

Marson, S. (1982) Ward Sister – teacher or facilitator? An investigation into the behavioural characteristics of effective ward teachers. *Journal of Advanced Nursing,* 7, 347–57.

Ministry of Health (1929) Report of the Departmental Committee on the training and employment of midwives (Chairman: Sir Robert Bolam), HMSO, London.

Ministry of Health (1959) Report of the maternity services committee (Chairman: The Earl of Cranbrook). HMSO, London.

Ministry of Health, Department of Health for Scotland, Ministry of Labour and National Service (1949) Report of the Working Party on Midwives (Chairman: Mrs M. Stocks), HMSO, London.

Murphy-Black, T. (1985) Antenatal Education: some aspects of the evaluation of a post-basic training course, in *Research and the Midwife Conference proceedings for 1984.* Nursing Research Unit, Kings College, London University, London.

Ogier, M. (1982) *An Ideal Sister: A study of the leadership style and verbal inter-actions of ward sisters with nurse learners in general hospitals.* Royal College of Nursing, London.

Opoku, D. and Davies, K. (1988) Exploring other perspectives in the midwifery curriculum. In *Research and the Midwife Conference proceedings for 1987.* Nursing Research Unit, Kings College, London University, London.

Orton, H.D. (1981) *Ward Learning Climate.* Royal College of Nursing, London.

Owen, H. and Robinson, S. (1990) Career Paths of Midwives in *Research and the Midwife Conference proceedings for 1989.* Department of Nursing Studies, University of Manchester, Manchester.

Parnaby, C. (1987) Surveying the opinions of midwives regarding the curriculum content of refresher courses. *Midwifery,* 3 (3), 133–42.

Pearson, J. (1979) Educational encounters in the ward. Unpublished M.Phil thesis. CNAA, London.

Pope, V.E. (1986) Midwifery training in Scotland: an opinion survey. *Midwives Chronicle,* 99, 198–200.

Prince, J. and Adams, M.E. (1979) *Minds, mothers and midwives.* Churchill Livingstone, Edinburgh.

Radford, N, and Thompson, A. (1988) *Direct Entry: A preparation for midwifery practice.* University of Surrey, Surrey.

Ramsden, D. and Radwanski, P. (1963) *Some aspects of the work of the midwife.*

Dan Mason Nursing Research Committee of the National Florence Nightingale Memorial Committee, London.

Robinson, S. (1980) Are there enough midwives? *Nursing Times,* **76**(17), 726–30.

Robinson, S. (1986a) Career intentions of newly qualified midwives. *Midwifery,* **2** (1), 25–36.

Robinson, S. (1986b) Midwifery training: the views of newly qualified midwives. *Nurse Education Today,* **6** (2), 49–59.

Robinson, S. (1986c) The 18 month training: what difference has it made? *Midwives' Chronicle,* **99**(1177), 22–9.

Robinson, S., Golden, J., and Bradley, S. (1983) *A study of the role and responsibilities of the midwife.* NERU report No. 1. Nursing Education Research Unit, King's College, London University, London.

Robinson, S. and Owen, H. (1989) Career intentions and career paths of midwives, in Wilson-Barnett, J. and Robinson S. (eds) *Directions in Nursing Research* Scutari Press, London.

Robinson, S., Owen, H., Jacka, K. and Dereky, C. (1988) *The Midwives Career Patterns Project. 1st Report on phase II of the Midwives Career Patterns Project.* King's College, London University, London.

Robinson, S., Thomson, A and Tickner, V. (1989) Midwives' views on directions and developments in midwifery research. In Robinson, S. and Thomson, A. *Research and the Midwife Conference Proceedings for 1988.* Nursing Research Unit, King's College, London University, London.

Royal College of Midwives (1964) *Statement of policy on the maternity services.* Royal College of Midwives, London.

Royal College of Midwives (1986a), Evidence to the Review Body for Nursing Staff, Midwives, Health Visitors and Professions allied to Medicine, 1986. *Midwives' Chronicle,* Vol. 99. no 1178.

Royal College of Midwives (1986b) *Comments by the Royal College of Midwives on UKCC Project 2000. A new preparation for practice.* Royal College of Midwives, London.

Royal College of Midwives (1987a), Evidence of the Review Body· for Nursing, Midwifery, Health Visiting and Professions allied to Medicine for 1987. *Midwives Chronicle,* Vol. 100. no 1,188.

Royal College of Midwives (1987b)*The role and education of the future midwife in the United Kingdom.* Royal College of Midwives, London.

Royal College of Midwives (1988) Evidence to the Review Body for Nursing Staff, Midwives, Health Visitors and Professions Allied to Medicine for 1988. *Midwives' Chronicle,* **101**(1200).

Runciman P.J. (1980) *Ward Sister at Work.* Churchill Livingstone, Edinburgh.

Standon-Batt, M. (1979) Where are the tutors? *Midwives' Chronicle and Nursing Notes,* **92**(1100), 304.

Stewart, A. (1981) The present state of midwifery training. *Midwife, Health Visitor and Community Nurse,* **17**(7), 270–2.

Sugarman, E. (1988) The case of the disappearing midwives. *Nursing Times,* **24**(8), 35–6.

Sweet, B. (1984) Midwives in clinical practice. *Nursing Times,* **80**(23), 60–2.

United Kingdom Central Council for Nursing, Midwifery and Health Visiting (1986) *Project 2000: A new preparation for practice, UKCC, London.*

Index